MW00714731

PERSONALIZED MEDICINE, IN RELATION TO REDOX STATE, DIET AND LIFESTYLE

Edited by **Faik Atroshi**

Personalized Medicine, in Relation to Redox State, Diet and Lifestyle

http://dx.doi.org/10.5772/intechopen.73582

Edited by Faik Atroshi

Contributors

Pekka Kaipainen, Roope Tikkanen, Erland Johansson, Arno Latvus, Mohamed Abdulla, Suthat Fucharoen, Somdet Srichairatanakool, Jerzy Majkowski, Shakir Ali, Tuomas Westermarck, Erkki Antila, Ananda S. Prasad, Markus Kaski, Pimpisid Koonyosying, Tijjani Salihu Shinkaf, Shirley Ekvall, Mari Havia

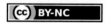
Notice

Statements and opinions expressed in the chapters are these of the individual contributors and not necessarily those of the editors or publisher. No responsibility is accepted for the accuracy of information contained in the published chapters. The publisher assumes no responsibility for any damage or injury to persons or property arising out of the use of any materials, instructions, methods or ideas contained in the book.

First published in London, United Kingdom, 2020 by IntechOpen
IntechOpen is the global imprint of INTECHOPEN LIMITED, registered in England and Wales, registration number: 11086078, 5 Princes Gate Court, London, SW7 2QJ, United Kingdom
Printed in Croatia

British Library Cataloguing-in-Publication Data
A catalogue record for this book is available from the British Library

Additional hard and PDF copies can be obtained from orders@intechopen.com

Personalized Medicine, in Relation to Redox State, Diet and Lifestyle, Edited by Faik Atroshi
p. cm.
Print ISBN 978-1-83880-369-8
Online ISBN 978-1-83968-846-1
eBook (PDF) ISBN 978-1-83968-847-8

We are IntechOpenOpen,
the world's leading publisher of
Open Access books
Built by scientists, for scientists

5,000+
Open access books available

125,000+
International authors and editors

140M+
Downloads

151
Countries delivered to

Our authors are among the

Top 1%
most cited scientists

12.2%
Contributors from top 500 universities

WEB OF SCIENCE™

Selection of our books indexed in the Book Citation Index
in Web of Science™ Core Collection (BKCI)

Interested in publishing with us?
Contact book.department@IntechOpenopen.com

Numbers displayed above are based on latest data collected.
For more information visit www.IntechOpenopen.com

Meet the editor

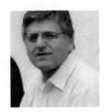 Dr. Faik Atroshi, PhD, is a docent and a senior research-er in Pharmacology and Toxicology at the University of Helsinki, Finland. With a licentiate in biomarkers of health and disease and as an adjunct professor in Clinical Genetics and Nutrition, he is both a senior researcher and a visiting professor in several interna-tional institutions and universities, including the Sleep Clinic andCancer Bio-Immunotherapy Institute, Helsinki, Finland. He is the director of Education and Research for the Finnish Satellite Center, UNESCO; the president of the International Global Society for Nutrition, Environment, and Health (GSNEH); an editorial board member of the Sci-entific World Journal; and the committee member of the Finnish Medical Physiological Society.

Contents

Preface

People falling ill will always want to get treatment for their ailment in the hope of becoming well again. The great advances in medical science have changed our outlook on the possibilities to conquer diseases and of life expectancy, especially in the western world. The developments that have led to this include the mapping of the human genome and the rapidly expanding application of this genetic knowledge to preventive medicine, the increasing knowledge of the role of hormones, the rapid pace of advancement in the field of immune-related diseases and their treatment, stem cell research, information technology and robotic techniques in surgery. A valuable approach is also provided by targeted therapies that are based on the gene environment and drugs that specifically target the diseases; it offers exciting new possibilities for understanding and managing health and disease.

Like all human skills the practice of medicine has evolved gradually, and from a craft using rather crude or ineffective measures it has transformed to include modern experimentally driven medicine and controlled standards of care. The completion of the Human Genome Project was a major landmark in this evolution. The collaborative efforts have realized the potential for a paradigm shift in clinical medicine. However, scientists soon found out that the sequenced genome was not the end point. The genetic code was no solution as such, and its implications were much more complex than could have been foreseen. Though some diseases can now be linked to a definitive genetic cause, other diseases are considered complex and multifactorial. As understanding of human biological variation deepens, hopes for a practice of medicine tailored for the individual and his genome grow stronger. The ideas behind such individualized medicine, widely called personalized medicine, are based on the understanding that individuals differ from each other genetically in ways that significantly impact disease processes. Though it is generally understood that individuals vary genetically more within a given continental population than between populations, different populations may have different predispositions for certain diseases. In addition, the efficacy of medications may vary by population.

DNA is identical up to 99% in the human population, yet each individual has a unique set of DNA. This uniqueness is maintained by over 30 million variants constituting a platform for researchers to discover, study and document their implications on our health and behavior. One field of this type of research aims to personalize the dosage of medicine according to the patient's unique genetic structure. Furthermore, drugs in standard dosages cannot be guaranteed to yield normal metabolic responses, and one of the important tasks of pharmacogenetics is to help end cases of adverse drug reactions that in the worst cases can result in death. DNA is constantly subject to mutations, i.e. accidental changes in its code. Mutations can lead to missing or malformed proteins, and that can lead to disease. Clinical studies have shown that molecular targeted therapies in lung cancer, such as EGFR tyrosine kinase inhibitors (TKIs), increase survival, lower toxicity and improve the quality of life in patients. Despite these advances, the realisation of personalized therapies for the non-small cell lung cancer (NSCLC) still faces a number of challenges. These include effective integration of clinical and genetic data and a lack of clinical decision support tools to assist physicians with patient selection.

Research in personalized medicine is producing new exciting information about the prediction and prevention of disease with respect to a particular patient and how to find the best possible treatment for this individual. The goal of this book, "Personalized Medicine, in Relation to Redox State, Diet and Lifestyle", was to function as an introduction to this field of research by describing the general principles and concepts and by reviewing the pertaining literature. We also tried to make the reading lighter by adding topics of general interest and curiosity.

Traditional medicines (TM) have been advised by World Health Organization (WHO) to be considered complementary or alternative to current classic medicine. Recently, targeted therapy has been proposed to be medical model for individualized healthcare, including all preventive, diagnostic, and therapeutic medical interventions according to genetic context. Personalized medicine is an evolving field in which physicians use diagnostic tests to determine which medical treatments will work best for each patient. By combining the data from those tests with an individual's medical history, circumstances and values, healthcare providers can develop targeted treatment and prevention plans. ersonalied medicine may revolutionize healthcare; it will, however, require great efforts.

Certain medications may cure or prevent the disease, whereas some drug interactions can even be harmful. Thus, for instance, administering too little of a drug or toxin can be harmful if poor results are achieved in the tumor cells targeted. Variation in drug metabolizing enzymes can lead to a situation in which individuals who are slow metabolizers are getting a lower dose and fast metabolizers a higher dose of the drug than required for optimal efficacy and reduced toxicity. Warfarin, for example, serves as a good example of how pharmacogenetics can be utilized before starting the therapy in order to achieve maximum efficacy and maximum toxicity (Holbrook et al. 2005, Arch. Intern. Med. 165 (10): 1095). Pharmacogenetics is a potential approach for establishing the guidelines for optimal quality in the use of medicines, and thus to improve the efficacy and safety of both prospective and licensed drugs. Pharmacogenetics and pharmacogenomics have been widely recognized as fundamental steps towards personalied medicine. They deal with genetically determined variants that affect the way in which individuals respond to drugs, and hold the promise to revolutionize drug therapy by tailoring it according to individual genotypes. Moreover, the application of pharmacogenetics and pharmacogenomics to therapies used in the treatment of osteoarticular diseases (e.g. rheumatoid arthritis, osteoporosis) is a respective method for tailoring therapies based on clinically relevant drugs (e.g. disease-modifying anti-rheumatic drugs, vitamin D, and estrogens).

This book also addresses differences and similarities among drugs, as well as the role of nutrients and dietary supplements. Advice on diet, exercise and cleanliness is found throughout the works of Hippocrates – the ancient Greeks understood some of the beneficial links between lifestyle, environment and health. Pharmacogenetics has the potential to produce knowledge for optimal quality use of medicines, and to improve the efficacy and safety of both prospective and licensed drugs. Pharmacogenetics and pharmacogenomics have been widely recognized as fundamental steps toward personalized medicine.

This book is intended to draw attention to the roles of food and nutrition in human/animal metabolism. Food and nutrition, which have a central role in maintaining health and preventing deficiencies, also play an intimate and inextricable role in all aspects of drug metabolism, effectiveness, and safety. Pharmacotherapy, on the other hand, is usually applied to combat some form of disease, trauma, or at least a medical complaint. However, the borders between these two disciplines are not always clear, and tend to dissolve. The role of specific foods of physiologically-active food components called functional foods as many fruits, vegetables, and unprocessed whole foods was introduced in Japan in the 1980s and these foods have properties that can benefit our health. Hippocrates, nearly 2,500 years ago, stressed the tent "Let food be thy medicine and medicine be thy food,". He taught that the first and foremost principle of medicine must be to respect nature's healing forces, which inhabit each living organism. Certain medications may cure or prevent the disease, whereas some drug interactions can even be harmful. William Gull said "I do not say no drugs are useful, but there is not enough discrimination in their use" (Pearce JMS. Sir William Gull (1816-1890)).

"I think for the history of man people have always wanted to see something about their future, and now, through the power of genetics and genomics, we are able to look into the future in a science-based way" (Lord J.U. Health, University of Miami, Miller School of Medicine, 01.11.2016.)

I wish to acknowledge the help of a number of people in the preparation of this book. Firstly, I wish to thank Allan Atroshi, a Director at the Global Society for Nutrition, Environment and Health (GSNEH), for the innumerable time he spent helping me edit this book. Secondly I must certainly express my gratitude towards Ilkka Linnankoski, PhD and Mrs Brenda Linnankoski, for their interest, as well as thoughtful reading and suggestions that helped to strengthen the book. Last, but certainly not least, this book would not have been possible without the support of the authors who contributed to this book. Thank you so very much for all your help in making the book a success.

Faik Atroshi

Pharmacology and Toxicology at the University of Helsinki
Helsinki, Finland

Note from the publisher

It is with great sadness and regret that we inform the contributing authors and future readers of this book that the Editor, Prof. Faik Atroshi, passed away shortly after finishing the book and before having a chance to see its publication. Prof. Faik Atroshi was IntechOpen's long term collaborator and edited 2 books with us in 2013. and 2017. ("Pharmacology and Nutritional Intervention in the Treatment of Disease" and "Cancer Causing Substances").

The fruitful collaboration continued until his final days when he was acting as an editor of the book "Personalized Medicine, in Relation to Redox State, Diet and Lifestyle". We would like to acknowledge Dr. Faik Atroshi's contribution to open access scientific publishing, which he made during the years of dedicated work on edited volumes and express our gratitude for his pleasant cooperation with us.

IntechOpen Book Department Team September, 2020

Helicobacter pylori Infection and Atrophic Corpus Gastritis on Patients with Intellectual Disability: Challenges in the Clinical Translation of Personalized Medicine

Pekka Kaipainen and Markus Kaski

Additional information is available at the end of the chapter

http://dx.doi.org/10.5772/intechopen.73585

Abstract

The purpose of this chapter is to clarify the prevalence of *Helicobacter pylori* infection (HPI) and atrophic corpus gastritis (ACG) in patients with intellectual disability (ID) and review the literature surrounding them. We measured the levels of pepsinogen I, pepsinogen II, gastrin-17b (basal), and *Helicobacter pylori* antibodies from 243 patients with intellectual disability living in Rinnekoti Research Centre at Lakisto area during 2009–2011. We determined the levels of hemoglobin, mean cell volume (MCV), hematocrit, and the mean amount (MCH) and concentration (MCHC) of red cell hemoglobin, the counts of erythrocytes, leucocytes, and thrombocytes. About 43% had high level of *Helicobacter pylori* antibodies and 6% ACG. Our results show that Helicobacter pylori infection occurs approximately twice the rate it appears in the normal population. Also, the incidence of ACG was higher among patients with ID than normal population. ID may be a risk of getting the *Helicobacter pylori* infection (HPI) and ACG. In addition, it was found that the level of thrombocytes was increased in HPI group compared to normal group and decreased in ACG group compared to normal group. This study shows that there is clearly a need to investigate (test) more stomach condition in patients with ID.

Keywords: helicobacter, *Helicobacter pylori*, pepsinogen, gastritis, atrophic corpus gastritis, intellectual disability, personalized medicine

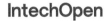

1. Literature review

1.1. *Helicobacter pylori* infection

Helicobacter pylori is a common Gram-negative bacterium, which may colonize the human stomach, wherein it can induce various gastroduodenal disorders (chronic gastritis, ulceration, atrophic corpus gastritis, and gastric cancer). However, only a small part of the people, who are colonized, develops associated diseases. It is estimated that *H. pylori* infection (HPI) affects more than half of the adult population worldwide [1] and is responsible for 75% of all gastric cancer cases [2]. In Finland and many other countries, the prevalence of *H. pylori* is decreased in last decades, in Finland to the level of approximately 15% of population [3]. Intellectually disabled children are a vulnerable subgroup and may experience higher rates of infections and morbidities [4]. *H. pylori* infection and gastric cancer occur at higher rates in subjects with ID than in the general population [5]. In institutionalized patients with intellectual disability (ID), *Helicobacter pylori* infection (HPI) occurs twice the rate it appears in the normal population [6–8]. It is suggested that the transmission of HPI occur via an oral-oral or fecal-oral pathway. Ohwada et al. [9] concluded that a high frequency of mild norm chromic anemia in institutionalized people with ID was observed. According to them, medications and chronic inflammation may increase the risk of anemia. Telaranta-Keerie et al. [10] noted the prevalence of 3.5 % of population for atrophic corpus gastritis (ACG) and also found that ACG may cause impairment in secretion of intrinsic factor, resulting in vitamin B12 deficiency. Because of these observations, we decided to evaluate the hematological values of our patients with ID. ACG can be autoimmune in origin or it can appear as multifocal atrophic gastritis (MAG) [11, 12]. According to Telaranta-Keerie et al. [10], MAG is always HPI-initiated. Achlorhydric or hypochlorhydric stomach with ACG may result in malabsorption of vitamin B12, micronutrients, and medicines [13]. It is well known that the stomach must be acid in order to absorb B12. Many people already suffer from borderline B12 deficiency—this is a difficult vitamin for the body to assimilate, but essential for normal biochemistry. Therefore, achlorhydria may be associated with vitamin B12 deficiency in the setting of pernicious anemia. Parenteral vitamin B12 may be important in selected patients. Achlorhydria is associated with thiamine deficiency in the setting of bacterial overgrowth [14–16]. In addition, increasing evidence accumulates that *H. pylori* infection may interfere with many biological processes and have a role in birth of several other extra-gastroduodenal manifestations including among others iron deficiency anemia, immune thrombocytopenic purpura, metabolic syndrome and diabetes mellitus, nonalcoholic fatty liver disease, coronary artery disease and cerebrovascular disorders [17]. Because of these facts, ACG is important disease to be diagnosed and recognized [18, 19]. It has been observed that *Helicobacter pylori* infection can cause rumination and numerous other behavioral disorders [20]. *Helicobacter pylori* are associated with gastric atrophy and gastric carcinoma [21].

1.2. The role of epidemiology in understanding the health effects of *Helicobacter pylori* in intellectual disability

H. pylori infection appears to be almost universal among certain groups of people with intellectual disability and appears to be a relatively silent condition in this population, even in those with more virulent strains [22]. The ID is potentially at risk of significant but preventable morbidity and mortality from the disease consequences of this infection [23]. The efficacy of standard treatment protocols appear lower than that in the general population, and in some, the side effects are more prominent [24]. The diagnosis of *H. pylori* infection can be made with reasonable clinical certainty using the fecal antigen test (and serology under some conditions) or, in those with greater abilities, using the urea breath test [25]. Although eradication of infection does not change the level of maladaptive behavior or intellectual disability, it may reduce the risk of the disease consequences of *H. pylori*. Given the clinical silence of the infection, the virulence of the strains, the acceptability of the diagnostic tests, and knowledge of the risk factors for infection, despite a possible lower eradication rate and higher rate of side effects, a strong argument can be made to proactively screen for and treat *H. pylori* infection among groups of people with intellectual disability who have a history of institutionalization, greater levels of intellectual disability or maladaptive behavior, or live with flatmates with hypersalivation or fecal incontinence [5].

Intellectually disabled children are a vulnerable subgroup and may experience higher rates of infections and morbidities [4]. *H. pylori* infection and gastric cancer occur at higher rates in subjects with ID than in the general population [5, 7]. Many children with ID and neurological impairments are not able to co-operate with performance of noninvasive test such as UBT [7]. In addition, because of limitations in their intellectual and adaptive functioning, such children are unable to report their symptoms. Behavior of people with ID is often difficult to explain and reactions may be similar on physical and emotional stress that is why they may be misunderstood and over medicated. One of the main reasons to begin this research study in our research center—Rinnekoti Research Centre—was the fact that patients with ID very often have difficulties to recognize, localize and indicate their symptoms. Although life-long *H. pylori* associated morbidities are well known, relatively few studies have addressed the status of *H. pylori* infection in people with ID [5].

1.3. Helicobacter infection and gastric neoplasia

As discussed above, *Helicobacter pylori* are one of the world's most common pathogens with a colonization of about 60% of the general population [26, 27]. It is estimated that *H. pylori* infection affects more than half of the adult population worldwide [1] and is responsible for 75% of all gastric cancer cases [2]. No mode of transmission is fully known, however, many factors may contribute such as socio-economic and poor living standards, poor nutrition and physical activity, and possibly poor access to health services. However, most individuals never develop clinical disease [28].

Gastrointestinal problems in handicapped children with neurodevelopmental disabilities are chronic and present long-term management problems. These conditions include dysphagia (60%), chronic pulmonary aspiration (41%), gastroesophageal reflux (32%), abdominal pain and gastritis (32%), constipation (74%), and malnutrition (33%) [29]. Growth failure and malnutrition are common in children with cerebral palsy, particularly in those with spastic quadriplegia, of which 85% report feeding problems [30, 31]. In addition, 20–30% of hemiplegic and diplegic cerebral palsy children are underweight for age [26, 32]. There are multifactorial causes:

insufficient food intake, feeding problems, increased nutrient losses from vomiting or diarrhea, and alterations in energy requirements in epileptic or metabolic syndromes where increased muscle tone or involuntary movements are seen. What is now clear is that undernutrition in cerebral palsy is often correctable and that providing a balanced diet and better nutrition can result in improvement in long-term spasticity, appearance, and effect of these children [33].

Good number of studies have been published in persons with intellectual disability, however, large-scale scientific studies have not been published with a population case-control study [22, 32, 34]. Harris et al. [35] (10) reported that hospital residents under 40 years of age had a 87% prevalence of HP compared with 24% for controls, whereas the overall prevalence for all ages was 87% for residents, and 43% for controls in hospital residents with severe learning disabilities. A larger study including 338 intellectually disabled and 254 controls from Holland (12) found a prevalence of 5% in children and 50% in the elderly in the general population, whereas 83% of the disabled and 27% of the healthy employees were infected. The presence of HP was significantly associated with male gender, longer duration of institutionalization, an IQ below 50, rumination, and a history of upper abdominal symptoms. Another study was conducted to determine the occurrence of HP infection in persons, who presented with severe dyspeptic symptoms and to monitor clinically the effect of treatment [36]. Over a 1-year period, a total of 43 persons (total population in care was 224) had severe dyspeptic symptoms and 42 persons (98%, 26 males, 16 females, mean age 45 years, mean institutionalization 20 years) had HP.

1.4. Treatment regimens used for *H. pylori* eradication

H. pylori infection is most likely acquired by ingesting contaminated food and water, and through person to person contact. *H. pylori* infections are usually treated with antibiotics to help prevent the bacteria from developing a resistance to any particular antibiotic. *Helicobacter pylori* infection causes progressive damage to gastric mucosa and results in serious disease such as peptic ulcer disease, MALT lymphoma, or gastric adenocarcinoma in 20–30% of patients [37]. Most persons who are infected with *H. pylori* never suffer any symptoms related to the infection; however, *H. pylori* causes chronic active, chronic persistent, and atrophic gastritis in adults and children. Infection with *H. pylori* also causes duodenal and gastric ulcers. Infected persons have a two- to six-fold increased risk of developing gastric cancer and mucosal-associated-lymphoid-type (MALT) lymphoma compared with their uninfected counterparts. The role of *H. pylori* in nonulcer dyspepsia remains unclear [38]. Therapy for *H. pylori* infection consists of 10 days to 2 weeks of one or two effective antibiotics, such as amoxicillin, tetracycline (not to be used for children <12 years), metronidazole, or clarithromycin, plus either ranitidine bismuth citrate, bismuth subsalicylate, or a proton pump inhibitor [39, 40]. H pylori eradication rates were higher for a 7-day antibiotic regimen containing lansoprazole, amoxicillin, and clarithromycin (LAC), when used as first-line therapy compared with levofloxacin, amoxicillin, and lansoprazole (LAL) [39]. Yoon et al. [40] investigated the efficacy of a moxifloxacin-containing triple therapy as second-line therapy for *H. pylori* infection as well as the effect of treatment duration and antibiotic resistance on the eradication rate [40].

Combination drug therapy regimens commonly used to treat *H. pylori* infection includes a proton pump inhibitor (PPI) plus clarithromycin plus amoxicillin or metronidazole and a proton pump inhibitor plus a bismuth compound plus metronidazole plus tetracycline. However, all medicines have side effects. But many people don't feel the side effects or they are able to deal with them [38, 41, 42].

1.5. *Helicobacter pylori* infection and oxidative stress

Oxidative stress results from the damaging action of reactive oxygen species. These molecules react with proteins, lipids, or DNA, altering their structure and causing oxidative damage to the cells. Reactive oxygen species (ROS) are produced during normal and physiological process, which inevitably leads to the generation of oxidative molecules: superoxide ($O_2\bullet^-$), hydrogen peroxide (H_2O_2), or hydroxyl radical ($\bullet OH$). Oxidative stress is implicated in a large number of diseases: cancer (oxidative damage to DNA causes mutations that can lead to carcinogenesis), atherosclerosis (atherosclerotic plaques are made from oxidized fat), and neurodegenerative diseases (oxidative damage is a central component of nerve cell destruction). Indicators of oxidative stress have been detected in muscles and blood of ID patients. Oxidative damage can alter the blood-brain barrier, which could explain some of the cognitive problems experienced by patients.

There is an increasing evidence that microbial pathogens induce oxidative stress in infected host cells [43–45] and this may represent an important mechanism leading to epithelial injury in *H. pylori* infection [46].

Oxidative stress could well play a role in the altered epithelial proliferation, increased apoptosis, and increased oxidative DNA damage [47–49] associated with *H. pylori* infection.

Evidence for this includes increased levels of reactive oxygen species (ROS) measured in the mucosae of infected patients [48, 50, 51]. While activated, ROS-releasing phagocytic leukocytes recruited to the gastric mucosa during infection represent one obvious source of oxidative stress [43, 50].

The mechanism of tissue damage and cell proliferation in H. Pylori infection remains unknown, although cytokines, chemokines, growth factors, including nitric oxide synthase and potent neutrophil. Derive reactive oxygen metabolism have all been proposed to contribute to such damage [52–54]. HP infection is associated with the increased production of free radicals in the gastric mucosa [50]. Accumulated free radicals in the tissue initiate lipid peroxidation of cell membranes and threaten cell integrity. Antioxidant may be useful in HP-related mucosal disease [47]. Evidence suggests that microbial pathogens induce oxidative stress in infected host cells [43–45], which represents an important mechanism causing damage to the epithelial in *H. pylori* infection [55]. *Helicobacter pylori* is the major cause of acute and chronic gastritis, gastric, and duodenal ulcer and increased incidence of gastric adenocarcinoma and elevated gastric mucosa lymph proliferation. Reactive oxygen species have been suggested as one of the main causes of cell injury in *H. pylori* associated gastritis. *H. pylori* mutants that are defective in RuvC have increased sensitivity to DNA-damaging agents and to oxidative stress, exhibit reduced survival within macrophages, and are unable to establish successful infection in a mouse model [56].

2. Research study

2.1. Material and methods

GastroPanel test (Biohit Oyj, Helsinki) was used. The test consisted of measurement of plasma pepsinogen I, pepsinogen II (PG I, PG II and PG I/PG II ratio), *H. pylori* IgG antibodies (HpAb) and gastrin-17-basal by the ELISA method. Test results, together with a short interpretation of the results are created by the GastroSoft software. The GastroSoft software uses an algorithm that is based on the levels of PG I, PG II, HpAb, and gastrin-17-basal in plasma as measured by GastroPanel. When the results showed a low PG I level (<30 µg/l) and/or a low PG I/PG II ratio (<3), the GastroSoft interpretation was "moderate or severe atrophic corpus gastritis". Cases fulfilling these criteria were considered to have advanced ACG. If PG I level and PG I/PG II ratio were normal but the patient had an elevated HpAb result (≥30 EIU), this was interpreted as "nonatrophic *H. pylori* gastritis". When the levels of all the biomarkers were within their reference ranges (PG I ≥ 30 µg/l and PG I/PG II ratio ≥ 3, HpAb below 30 EIU), the GastroSoft interpretation was "healthy, normal stomach mucosa".

2.2. Laboratory determinations and reagents

Vacuette serum tubes were used to obtain serum samples and vacuette K2EDTA tubes were used to obtain hematological samples. Hemoglobin, mean cell volume (MCV), hematocrit, erythrocytes, thrombocytes, and leukocytes were assayed with Sysmex KX-21 N analyzer. All used reagents were reagent grade. All laboratory determinations were controlled with the control samples from Labquality Ltd., Helsinki, Finland. All enzyme immunoassays were done with BP 800 reader.

2.3. Study population

The study material consisted of blood samples from patients with intellectual disability (243 individuals). Patients with ID lived in groups containing 6–8 persons during 2009–2011. Age was from 10 to 80. The whole group consisted 157 male and 86 female patients with ID. Sanitary facilities were common for each group as normal family living. The personnel taking care of these patients was living with them for 24 hours per day with 8–10 hours shifts.

3. Results

We measured the levels of pepsinogen I, pepsinogen II, gastrin 17-beta, and *Helicobacter pylori* antibodies from 243 patients with intellectual disability (157 male patients and 86 female patients). Results are shown in **Tables 1** and **2** and **Figures 1–4**. The prevalence of subjects with ACG, HPI, and normal stomach mucosa is shown in **Table 1**. Among male patients, 7% had ACG, while among female patients, 4.7% had ACG. 6.2% of all patients had ACG. Among male patients, 45.2% had HPI, while among female patients, 39.5% had HPI. About 43.2% of all

Populations	Number of patients	Advanced corpus gastritis	Elevated helicobacter pylori antibodies	Healthy stomach mucosa
	No.	No. (%)	No. (%)	No. (%)
Patients (male)	157	11 (7,0%)	71 (45,2%)	75 (47,8%)
Patients (female)	86	4 (4,7%)	34 (39,5%)	48 (55,8%)
Total	243	15 (6,2%)	105 (43,2%)	123 (50,6%)

Table 1. Prevalence of subjects with advanced atrophic corpus gastritis (ACG), elevated *Helicobacter pylori* antibodies, and normal stomach mucosa in male and female patients with ID.

patients had HPI. Among male patients, 47.8% had normal stomach mucosa, while among female patients, 55.8% had normal stomach mucosa. About 50.6% of all patients had normal stomach mucosa (**Table 1**). Differences in the levels of pepsinogen II, PG I/PG II, and *Helicobacter pylori* antibodies between HPI group and normal group were statistically extremely significant. Differences in the levels of pepsinogen I, PG I/PG II, and *Helicobacter pylori* antibodies between ACG group and normal group were also statistically extremely significant. Differences in the levels of hemoglobin, hematocrit, erythrocytes, and leucocytes between HPI group and normal group were not statistically significant. The level of thrombocytes was increased in HPI group compared to normal group and decreased in ACG group compared to normal group. These differences were statistically significant. Differences in the MCHC, MCH, and MCV were not statistically significant between these groups. Same results were between ACG group and normal group (**Table 2**).

Determinations	ACG	HPI	Normal	Reference values	Unit	p-value	p-value
	(N=13)	(N=87)	(N=100)			ACG vs Normal	HPI vs Normal
	(M ±SD)	(M ±SD)	(M ±SD)				
Age	50 ±11	43 ±16	35 ±21			0,0003	0,0056
Pepsinogen I	25 ±12	127 ±68	103 ±60	30-165	µg/l	6,99 E-21	0,01
Pepsinogen II	15,2 ±8,5	21,0 ±14,9	9,6 ±6,9	3-15	µg/l	0,02	1,27 E-09
PEP I/PEP II	2,4 ±2,2	7,7 ±4,5	12,3 ±6,6	3-20		9,22 E-17	8,24 E-08
Gastrin 17-beta	44 ±81	14 ±20	9 ±14	5-30	pmol/l	0,12	0,06
H.pylori antibodies	77 ±45	85 ±26	12 ±10	<30	EIU	5,99 E-05	3,35 E-45
B-Hb	138 ±16	136 ±16	134 ±14	male 134-167 female 117-155	g/l	0,39	0,47
B-Hkr	0,41 ±0,04	0,39 ±0,04	0,39 ±0,04	male 0,39-0,5 female 0,35-0,46		0,24	0,96
B-Eryt	4,5 ±0,5	4,5 ±0,5	4,4 ±0,4	male 4,3-5,7 female 3,9-5,3	E12/L	0,77	0,52
E-MCV	92 ±5	88 ±4	89 ±5	82-98	fl	0,11	0,28
E-MCH	31 ±2	30 ±2	31 ±2	27-33	pg	0,53	0,78
E-MCHC	339 ±11	346 ±13	341 ±12	320-360	g/l	0,42	0,03
B-Tromb	167 ±52	225 ±88	201 ±70	150-360	E9/L	0,04	0,04
B-Leuk	5,7 ±2,3	6,1 ±2,1	6,0 ±2,4	3,4-8,2	E9/L	0,62	0,77

Table 2. Five gastro and eight hematological parameters in groups with advanced corpus gastritis (ACG), *Helicobacter pylori* antibodies (HPI), and healthy stomach mucosa (normal).

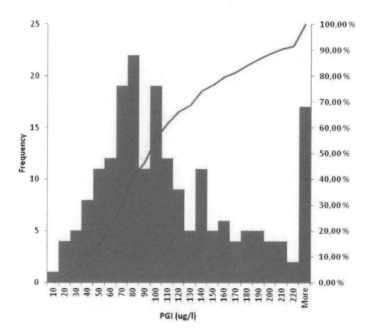

Figure 1. The levels of pepsinogen I on 243 patients with ID.

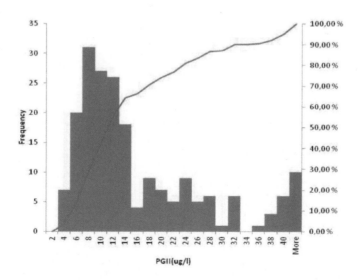

Figure 2. The levels of pepsinogen II on 243 patients with ID.

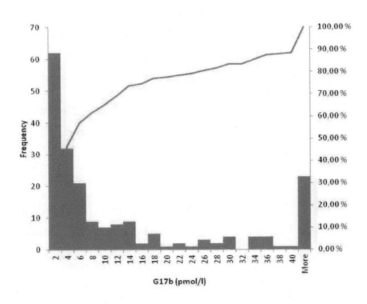

Figure 3. The levels of Gastrin 17-b on 243 patients with ID.

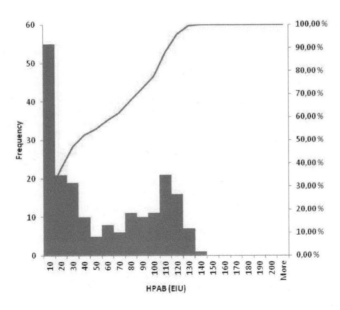

Figure 4. The levels of H. pylori antibodies on 243 patients with ID.

4. Discussion

This study provides an overview of the best available evidence on the prevalence of *H. pylori* infection obtained from patients with intellectual disability.

The level of ID and environmental factors may be related to the risk of infection with *H. pylori* [7]. According to Merrick, 43 persons (total population in care was 224) had severe dyspeptic symptoms. Wallace et al. [7] showed that adults with ID may be at risk of infection with HPI. According to their results, a long period of institutionalization living with other patients predisposes to HPI. *Helicobacter pylori* among patients with ID living in hospitals are common [7]. In institutionalized patients with intellectual disability (ID), *Helicobacter pylori* infection (HPI) occur twice the rate it appears in the normal population [6–8]. However, this trend has not been before observed in Finland. The patients with ID lived in groups containing 6–8 persons. Sanitary facilities were common for each group as normal family living. It is suggested that the transmission of HPI occur via an oral-oral or fecal-oral pathway. The mechanism of transmission of this pathogen is not known exactly. But it is known that the rate of this disease is increased with age and other living conditions. According to our findings, patients with ID and age of 50 and living for a long time in group residences are high at risk to get *Helicobacter pylori* infection and also so atrophic corpus gastritis. Because well-being of patients with ID is important, we decided to determine also the hematological values of these people. We did not find any big differences between the patients with healthy and sick stomach mucosa. The count of thrombocytes was increased in HPI group and decreased in ACG group. Thrombocytes have an important role in inflammation [57]. They participate in inflammatory response to *H. pylori* infection by activation and aggregation as well as acting as a source of inflammatory mediators and modulating the activity of other inflammatory cells in stomach mucosa [58]. The volume of thrombocytes may be increased during infection. Their persistent activation and enhanced destruction production process during infection may lead to decreased amounts of them [59]. However, it seems that there lacks association between *H. pylori* infection and various markers of systemic inflammation including thrombocyte/lymphocyte ratio in adults with chronic asymptomatic *H. pylori* infection [60]. *Helicobacter pylori* infection and its consequences may be severe to people with ID. Wallace et al. [7] concluded that if this infection leads to increased levels of maladaptive behavior, this could result in loss of social opportunities, sedative drug use and so decrease of well-being. The mental pressure among workers in institutions for people with ID will increase. Böhmer et al. [61] and Schryver et al. [62] found that *Helicobacter pylori* infection is an occupational risk in healthcare workers working in institutions for people with ID. This observation gives the reason to also investigate all workers taking care of patients with ID.

Proujansky et al. [20] stated that rumination may be a possible symptom of *Helicobacter pylori* infection. Rumination occurs more frequently in patients with ID. Dentists play the important role in finding patients with rumination. From these patients, it is important to investigate *Helicobacter pylori* infection and treat it. Ohwada et al. [9] found that the prevalence of anemia was increased on patients with ID. According to their results, most patients showed a normocytic norm chromic anemia pattern. They say that medications and inflammation may increase the risk of anemia. We did not find differences on hemoglobin levels between the patients with normal and sick mucosa of stomach. We need more research on this field.

Wallace et al. [63, 64] reported that 7% of institutionalized adults with ID treated for *Helicobacter pylori* infection and test negative at the end of treatment are at risk of reinfection. They suggest that patients with ID should retest at an interval of approximately 3–5 years after apparent eradication. More research is needed to evaluate the effects of *Helicobacter pylori* infection on pain and use of drugs on patients with ID. Taking care of this infection, we can probably increase the level of well-being of these patients and so to decrease the physical and physiological pressure of workers in institutions for people with ID. Many studies have explored the association of *H. pylori* with hypermethylation of specific genes [65, 66] as well as hypomethylation of genes [67, 68]. Further research is required to elucidate the exact mechanisms of inflammation and tumor suppression, which might provide new opportunities for personalized treatment options.

The poor prognosis of patients with a negative *H. pylori* status might be the result of a more aggressive form of gastric cancer [69, 70]. The present study demonstrates that *H. pylori* positivity is a beneficial prognostic indicator in patients with intellectual disability, independent of other clinic pathologic variables. In clinical practice, patients with curatively resected gastric cancer who are negative for *H. pylori* may need more careful follow-up and more aggressive antitumor treatment to prolong life expectancy. Further research is required to elucidate the exact mechanisms of inflammation and tumor suppression, which might provide new opportunities for personalized treatment options. We believe that the current prospective study is the first to confirm *H. pylori* status as a favorable prognostic factor in a large number of intellectual disability patients with *Helicobacter pylori* infection and atrophic corpus gastritis in Finland, thus validating the effect of *H. pylori* infection status on survival in intellectual disability patients.

Antibiotic susceptibility should be checked in all patients, ideally, before the start of eradication treatment. The knowledge of local antibiotic resistance and consumption pattern is important in selecting a reliable regimen [71–73]. Future development for *H. pylori* therapy should be directed to overcome individualized antibiotic resistance. Warneke et al. [74] investigated various phenotypic and genotypic biomarkers of gastric cancer (GC) and concluded whether these biomarkers are suitable for the identification of GC subtypes, are they of prognostic significance, and should any of these biomarkers be considered to tailor patient treatment in the future. There remains a need to better understand the prognostic factors affecting the cure rate of *Helicobacter pylori* infection might lead to the development of novel prevention strategies and therapeutic targets. Therefore, personalized medical approach will likely increase the cure rate of *H. pylori* infection [75].

A complete history could also do away with the need for additional testing and increased medical expenses for the patient and the healthcare system as a whole.

Acknowledgements

We would like to thank all the patients who lived at Rinnekoti Research Centre during 2009–2011. Also we want to thank the laboratory workers of Rinnekoti and we are grateful for a financial help of Rinnekoti Foundation and Finnish Brain Foundation.

Author details

Pekka Kaipainen[1]* and Markus Kaski[2]

*Address all correspondence to: pekka.kaipainen@nordlab.fi

1 Nordlab Kokkola, Kokkola, Finland

2 Rinnekoti Research Centre, Espoo, Finland

References

[1] Parkin DM. International variation. Oncogene. 2004;**23**:6329-6340

[2] de Martel C, Ferlay J, Franceschi S, Vignat J, et al. Global burden of cancers attributable to infections in 2008: A review and synthetic analysis. The Lancet Oncology. 2012;**13**: 607-615

[3] Rehnberg-Laiho L, Rautelin, H, Koskela P, Sarna S, Pukkala E, Aromaa A, Knekt P, Kosunen U. Decreasing prevalence of helicobacter antibodies in Finland, with reference to the decreasing incidence of gastric cancer. Epidemiology and Infection. 2001;**126**(1):37-42

[4] Jeevanandam L. Perspectives of intellectual disability in Asia: Epidemiology, policy, and services for children and adults. Current Opinion in Psychiatry. 2009;**22**:462-468

[5] Kitchens DH, Binkley CJ, Wallace DL, Darling D. *Helicobacter pylori* infection in people who are intellectually and developmentally disabled: A review. Special Care in Dentistry. 2007;**27**:127-133

[6] Merrick J, Aspler S, Dubman I. *Helicobacter pylori* infection in persons with intellectual disability in residential care in Israel. ScientificWorldJournal. 2001;**6**:1264-1268

[7] Wallace RA, Webb PM, Schluter PJ. Environmental, medical, behavioural and disability factors associated with *Helicobacter pylori* infection in adults with intellectual disability. Journal of Intellectual Disability Research. 2002;**46**(Pt 1):51-60

[8] Wallace RA, Schluter PJ, Forgan-Smith R, Wood R, Webb PM. Diagnosis of *Helicobacter pylori* infection in adults with intellectual disability. Journal of Clinical Microbiology. 2003; **41**(10):4700-4704

[9] Ohwada H, Nakayama T, Nara N, Tomono Y, Yamanaka K. An epidemiological study on anemia among institutionalized people with intellectual and/or motor disability with special reference to its frequency, severity and predictors. BMC Public Health. 2006;**6**:85. DOI: 10.1186/1471-2458/6/85

[10] Telaranta-Keerie A, Kara R, Paloheimo L, Härkönen M, Sipponen P. Prevalence of undiagnosed advanced atrophic corpus gastritis in Finland: An observational study among 4256 volunteers without specific complaints. Scandinavian Journal of Gastroenterology. 2010;**45**(9):1036-1041

[11] Correa P. *Helicobacter pylori* and gastric carcinogenesis. The American Journal of Surgical Pathology. 1995;**19**(Suppl 1):37-43

[12] Valle J, Kekki M, Sipponen P, Ihamäki T, Siurala M. Longterm course and consequences of *Helicobacter pylori* gastritis. Results of a 32-year follow-up study. Scandinavian Journal of Gastroenterology. 1996;**31**:546-550

[13] Cater RE 2nd. The clinical importance of hypochlorhydria (a consequence of chronic Helicobacter infection): Its possible etiological role in mineral and amino acid malabsorption, depression, and other syndromes. Medical Hypotheses. 1992;**39**(4):375-383. PMID: 1494327

[14] Iijima K, Sekine H, Koike T, Imatani A, Ohara S, Shimosegawa T. Long-term effect of *Helicobacter pylori* eradication on the reversibility of acid secretion in profound hypochlorhydria. Alimentary Pharmacology and Therapeutics. 2004;**19**(11):1181-1188

[15] Drake WM, Innes DF. Primary gastric lymphoma presenting with vitamin B12 deficiency and achlorhydria. The American Journal of Gastroenterology. 1996;**91**(12):2605-2606

[16] Svendsen JH, Dahl C, Svendsen LB, Christiansen PM. Gastric cancer risk in achlorhydric patients. A long-term follow-up study. Scandinavian Journal of Gastroenterology. 1986; **21**(1):16-20

[17] Tsay FW, Hsu PI. *H. pylori* infection and extra-gastroduodenal diseases. Journal of Biomedical Science. 2018;**25**(1):65

[18] Correa P, Haenszel W, Cuello C, Zavala D, Fontham E, Zarama G. Gastric precancerous process in a high risk population: Cohort follow-up. Cancer Research. 1990;**50**:4737-4740

[19] Sipponen P, Kekki M, Haapakoski J, Ihamäki T, Siurala M. Gastric cancer risk in chronic atrophic gastritis: Statistical calculations of cross-sectional data. International Journal of Cancer. 1985;**35**:173-177

[20] Proujansky RM, Shaffer SE, Vinton NE, Bachrach SJ. Symptomatic *Helicobacter pylori* infection in young patients severe neurologic impairment. The Journal of Pediatrics. 1994;**125**:750-752

[21] Howden CW. Clinical expressions of *Helicobacter pylori* infection. American Journal of Medicine. 1996;**100**:27-32

[22] Kindermann A, Lopes AI. *Helicobacter pylori* infection in pediatrics. Helicobacter. 2009;**14** (Suppl 1):52-57

[23] Mauk JE. *Helicobacter pylori* infection in neurologically impaired children. The Journal of Pediatrics. 1995;**126**(5Pt1):849

[24] Redeen S, Petersson F, Tornkrantz E, Levander H, Mardh E, Borch K. Reliability of diagnostic tests for *Helicobacter pylori* infection. Gastroenterology Research and Practice. 2011; **2011**:940650

[25] Bytzer P, Dahlerup JF, Eriksen JR, Jarbol DE, Rosenstock S, Wildt S. Diagnosis and treatment of *Helicobacter pylori* infection. Danish Medical Bulletin. 2011;**58**:C4271

[26] Cave DR. How is *Helicobacter pylori* transmitted? Gastroenterology. 1997;**113**(6 Suppl): S9-14

[27] Cilley RE, Brighton VK. The significance of *Helicobacter pylori* colonization of the stomach. Seminars in Pediatric Surgery. 1995;**4**(4):221-227

[28] Mitchell H. The epidemiology of *Helicobacter pylori*. Current Topics in Microbiology and Immunology. 1999;**241**:11-30

[29] Del Giudice E, Staiano A, Capano G, et al. Gastrointestinal manifestations in children with cerebral palsy. Brain & Development. 1999;**21**:307-311

[30] Stallings VA, Cronk CE, Zemel BS, et al. Body composition in children with spastic quadriplegic cerebral palsy. The Journal of Pediatrics. 1995;**126**:833-839

[31] Stallings VA, Zemel BS, Davies JC, et al. Energy expenditure of children and adolescents with severe disabilities: A cerebral palsy model. American Journal of Clinical Nutrition. 1996;**64**:627-634

[32] Lubani MM, Al-Saleh QA, Teebi AS, Moosa A, Kalaoui MH. Cystic fibrosis and *Helicobacter pylori* gastritis, megaloblastic anaemia, subnormal mentality and minor anomalies in two siblings: A new syndrome ? European Journal of Pediatrics. 1991;**150**(4):253-255

[33] Patrick J, Boland M, Stoski D, et al. Rapid correction of wasting in children with cerebral palsy. Developmental Medicine and Child Neurology;**1986**(28):734-739

[34] Dellavecchia C, Guala A, Olivieri C, et al. Early onset of gastric carcinoma and constitutional deletion of 18p. Cancer Genetics and Cytogenetics. 1999;**113**(1):96-99

[35] Harris AW, Douds A, Meurisse EV, Dennis M, Chambers S, Gould SR. Seroprevalence of *Helicobacter pylori* in residents of a hospital for people with severe learning difficulties. European Journal of Gastroenterology & Hepatology. 1995;**7**(1):21-23

[36] Morad M, Merrick J, Nasri Y. Prevalence of *Helicobacter pylori* in persons with intellectual disability in a residential care center in Israel. Journal of Intellectual Disability Research. 2002;**46**(2):141-143

[37] Graham DY, Qureshi WA. Antibiotic-resistant *H. pylori* infection and its treatment. Current Pharmaceutical Design. 2000;**6**(15):1537-1544

[38] Soll AH. Medical treatment of peptic ulcer disease. Practice guidelines. [Review]. JAMA. 1996;**275**:622-629. [published erratum appears in JAMA 1996 May 1;275:1314]

[39] Liou JM, Lin JT, Chang CY, et al. Levofloxacin-based and clarithromycin-based triple therapies as first-line and second-line treatments for *Helicobacter pylori* infection: A randomised comparative trial with crossover design. Gut. 2010;**59**(5):572-578

[40] Yoon H, Kim N, Lee BH, et al. Moxifloxacin-containing triple therapy as second-line treatment for *Helicobacter pylori* infection: Effect of treatment duration and antibiotic resistance on the eradication rate. Helicobacter. 2009 Oct;**14**(5):77-85

[41] European *Helicobacter pylori* Study Group. Current European concepts in the management of *H. pylori* information. The Maastricht consensus. Gut. 1997;**41**:8-13

[42] Hunt RH. *Helicobacter pylori*: from theory to practice. Proceedings of a symposium. The American Journal of Medicine. 1996;**100**(5A) supplement

[43] Giri DK, Mehta RT, Kansal RG, Aggarwal BB. Mycobacterium avium-intracellulare complex activates nuclear transcription factor-κB in different cell types through reactive oxygen intermediates. Journal of Immunology. 1998;**161**:4834-4841

[44] Schweizer M, Peterhans E. Oxidative stress in cells infected with bovine viral diarrhoea virus: A crucial step in the induction of apoptosis. The Journal of General Virology. 1999;**80**:1147-1155

[45] Sipowicz MA, Chomarat P, Diwan BA, Anver MA, Awasthi YC, Ward JM, Rice JM, Kasprzak KS, Wild CP, Anderson LM. Increased oxidative DNA damage and hepatocyte overexpression of specific cytochrome p450 isoforms in hepatitis of mice infected with Helicobacter hepaticus. The American Journal of Pathology. 1997;**151**:933-941

[46] Smoot DT, Elliott TB, Verspaget HW, Jones D, Allen CR, Vernon KG, Bremner T, Kidd LC, Kim KS, Groupman JD, Ashktorab H. Influence of *Helicobacter pylori* on reactive oxygen-induced gastric epithelial cell injury. Carcinogenesis. 2000;**21**:2091-2095

[47] Baik S-C, Youn H-S, Chung M-H, Lee W-K, Cho M-J, Ko G-H, Park C-K, Kasai H, Rhee K-H. Increased oxidative DNA damage in *Helicobacter pylori*-infected human gastric mucosa. Cancer Research. 1996;**56**:1279-1282

[48] Clement MV, Pervaiz S. Reactive oxygen intermediates regulate cellular response to apoptotic stimuli: An hypothesis. Free Radical Research. 1999;**30**:247-252

[49] Farinati F, Cardin R, Degan P, Rugge M, Mario FD, Bonvicini P, Naccarato R. Oxidative DNA damage accumulation in gastric carcinogenesis. Gut. 1998;**42**:351-356

[50] Davies GR, Simmonds NJ, Stevens TRJ, Sheaff MT, Banatvala N, Laurenson IF, Blake DR, Rampton DS. *Helicobacter pylori* stimulates antral mucosal reactive oxygen metabolite production in vivo. Gut. 1994;**35**:179-185

[51] Drake IM, Mapstone NP, Schorah CJ, White KLM, Chalmers DM, Dixon MF, Axon ATR. Reactive oxygen species activity and lipid peroxidation in *Helicobacter pylori* associated gastritis: Relation to gastric mucosal ascorbic acid concentrations and effect of *H. pylori* eradication. Gut. 1998;**42**:768-771

[52] Harris PR, Mobley HL, Perez-Perez GI, Blaser MJ, Smith PD. *Helicobacter pylori* urease is a potent stimulus of mononuclear phagocyte activation and inflammatory cytokine production. Gastroenterology. 1996;**111**(2):419-425

[53] Gionchetti P, Vaira D, Campieri M, Holton J, Menegatti M, Belluzzi A, Bertinelli E, Ferretti M, Brignola C, Miglioli M, et al. Enhanced mucosal interleukin-6 and -8 in *Helicobacter pylori*-positive dyspeptic patients. The American Journal of Gastroenterology. 1994;**89**(6): 883-887

[54] Mannick EE, Bravo LE, Zarama G, Realpe JL, Zhang XJ, Ruiz B, Fontham ET, Mera R, Miller MJ, Correa P. Inducible nitric oxide synthase, nitrotyrosine, and apoptosis in *Helicobacter pylori* gastritis: Effect of antibiotics and antioxidants. Cancer Research. 1996; **56**(14):3238-3243

[55] Ding SZ, Minohara Y, Fan XJ, Wang J, Reyes VE, Patel J, Dirden-Kramer B, Boldogh I, Ernst PB, Crowe SE. *Helicobacter pylori* infection induces oxidative stress and programmed cell death in human gastric epithelial cells. Infection and Immunity. 2007 Aug;**75**(8):4030-4039

[56] Loughlin MF, Barnard FM, Jenkins D, Sharples GJ, Jenks PJ. *Helicobacter pylori* mutants defective in RuvC Holliday junction resolvase display reduced macrophage survival and spontaneous clearance from the murine gastric mucosa. Infection and Immunity. 2003; **71**(4):2022-2031

[57] Thomas MR, Storey RF. The role of platelets in inflammation. Thrombosis and Haemostasis. 2015;**114**:3449-458

[58] Kalia N, Bardhan KD. Of blood and guts: Association between *Helicobacter pylori* and the gastric microcirculation. Journal of Gastroenterology and Hepatology 2003;**18**(9):1010-1017

[59] Umit H, Umit EG. *Helicobacter pylori* and mean platelet volume: A relation way before immune thrombocytopenia? European Review for Medical and Pharmacological Sciences. 2015;**19**(15):2818-2823

[60] Kim TJ, Pyo JH, Lee H, Baek SY, Ahn SH, Min YW, Min BH, Lee JH, Son HJ, Rhee PL, Kim JJ. Lack of association between helicobacter pylori infection and various markers of systemic inflammation in asymptomatic adults. Korean Journal of Gastroenterology. 2018;**72**(1):21-27

[61] Böhmer CJM, Klinkenberg-Knol EC, Kuipers EJ, Niezen-de Boer MC, Schreuder H, Schuckink-Kool F, Meuwissen GM. The prevalence of *Helicobacter pylori* infection among inhabitants and healthy employees of institutes for the intellectual disabled. The American Journal of Gastroenterology. 1997;**92**:1000-1004

[62] Schryver ADE, Cornelis K, Winckel M, Moens G, Devlies G, Derthoo D, Van SM. The occupational risk of *Helicobacter pylori* infection among workers in institutions for people with intellectual disability. Occupational and Environmental Medicine. 2008;**65**:587-591

[63] Wallace RA, Schluter PJ, Webb PM. Recurrence of *Helicobacter pylori* infection in adults with intellectual disability. Internal Medicine Journal. 2004a;**34**:131-133

[64] Wallace RA, Schluter PJ, Webb PM. Effects of *Helicobacter pylori* eradication among adults with intellectual disability. Journal of Intellectual Disability Research. 2004b;**48**(7):646-654

[65] Shin CM, Kim N, Lee HS, et al. Changes in aberrant DNA methylation after *Helicobacter pylori* eradication: A long-term follow-up study. International Journal of Cancer. 2013;**133**: 2034-2042

[66] Shin CM, Kim N, Park JH, et al. Prediction of the risk for gastric cancer using candidate methylation markers in the non-neoplastic gastric mucosae. The Journal of Pathology. 2012;**226**:654-665

[67] Yoshida T, Kato J, Maekita T, et al. Altered mucosal DNA methylation in parallel with highly active *Helicobacter pylori*-related gastritis. Gastric Cancer. 2013;**16**:488-497

[68] Yuasa Y, Nagasaki H, Oze I, et al. Insulin-like growth factor 2 hypomethylation of blood leukocyte DNA is associated with gastric cancer risk. International Journal of Cancer. 2012;**131**:2596-2603

[69] Hur H, Lee SR, Xuan Y, et al. The effects of *Helicobacter pylori* on the prognosis of patients with curatively resected gastric cancers in a population with high infection rate. Journal of the Korean Surgical Society. 2012;**83**:203-211. DOI: 10.4174/jkss.2012.83.4.203

[70] McColl KE. Clinical practice. *Helicobacter pylori* infection. The New England Journal of Medicine. 2010;**362**:1597-1604

[71] Bang CS, Baik GH. Attempts to enhance the eradication rate of *Helicobacter pylori* infection. World Journal of Gastroenterology. 2014 May 14;**20**(18):5252-5262

[72] De Francesco V, Giorgio F, Hassan C, et al. Worldwide *H. pylori* antibiotic resistance: A systematic review. Journal of Gastrointestinal and Liver Diseases. 2010;**19**:409-414

[73] Duck WM, Sobel J, Pruckler JM, et al. Antimicrobial resistance incidence and risk factors among *Helicobacter pylori*-infected persons, United States. Emerging Infectious Diseases. 2004;**10**:1088-1094

[74] Warneke VS, Behrens HM, Haag J, Balschun K, Böger C, Becker T, Ebert MP, Lordick F, Röcken C. Prognostic and putative predictive biomarkers of gastric cancer for personalized medicine. Diagnostic Molecular Pathology. 2013;**22**(3):127-137

[75] Uotani T, Miftahussurur M, Yamaoka Y. Effect of bacterial and host factors on *Helicobacter pylori* eradication therapy. Expert Opinion on Therapeutic Targets. 2015;**6**:1-14

Personalized Treatment of Antisocial Personality Disorder with Inherent Impulsivity and Severe Alcoholism: A Brief Review of Relevant Literature

Roope Tikkanen

Additional information is available at the end of the chapter

http://dx.doi.org/10.5772/intechopen.73586

Abstract

Antisocial personality disorder (ASPD) is a persistent psychiatric disorder. Behaviors and emotions deviate from the norm. Inherent impulsivity, comorbid alcohol dependence, and violation of laws cause severe challenges at individual and societal levels. Both environment and heritability alter the risk for ASPD. Research shows that specific biologic changes predispose to this disorder. Biological factors may lead to novel possibilities to treat and alleviate symptoms with medications or nutritional means. However, treatment of ASPD meets particular challenges due to the inherent symptoms of the disorder, and firm evidence-based personalized treatments are scant. This chapter describes the disorder and associated adverse outcomes in life such as recurrent violent behavior and increased mortality. Moreover, treatment possibilities are discussed covering risk assessment, medication, psychotherapy, and nutrition.

Keywords: antisocial personality disorder, ASPD, alcoholism, impulsivity, violent behavior

1. Introduction

Antisocial personality disorder (ASPD) is a psychiatric disorder, which despite being probably heavily under diagnosed has at least a prevalence of 1 in 100 persons [1]. The golden standard of treatment of psychiatric disorders is a combination of pharmacological treatment and psychotherapy. To date, there are no specific golden standards of pharmacological or psychotherapeutic treatments of ASPD, but in the future, treatment results may improve

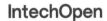

after careful selection of whom to treat. ASPD forms a patient group, which has a poor treatment compliance in general due to inherent diagnostic symptoms of unplanned lifestyle and impulsive decision-making.

2. What is ASPD: what to treat

The core symptoms of ASPD are antisocial attitudes that lead to generally destructive behavior in part due to the inherent impulsive behavior and severe alcoholism (early-onset type II alcoholism) associated with this disorder. ASPD is diagnosed among adults, but it is preceded by conduct disorder symptoms before age 15, symptoms such as running away from home, initiation of physical fights, usage of weapons in fights, forcing others into sexual activity, cruelty to animals, destruction of other persons' property, deliberately engaged in fire-setting, frequent lying, and stealing. An extensive description of conduct disorder, however, is beyond the scope of this article.

Diagnostic symptoms of ASPD have not changed much over time. The symptom cluster includes the following type of items [2]:

- Inability to sustain consistent work or studies due to lack of motivation, repeated absence from work, impulsive abandonment of several jobs without realistic plans of future jobs or education.

- Failure to conform to social norms with respect to lawful behavior, as indicated by repeatedly performing acts that are grounds for arrest (whether arrested or not), e.g., destroying property, harassing others, stealing, and pursuing an illegal occupation.

- Irritability and aggressiveness, as indicated by repeated physical fights or assaults.

- Repeatedly failing to honor financial obligations, as indicated by defaulting on debts or failing to provide child support on regular basis.

- Impulsive behavior and inability to plan ahead, as indicated by, e.g., traveling from place to place without a prearranged job or clear goal for the period of travel or clear idea about when the travel will terminate and lack of a fixed address for a long period.

- No respect for the truth as indicated by repeated lying, use of aliases, and "conning" others for personal profit or pleasure.

- Recklessness regarding own or others' safety, as indicated by driving while intoxicated or recurrent speeding.

- If being a parent or guardian, lacks ability to function as a responsible parent, as indicated by, for instance, malnutrition of child, child's illness resulting from lack of minimal hygiene, child's dependence on neighbors or nonresident relative for food or shelter, failure to arrange for a caretaker for your child when parent is away from home, and repeated squandering on personal items or of money required for household necessities.

- Never sustained a totally monogamous relationship for more than 1 year.

- Lacks remorse (feels justified in having hurt, mistreated, or stolen from others).

Realistic foci of treatment for persons diagnosed with ASPD are (i) modulation of attitudes, (ii) decrease of impulsive behavior, and (iii) treatment of alcoholism.

3. Personalized focus and selection of whom to treat

As patient care resources and skills to treat specifically ASPD are limited, there is a strong rationale to carefully choose the target groups of individuals suffering from ASPD, whom should persistently be encouraged and motivated to treatment. For this, two separate ways of selective approach may be adapted, each focusing on different criteria. One alternative for selection of whom to treat in this patient group would be a focus in primary prevention when the first symptoms appear and accumulate (early interventions). Another focus is secondary prevention and treatment when the first tangible severe consequences of having ASPD appear.

Some of the more obvious measurement tools that could be considered for the decision-making on whether to start an intervention or not would be presence of persistent alcohol consumption and conduct disorder symptoms appearing at an early age (age 10–14) or acts leading to a prison sentence. An act of violence that leads to a prison sentence is unfortunately frequent among ASPD patients in early adulthood preceded by several smaller violations of the law not leading to incarceration. However, in the incarcerated environment, a meaningful secondary prevention effort can be arranged. As 50% of prison populations are diagnosed with ASPD [3], it is unrealistic to provide treatment for all ASPD patients, but a good rationale for focus would be those individuals who are at an increased risk for reoffenses.

Decisions for offering treatments are dichotomous but symptoms and risk are often measured on a continuum from mild to severe. However, scales of symptom and risk severity can easily be constructed, and often a meaningful cutoff point, depending on the size of the selection population, is the 75–90% percentile. Continuums such as alcohol consumption quantity, trait impulsivity, and accumulation of acts of violent can be transformed into categories of high-low expected efficacy of treatment for the individual or high-low expectancy of benefit for society. Both interests are often in line with each other.

4. Risk assessment for recurrent violent behavior or premature death

The tools for assessing risk for future acts of violence in previously violent populations have been criticized as an inexact science [4]. Many attempts of constructing assessment tools have been made, but their accuracy is far from satisfactory. For instance, the risk assessment tools HCR-20 and PCL-R rely on psychological assessments and historical data on life events, which may be difficult to assess. Moreover, application of such tool needs highly trained professionals. The accuracy of such assessments suffers from several sources of bias such as underlying biologic individual variation [5]. Likewise, childhood maltreatment may also have ambiguous inter-rater variations and compromised data source reliability. However, childhood maltreatment has been unambiguously assessed to increase the risk for antisocial behavior, recurrent violent behavior, and premature death at the age of 40, especially in combinations with biological variations (e.g., different monoamine oxidase A genotypes) leading to alteration of risk [6–8]. Alcohol consumption has shown a positive correlation with increase in risk for recurrent acts of violence, whereas aging has shown to have a negative correlation to this outcome measure [9]. The biologic field of research may have most new tools to contribute to risk assessments in the future.

The biological research in violent reconvictions may reveal new possibilities to pharmacological treatments of ASPD and support decisions on whom to treat. The method for obtaining reliable scientific evidence of causalities leading to recurrent violent behavior is conducting long follow-up study settings in large cohorts. Both ASPD and severe alcoholism are considered hereditary. A consensus approximation of the hereditary component of alcoholism is 50% [10]. Impulsivity, composed of a persistent tendency to act on the spur of the moment and locomotive restlessness, is also partly hereditary [11]. Detection of genetic causalities underlying ASPD, severe alcoholism, and impulsivity has to date resulted in a handful of robust findings mainly through utilization of violent alcoholics in a young Finnish founder population. Genetic research in founder population allows an increased power to detect specific genetic risk for complex disorders due to a relatively homogenous gene pool caused by geographic isolation [12]. Six functional genetic loci associated with ASPD, impulsivity, alcoholism, and violent behavior, have been detected in the Finnish founder population. These genes comprise the serotonin 2B receptor (HTR2B) [13], tryptophan hydroxylase 2 (TPH2) [14], serotonin 1B receptor (HTR1B) [15], serotonin 3B receptor (HTR3B) [16], monoamine oxidase A (MAOA) [7, 9, 17], and T-cadherin [17].

Apart from specific genes, variation in glucose and insulin metabolism, which could be regarded as biomarkers, has also been shown to robustly predict recurrent violent behavior [18, 19]. Likewise, low serotonin levels have also been robustly associated with impulsive-aggressive behavior [20, 21].

Detection of individuals with high risk, especially due to biologic reasons, may raise ethical issues whether to treat or isolate individuals with increased risk for recurrent violent behavior. However, for medical professionals, the importance of treatment efforts of the psychiatric disorder ASPD, alcoholism, and overt impulsivity is clear as treatment is offered for other diseases with underlying biologic causalities such as diabetes or strokes, as well.

5. Medication

Impulsivity and alcoholism frequently coexist. Consequently, treatment of either symptom or disorder alleviates the other. The treatment of alcoholism is more advanced compared with treatment of impulsivity. At best, specific genetic data may reveal who will benefit from a specific treatment in a dichotomous manner. A prime example of this is that individuals having a specific gene variant (Asp40) in the μ-opioid receptor (OPRM1) seem to clearly benefit from naltrexone treatment of alcoholism, whereas individuals with another genetic variant do not benefit from this medication [22]. Although there is a paucity of studies with such clear evidence of one gene's effect on a particular pharmacological treatment, this is the direction research should move into. Kupila et al. [23] recently found that the severity of alcoholism (Cloninger's type I vs. type II) alters pharmacological binding to the glutamate system, which is associated with addictions. Such findings give clues for meaningful study-setting which could contribute to future evidence-based personalized medical management. The severity of alcoholism has also been examined as a predictor in some pharmacological studies. It seems that patients with severe alcohol dependence (type II), which is associated with ASPD, may react differently to medications as compared with patients with the less severe form of alcoholism (type I), which is the type of alcohol dependence that the majority of "alcoholics" suffer from. For instance, antagonism of the serotonin 3 receptor with ondansetron has shown beneficial in the treatment of early onset severe alcoholism (type II), whereas no considerable therapeutic effect appears among patients with less severe alcoholism [24].

Moreover, carriers of a loss-of-function point mutation allele of the serotonin 2B receptor (HTR2B Q20*) may benefit from focused treatment of alcoholism and impulsivity as this mutation has been shown to make the carriers of this mutation more susceptible for problem-behavior especially while under the influence of alcohol, but also while sober [25]. However, this point mutation in the serotonin 2B receptor has only been found among Finns at this point, but this may serve as an example of a functional genetic discovery, which may lead to development of personalized treatments. Widely used serotonin selective reuptake inhibitors (SSRIs), such as fluoxetine and citalopram, do not seem to decrease depression or suicide rates among human HTR2B Q20* carriers or Htr2b knockout mice [26, 27]. Therefore, SSRIs likely show no effect on HTR2B Q20* ASPD carriers, but new pharmacological strategies are being currently developed [28].

Due to a lack of highly efficient pharmacological treatment of impulsivity and aggression, a vast variety of psychotropic medications have been used for treatment of impulsivity and aggression. However, recent research both in animal study settings [29] and large human follow-up cohorts [30] suggests that lithium could be the drug of choice for preventative treatment of impulsive behavior, due to the associated lower risk of suicide attempts and significantly decreased suicide mortality, in comparison to valproic acid and benzodiazepines, in high-risk bipolar patients [30].

6. Psychotherapy

Psychotherapy aims at alleviating various symptoms, modulate thought constructs, and to gain control of behavior such as antisocial attitudes, drinking alcohol, or acting impulsively. A slight pessimism regarding the efficacy of psychotherapy in treating ASPD is frequent among clinicians, which is partly justified as antisocial thought constructs and impulsive behavior decrease treatment compliance. Persons suffering from personality disorders tend to have difficulties to realize or admit that they have a mental health problem that would need treatment. This is especially true for ASPD. However, this pessimism for the efficacy of treatment is not justified for all ASPD patients. For instance, group-based cognitive and behavioral interventions focused on reducing offending and other antisocial behaviors in an optimistic and trusting context have shown some good results [31]. It is also important not to have to ambitious goals, but to aim at alleviating some symptoms such as impulsive behavior, decrease in alcohol consumption, and decrease in disrespect of the rights of others. Clinical experience in the field of forensic psychiatry suggests that life events such as coming into religious faith and commitment to a strong-willed spouse would represent a "natural" psychotherapy altering thought constructs and behavior, and it has proved to be helpful for some ASPD patients. Consequently, simple psychotherapeutic themes in treatment of ASPD would be discussing religious interests and the benefits of being in a stable long-term relationship.

7. Nutrition

There is no convincing robust scientific evidence for treating ASPD with specific diets alone, but the inherent impulsivity and lack of persistence in ASPD certainly cause poor dietary habits. Many vitamins and other compounds received through food are vital for the proper biologic and physiologic functioning of the body. Thus, it is likely—and a fair hypothesis—that specific diets and supplements may show beneficiary for the treatment of ASPD with associated symptoms in the future as a part of the treatment strategy. One randomized placebo-controlled study suggests that the influence of supplementary vitamins, minerals, and essential fatty acid would decrease antisocial behavior and violence in an incarcerated context [32]. These kinds of study settings should be replicated and performed in outpatient study settings.

Some general advice, although speculative, on what diet to recommend for ASPD individuals could be mentioned. As low serotonin levels have been coupled with impulsivity and aggression [20, 21], a tangible means of ensuring a sufficient supply of tryptophan in the diet would be consumption of cheese and peanuts. When an alcoholic is being in a prolonged relapse period of drinking, it may be a good advice to make sure to eat glucose-rich food, as low glucose levels have been associated to violent and irritable behavior [20]. On the other hand, a glucose-rich diet may be harmful in the long run as it increases the risk for type 2 diabetes, and high insulin levels have been associated with increased risk for acts of violence [18].

8. Conclusions and future direction

As most of the acts of violence in the western world are attributable to individuals having ASPD, enhancement of the treatment of ASPD will have tangible effects in terms of reduction of violence in society. Most new ground is expected to be gained through an increasing understanding of biological causalities underlying ASPD will help to personalize treatments, including the therapeutic areas such as redox state and diet. Combination of several treatment strategies likely amounts in best treatment results. As treatment is challenging, professionals should be trained to treat this specific patient group. Furthermore, clinicians—including general practitioners—would need education in recognizing symptoms associated with ASPD and encouragement to refer these patients to specialized treatment, although the problem remains that ASPD patients rarely seek treatment due to the inherent nature of the disorder. Conclusively, it should be noted that research supporting evidence-based personalized treatment of ASPD is sparse. This review therefore reflects the clinical and theoretical expertise of the author, which hopefully could initiate further research.

Author details

Roope Tikkanen

Address all correspondence to: roope.tikkanen@helsinki.fi

Department of Psychiatry, University of Helsinki and Laboratory of Neurogenetics, National Institute on Alcohol Abuse and Alcoholism, National Institute of Health, Rockville, MD, USA

References

[1] Lenzenweger MF, Lane MC, Loranger AW, Kessler RC. DSMIV personality disorders in the national comorbidity survey replication. Biological Psychiatry. 2007;**62**(6):55364

[2] American Psychiatric Association. Diagnostic and Statistical Manual of Mental Disorders. 3rd revised ed. Washington, DC: American Psychiatric Press; 1987

[3] Fazel S, Danesh J. Serious mental disorder in 23000 prisoners: A systematic review of 62 surveys. Lancet. 2002;**359**(9306):54550

[4] Doyle M, Dolan M. Violence risk assessment: Combining actuarial and clinical information to structure clinical judgements for the formulation and management of risk. Journal of Psychiatric and Mental Health Nursing. 2002;**9**(6):64957

[5] Tikkanen R, AuvinenLintunen L, Ducci F, Sjoberg RL, Goldman D, Tiihonen J, Ojansuu I, Virkkunen M. Psychopathy, PCLR, and MAOA genotype as predictors of violent reconvictions. Psychiatry Research. 2011;**185**(3):3826

[6] Caspi A, McClay J, Moffitt TE, Mill J, Martin J, Craig IW, Taylor A, Poulton R. Role of genotype in the cycle of violence in maltreated children. Science. 2002;**297**(5582):8514

[7] Tikkanen R, Ducci F, Goldman D, Holi M, Lindberg N, Tiihonen J, Virkkunen M. MAOA alters the effects of heavy drinking and childhood physical abuse on risk for severe impulsive acts of violence among alcoholic violent offenders. Alcoholism: Clinical and Experimental Research. 2010;**34**(5):85360

[8] Tikkanen R, Holi M, Lindberg N, Tiihonen J, Virkkunen M. Recidivistic offending and mortality in alcoholic violent offenders: A prospective follow-up study. Psychiatry Research. 2009;**168**(1):1825

[9]   Tikkanen R, Sjoberg RL, Ducci F, Goldman D, Holi M, Tiihonen J, Virkkunen M. Effects of MAOA genotype, alcohol consumption, and aging on violent behavior. Alcoholism: Clinical and Experimental Research. 2009;**33**(3):42834

[10] Ducci F, Goldman D. The genetic basis of addictive disorders. The Psychiatric Clinics of North America. 2012;**35**(2):495519

[11] Bevilacqua L, Goldman D. Genetics of impulsive behaviour. Philosophical Transactions of the Royal Society of London Series B: Biological Sciences. 2013;**368**(1615):20120380

[12] Lim ET, Wurtz P, Havulinna AS, Palta P, Tukiainen T, Rehnstrom K, Esko T, Magi R, Inouye M, Lappalainen T, et al. Distribution and medical impact of loss-of-function variants in the Finnish founder population. PLoS Genetics. 2014;**10**(7):e1004494

[13] Bevilacqua L, Doly S, Kaprio J, Yuan Q, Tikkanen R, Paunio T, Zhou Z, Wedenoja J, Maroteaux L, Diaz S, et al. A population specific HTR2B stop codon predisposes to severe impulsivity. Nature. 2010;**468**(7327):10616

[14] Zhou Z, Roy A, Lipsky R, Kuchipudi K, Zhu G, Taubman J, Enoch M, Virkkunen M, Goldman D. Haplotype-based linkage of tryptophan hydroxylase 2 to suicide attempt, major depression, and cerebrospinal fluid 5hydroxyindoleacetic acid in 4 populations. Archives of General Psychiatry. 2005;**62**(10):110918

[15] Lappalainen J, Long JC, Eggert M, Ozaki N, Robin RW, Brown GL, Naukkarinen H, Virkkunen M, Linnoila M, Goldman D. Linkage of antisocial alcoholism to the serotonin 5HT1B receptor gene in 2 populations. Archives of General Psychiatry. 1998;**55**(11):98994

[16] Ducci F, Enoch M, Yuan Q, Shen P, White KV, Hodgkinson C, Albaugh B, Virkkunen M, Goldman D. HTR3B is associated with alcoholism with antisocial behavior and alpha EEG power: An intermediate phenotype for alcoholism and comorbid behaviors. Alcohol. 2009;**43**(1):7384

[17] Tiihonen J, Rautiainen M, Ollila HM, RepoTiihonen E, Virkkunen M, Palotie A, Pietilainen O, Kristiansson K, Joukamaa M, Lauerma H, et al. Genetic background of extreme violent behavior. Molecular Psychiatry. 2015;**20**(6):78692

[18] Ojala KP, Tiihonen J, RepoTiihonen E, Tikkanen R, Virkkunen M. Basal insulin secretion, PCLR and recidivism among impulsive violent alcoholic offenders. Psychiatry Research. 2015;**225**(3):4204

[19] Virkkunen M, Rissanen A, FranssilaKallunki A, Tiihonen J. Low nonoxidative glucose metabolism and violent offending: An 8 year prospective follow-up study. Psychiatry Research. 2009;**168**(1):2631

[20] Virkkunen M, Linnoila M. Brain serotonin, type II alcoholism and impulsive violence. Journal of Studies on Alcohol Supplement. 1993;**11**:163-169

[21] Virkkunen M, Rawlings R, Tokola R, Poland RE, Guidotti A, Nemeroff C, Bissette G, Kalogeras K, Karonen SL, Linnoila M. CSF biochemistries, glucose metabolism, and diurnal activity rhythms in alcoholic, violent offenders, fire setters, and healthy volunteers. Archives of General Psychiatry. 1994;**51**(1):207

[22] Anton RF, Oroszi G, O'Malley S, Couper D, Swift R, Pettinati H, Goldman D. An evaluation of mu-opioid receptor (OPRM1) as a predictor of naltrexone response in the treatment of alcohol dependence: Results from the combined pharmacotherapies and behavioral interventions for alcohol dependence (COMBINE) study. Archives of General Psychiatry. 2008;**65**(2):13544

[23] Kupila J, Karkkainen O, Laukkanen V, Hakkinen M, Kautiainen H, Tiihonen J, Storvik M. [3H]Ifenprodil binding in postmortem brains of Cloninger type 1 and 2 alcoholics: A whole hemisphere autoradiography study. Psychiatry Research. 2015;**231**(3):197201

[24] Johnson BA. Update on neuropharmacological treatments for alcoholism: Scientific basis and clinical findings. Biochemical Pharmacology. 2008;**75**(1):3456

[25] Tikkanen R, Tiihonen J, Rautiainen MR, Paunio T, Bevilacqua L, Panarsky R, Goldman D, Virkkunen M. Impulsive alcohol-related risk-behavior and emotional dysregulation among individuals with a serotonin 2B receptor stop codon. Translational Psychiatry. 2015;**5**:e681

[26] Diaz SL, Narboux-Neme N, Boutourlinsky K, Doly S, Maroteaux L. Mice lacking the serotonin 5-HT2B receptor as an animal model of resistance to selective serotonin reuptake inhibitors antidepressants. European Neuropsychopharmacology. 2016;**26**(2):265-279

[27] Rahikainen AL, Majaharju S, Haukka J, Palo JU, Sajantila A. Serotonergic 5HTTLPR/rs25531 s-allele homozygosity associates with violent suicides in male citalopram users. American Journal of Medical Genetics. Part B, Neuropsychiatric Genetics. 2017;**174**(7):691-700

[28] Maroteaux L, Ayme-Dietrich E, Aubertin-Kirch G, Banas S, Quentin E, Lawson R, et al. New therapeutic opportunities for 5-HT2 receptor ligands. Pharmacology & Therapeutics. 2017;**170**:14-36

[29] Halcomb ME, Gould TD, Grahame NJ. Lithium, but not valproate, reduces impulsive choice in the delay discounting task in mice. Neuropsychopharmacology. 2013;**38**(10):193744

[30] Toffol E, Hatonen T, Tanskanen A, Lonnqvist J, Wahlbeck K, Joffe G, Tiihonen J, Haukka J, Partonen T. Lithium is associated with decrease in all-cause and suicide mortality in high-risk bipolar patients: A nationwide registry-based prospective cohort study. Journal of Affective Disorders. 2015;**183**:15965

[31] Kendall T, Pilling S, Tyrer P, Duggan C, Burbeck R, Meader N, Taylor C, Guideline Development Groups. Borderline and antisocial personality disorders: Summary of NICE guidance. BMJ. 2009;**338**:b93

[32] Gesch CB, Hammond SM, Hampson SE, Eves A, Crowder MJ. Influence of supplementary vitamins, minerals and essential fatty acids on the antisocial behaviour of young adult prisoners. Randomised, placebo controlled trial. British Journal of Psychiatry. 2002;**181**:228

Comparison of Erythrocytes for Individual Indications of Metabolism Changes in Parkinson's and Alzheimer's Diseases

Erland Johansson, Tuomas Westermarck, Paul Ek,
Arno Latvus and Faik Atroshi

Additional information is available at the end of the chapter

http://dx.doi.org/10.5772/intechopen.91660

Abstract

Alzheimer's and Parkinson's diseases are neurodegenerative diseases where several biomarkers have suggested that a single measurement is not a sufficient biomarker. The observation of increased concentration of cadmium (Cd), lead (Pb), and silver (Ag) in erythrocytes by inductively coupled plasma mass spectrometry (ICP-MS) shows a need to look for new approaches to understand the complex synchronistic effects of the cell metabolism. We have used a simplified scheme to follow some of the effects by following a hierarchy of reactions simplified to monitor elements in peripheral blood cells, e.g., erythrocytes. Erythrocytes carry oxygen to cells and carbon dioxide and waste to the lungs and back when passing from different organs including the brain. Erythrocytes also have the capacity to carry metal ions, which may be transferred to other organs, e.g., brain, despite the blood-brain barrier (BBB) and choroid plexus filter. If transfer of Cd, Pb, and Ag is continued too long, the repair systems may not be sufficient, and epigenetic effects on DNA and RNA may begin. Peripheral blood cells, e.g., erythrocytes, may help get earlier individual indications of changes at the cell level by using ICP-MS.

Keywords: hierarchy, cells, Cd, Pb, Ag, erythrocytes, Alzheimer's disease, Parkinson's disease, epigenetic changes, element profile, ICP-MS

1. Introduction

The cell metabolism is a complex balance of proteins, fatty acids, carbohydrates, metal ions, and trace elements regulated by DNA and RNA in nucleus. The metabolism of proteins is

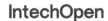

further influenced by a noncoding RNA, e.g., siRNA, which involves molecular reactions and metal ions. Reactions involving metal ions and molecules may create difficulties in interpreting which components are involved due to similar symptoms that may be created by different reactions at the cellular level, masking symptoms. A simplified summary of reactions is given in **Figure 1**.

In **Figure 1**, it is suggested that cell reactions proceed in a hierarchical manner, along with three main pathways [1]. The first pathway involves metal ions associated with ligands with different strengths due to properties of metal ions, binding compounds, pH, redox state, and medium where this reaction takes place. The second pathway involves organic compounds with nucleophilic or electrophilic properties resulting in products favoring the most reactive partner. The third pathway involves radical reactions which may be fast or slow depending on cell demand. The brain has high needs for oxygen and uses about 20% of the total oxygen. Oxygen is important for many reactions but can produce H_2O_2 or OH^*- radicals that can cause severe damage when not under control. The reaction pathway used for processing a component will be dependent on DNA, RNA, and cell demand.

According to the Food and Drug Administration (FDA) [2], as many as 70% of drugs for Alzheimer's disease, 75% cancer diseases, 50% arthritis diseases, and 40% asthma diseases are

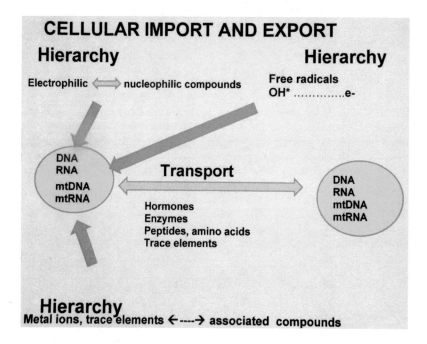

Figure 1. The flow of compounds and metal ions between cells is dependent on the three main chemical pathways in a hierarchy. The first path involves free radical-induced production of compounds where hydroxyl radical and solvated electron reactions may be involved. The second path involves electrophilic and nucleophilic compounds forming products adequate to the cells. The third path involves metal ions and ligands dependent on the previous two pathways but adapted to cell demand. The symbolic schedule indicates that compounds and metal ions may reach DNA and RNA not controlled by evolutionary developed genome adapted to cell demand. Small changes of DNA and RNA may take place, an epigenetic change, which may be restored or adapted, but large damages will present symptoms and are difficult to restore.

not effective. The report may indicate compliance problems and difficulties with translating symptoms from reactions, but above all there is a need of more sensitive and selective systems to handle diseases.

Personalized medicine may be one way to improve systems by better diagnostic tools, designing drugs, etc. Peripheral blood has been used in medical diagnosis for a very long time, because, among other things, it is easily accessible. In the search for signs of lack or excess of minerals and trace elements in the disease, the interest has been focused mainly on blood, plasma, or serum. The utilization of blood cells as a marker model is proposed here. The element profile of blood cells may be one part to improve the present systems.

It is a challenge to separate normal reactions of cell metabolism from early pathophysiological differences. The identification of early changes in cells is important for correct diagnosis and optimal treatment when symptoms indicate the beginning of a disease. Blood cells which pass through several organs may be useful as they exchange information between systems involved. One example is the erythrocytes which transport oxygen from the lungs to different recipients and waste products back, e.g., CO_2 and hemoglobin, for decomposition and excretion. Besides the important transport of oxygen to oxygen-dependent organs, e.g., the brain, liver, and kidneys, they carry metal ions. When cells are growing old or have accumulated metal ions, the metabolism capacity of oxygen or transfer process of metal ions may be changed. By following the variations in the metal concentrations of the erythrocytes, summarized in an element profile, multifactorial diseases may be identified earlier. Observations of increased concentrations of metal ions, e.g., lead (Pb), (cadmium) Cd, and (silver) Ag, in the erythrocytes of patients with Alzheimer's and Parkinson's diseases by inductively coupled plasma mass spectrometry (ICP-MS) indicate possibilities to observe early steps in the pathophysiological processes and early epigenetic changes [3–5].

An early indication of changed metal ion homeostasis by an element profile is the change of important cell reactions. The element profile may be looked upon as the integrated results of reactions of metal ions and ligands. Cells with different life span, e.g., erythrocytes and platelets, help in the interpretation of possible changes. Changes in the element profile may give early biochemical, physiological, and pathophysiological information of changed cell metabolism and indicate defects in vulnerable organs.

2. Comparison of significant increased concentrations of Pb, Cd, and Ag in the erythrocytes of patients with Alzheimer's and Parkinson's diseases

Patients with Alzheimer's disease were selected in Finland [3] and patients with Parkinson's disease in Sweden [4, 5]. The mean concentrations of Pb in patients with Alzheimer' disease [3] and Parkinson's disease were 157 µg/kg (wet weight) and 67.8 µg/kg, respectively, about two times higher than that of Parkinson's disease [5]. The concentration of Cd in erythrocytes of patients with Alzheimer's disease was 11.5 µg/kg (wet weight) and 1.9 µg/kg in Parkinson's disease, about five times higher in Alzheimer's disease. An increased concentration of Ag was observed in both Alzheimer's and Parkinson's diseases 7.4 µg/kg (wet weight) and 2.8 µg/kg, respectively, about two times higher in Alzheimer's disease. Pb, Cd, and Ag maintain the hierarchical effects on weaker associated metal ions in relation to association constants and not to DNA control when the balance of metal ions or binding compounds cannot be controlled [1]. It is important to identify early changes to understand the pathophysiological mechanisms and find proper treatments. Some effects will be discussed in relation to the imbalance of metal ion homeostasis and significant concentration changes of Pb, Cd, and Ag in the erythrocytes.

3. Reduced filter capacity of the kidneys and control of adrenal glands may promote the uptake of Pb, Cd, and Ag in erythrocytes

The reasons for the significant increased concentration of Pb, Cd, and Ag in erythrocytes of patients with Alzheimer's and Parkinson's diseases are not well understood. The absorption of essential elements starts in the small intestine, e.g., duodenum, less in the jejunum, and ileum, and large intestine. It is a complex interplay between intestinal bacteria and the liver, kidneys, pancreas, and bone. It is probable that Pb, Cd, and Ag may use the same carrier systems as essential elements in the blood. After the uptake of Pb, Cd, and Ag, they are transported to other organs for use or storage in the bone and also balanced by the kidneys and adrenal glands. The absorbed Pb, Cd, and Ag may not be properly controlled by the kidneys and adrenal glands. Excretion of Cd is very low and thus Cd is accumulated. The half-life of Cd in humans is about 20–35 years [6]. Most of the Cd is deposited in the kidneys, liver, pancreas, and lungs. Excess Pb is also accumulated often in the bone with a half-life of about 5–19 years [7]. The half-life of Ag in humans is not well documented, but an indicative value may be about 50 days [8]. Erythrocytes have a half-life of about 120 days. The accumulated silver in the erythrocytes may indicate a leakage of silver from root tips with silver amalgam [1, 9]. The contribution of Ag from food, drinking water, and vaccines is probably low. An imbalance of metal ion homeostasis in cell membrane carrier systems may interfere with essential element metabolism in favor of an epigenetic change. The decreased filter capacity of the kidneys and decreased control by parathyroid and adrenal glands can to some extent explain the accumulation of elements in the erythrocytes and the transport to other organs, e.g., brain. If imbalance of metal ion homeostasis in the erythrocytes is lasting too long, DNA control may decrease. The kidneys and adrenal glands in collaboration with the hypothalamus, pineal gland, pituitary glands, and choroid plexus are known to involve in the control of electrolyte and water balance [10, 11]. Chronic exposure to low concentrations of compounds with Pb, Cd, and Ag and loss of binding compounds, e.g., decreased available selenium and compounds with low metal binding capacity, may decrease the filter selectivity and disrupt DNA control. The background of decreased filter capacity is of course complex, but a part of the problem may be found in nutrition, e.g., lack of adequate selenium, phytate (inositol hexakisphosphate), flavonoids, and tannins balancing metal ion flux. In addition, environmental exposure, lack of exercise, smoking habit, and genetic factors may contribute. The decreased filter capacity of the kidneys and decreased brain control may promote the transport of metal ions and compounds not controlled by DNA, thus opening for epigenetic changes. Besides the transport of Pb, Cd, and Ag by erythrocytes in the blood, carriers like albumin, metallothionein, transferrin, and ceruloplasmin carry metal ions to recipients in the body. It is possible that the kidneys provide Pb, Cd, and Ag to erythrocytes, thus disturbing other carrier systems of elements, e.g., Na, K, Mg, Ca, and Se. It is not known if the imbalance of metal ion homeostasis in erythrocytes of patients with Alzheimer's and Parkinson's diseases starts in the kidneys and adrenal glands or how the imbalance of metal ions in the erythrocytes is transferred to other organs. The transport of Pb, Cd, and Ag from the membranes and further selection of metal ions are provided by different systems, e.g., transient receptor protein (TRP) channels [12–14], solute carrier (SLC) protein families [15, 16], and ATP binding cassette (ABC) families [17, 18] and calmodulin families [19, 20]. Interestingly, difference in binding capacity of the membranes gives an additional way to regulate metal ion flow controlled by DNA.

4. Increased concentration of Pb, Cd, and Ag in the erythrocytes and effects of messengers and cellular overload in metal ion homeostasis with reference to calcium homeostasis

The discussion will be limited to some effects of elements, which involve the important messengers in Alzheimer's and Parkinson's diseases: calcium, selenium, and inosine 1,4,5-triphosphate (IP3), the latter being an example of an organic messenger [21]. Calcium is an important intracellular messenger involved in the release of, e.g., [Ca^{2+}], from the rough and smooth endoplasmic reticulum (ER), ryanodine receptor, TRP, mitochondria, and calmodulin family, and apoptosis. Alterations in [Ca^{2+}] homeostasis have been suggested in neurological diseases, such as Parkinson's and Alzheimer's diseases [22–24]. The metabolism and flux of calcium in the ER are suggested to be dependent on, e.g., selenoprotein N, selenoprotein S, and selenoprotein T, critical for maintaining [Ca^{2+}] [25–27]. Microglia were implicated in Alzheimer's disease [28]. If Pb, Cd, and Ag enter in the microglia local defense systems, they may be decreased. Sodium and potassium ions are important for nerve signals and in glucose metabolism [29]. O'Brien and Legge [30] showed that erythrocytes may be mapped by using potassium ions with μ-PIXE technique resulting in a disclike structure indicating high concentration of potassium in the erythrocytes. Erythrocytes and neuron cells carry insulin receptors [31, 32]. Insulin facilitates the introduction of sodium-potassium pumps, indicating that insulin and insulin receptors also support the distribution of Na and K in membranes [33]. As Li, Na, and K often have lower affinity to receptors and carriers than Pb, Cd, and Ag, interactions can be expected in the uptake and transport of channels. In many cells, transport of K can be made in Ca channels, e.g., Gardos channels [34, 35], by SLC family [36]. Insulin facilitates the introduction of sodium-potassium pumps indicating that insulin and insulin receptors also support the distribution of these elements in neuron cells. Cd may interact with Na and K-ATPase, indicating a possible interaction with Na and K ions [37]. Ca and Mg in cells often are carried by members of calmodulin families [38]. Similar size of ionic radius of cadmium 0.97 A and Ca 0.99 A may explain competition of binding sites. Cd in calmodulin molecule causes conformational changes of calmodulin [39]. The binding constants for Pb and Cd in calmodulin are higher than those of Mg and Ca. When cells are not controlled by DNA, Pb, Cd, and Ag may change the metabolism of Mg and Ca. It is not known if and how Pb, Cd, and Ag of erythrocytes compete with carrier systems of patients with Alzheimer's and Parkinson's diseases. In Alzheimer's disease acetylcholine receptors involve Ca [21, 40] which may be repressed by Pb, Cd, and Ag. In cells the calcium concentration is low and kept under strong control because correct concentration of Ca is important for the regulation of ATP synthesis in mitochondria and organelle functions. Uncontrolled release of Ca in cells disturbs ATP synthesis and apoptosis regulation. Cellular overload of Pb, Cd, and Ag is interesting in view of possible interactions of cell metabolism in three ways: (1) competition of Pb, Cd, and Ag with weaker associated metal ions as K, Mg, and Ca; (2) interaction of Pb, Cd, and Ag with selenium compounds in mitochondria and ER; and (3) reaction with phosphate groups in ATP and IP3. Reactive selenium compounds may be identified in different parts of ER important in the regulation of Ca [25]. Studies on harmful effects of metal ions often refer to one element at a time; very little is known about the effects of accumulated Pb, Cd, and Ag and their synchronistic damage. Dementia in Alzheimer's and Parkinson's diseases has been demonstrated in several studies [41]. The effects of Pb and Cd were demonstrated in mentally retarded children [42]. Pb, Cd, and Ag may also "hitchhike" endogenous carriers of essential metal ions making the interpretation of metal ion homeostasis not controlled by DNA reactions more complex. It is likely that Pb, Cd, and Ag may be able to repress Mg and Ca in cell DNA and disrupt DNA and RNA control due to synchronistic damaging effects.

5. Possible effects of Pb, Cd, and Ag on blood-brain barrier (BBB) filter and choroid plexus in relation to metal ion imbalance and selenium homeostasis

In Alzheimer's and Parkinson's diseases, malfunctions may be attributed to damage in different regions. The transport of compounds and metal ions to the brain is controlled by blood-brain barrier and by CSF in the choroid plexus [43–45]. The blood-brain barrier is constructed of endothelial cells, astrocyte end-feet, and pericytes forming diffuse barriers, tight junctions, receptors, and channels for carrier-mediated transport [46]. Leukocytes and larger molecules cannot pass into the BBB as well as in other vessels, but, e.g., oxygen, carbon dioxide, iron, glucose, and certain amino acids can pass. If Pb, Cd, and Ag from erythrocytes enter the BBB, an imbalance may be expected of metal ions and compounds in regions of, e.g., the hippocampus, hypothalamus, pituitary gland, pineal gland, and cortex. Part of Pb, Cd, and Ag in the erythrocytes may "hitchhike" tight junctions, channels, and carriers for essential elements in BBB and enter neuron cells, astrocytes, and microglia in a way not controlled by DNA. Pericytes and endothelial cells have mitochondria and ER which need selenium for proper function of, e.g., Ca and Mg. Mitochondria synthesize ATP, and lowered selenium and Mg may decrease the production of ATP and complicate synthesis systems in ER for the control of Ca and Mg. Activated neutrophil granulocytes can produce (H_2O_2) damage in tight junctions and receptors in membranes of pericytes and endothelial cells when there are local low selenium status and low activity of protecting GSH-Px (GPx1 and GPx4). The ER stores selenium [25] and metal ions for maintaining calcium metabolism. Imbalance in metal ion homeostasis and selenium homeostasis can hamper DNA control of metal flux to different organelles, e.g., ER, mitochondria, Golgi, and nuclei. Besides erythrocyte transport of Pb, Cd, and Ag, albumin may carry Pb, Cd, and Ag which can react with tight junctions and receptors on pericytes and pass, loaded with Pb, Cd, and Ag producing reactive oxygen species (ROS). Pb, Cd, and Ag can interact with elements in mitochondria, e.g., Mg, Ca, Mn, and Se, and disturb ER storage of calcium and action of selenophosphate synthetase. The introduction of selenium in amino acids and UGA (stop codon) is very important for cell metabolism. Albumin may carry heme groups having an antioxidant effect, which decreases the risk of ROS production [47]. Microglia can attack receptors and tight junctions on pericytes around the endothelial cells producing ROS damage and perhaps open for albumin entrance carrying Pb, Cd, and Ag. The brain is composed of 80% water and uses aquaporin, AQ1, AQ4, and AQ9, for water balance [10]. Apart from water control, Pb, Cd, and Ag can use aquaporin for passage [11]. If Pb and Cd can pass into the mitochondria, Mn may be displaced and trigger SOD to produce ROS. Pb, Ca, and Ag may use the SLC system [48], "hitchhike," and transfer elements through the BBB in a way not controlled by DNA. Choroid plexus epithelial cells are rich in selenium [25] and may act as an additional barrier against metal ions and toxic compounds [43]. If erythrocytes are overloaded with Cd, Pb, and Ag, some ions may pass the BBB in other regions of the brain, e.g., hippocampus and cortex, and produce local imbalance of metal ions and selenium homeostasis in the brain.

6. Effects of Pb, Cd, and Ag on insulin receptors in brain cells and energy homeostasis

Increased concentrations of Pb, Cd, and Ag do not only affect the transfer of metal ions but also may influence the metabolism of proteins and peptides [49–51]. In plasma about 30% of Ca and about 40% Zn may be carried by albumin, but albumin also carries other elements and organic compounds [47, 52–54]. In the study of albumin, Pb and Cd decreased the transport of taxifolin [55]. Albumin in the blood carries 1–10% of glucose. If Pb, Cd, and Ag bind to albumin, transport of organic compounds, e.g., glucose, may be decreased. Many peptides and proteins in the BBB are transported by carrier in membranes, e.g., SLC and ABC families, which can be blocked by Pb, Cd, and Ag. T4 (thyroxin) in the blood is transported by transthyretin to the BBB [56]. T4 is dependent on selenium deiodinases for transfer to active T3 (thyronine) [57]. As both deiodinases and T4 and T3 have reactive selenium and iodine groups can Pb, Cd, and Ag disturb selenium homeostasis. Insulin present in the brain is not known to be directly involved in glucose metabolism but may assist in the regulation of energy homeostasis [49, 50]. The brain has many insulin receptors, which is highest in the hippocampus. The association of metal ions to insulin receptors in neuron cells may be similar as that of erythrocytes when Cd, Pb, and Ag interact with K^+ and Na^+ ions with insulin receptors [32]. Insulin binding sites to insulin receptor may be occupied by Pb, Cd, and Ag and decrease transport. Memory problems connected to the hippocampus may be explained to some extent by a decreased transport of insulin, availability of glucose, and the antioxidant capacity of the brain involved in energy homeostasis [49, 50]. If the concentration of Pb, Cd, and Ag of the erythrocytes is too high, insulin transport in the brain may be decreased with less capacity to control energy homeostasis and hormone balance of insulin, leptin, and serotonin [49].

7. Axonal transport and possible interactions of Pb, Cd, and Ag

The axonal transport of mitochondria [58, 59] may be blocked by Pb, Cd, and Ag. Mitochondria were transported by kinesin, dynein, and myosin motors. Accumulation of Pb, Cd, and Ag in the erythrocytes may interact with transport in neurons due to carry-over effects.

In the synapse dopamine and acetylcholine are transported in the vesicles. The observed accumulation of Pb, Cd, and Ag in the erythrocytes may present two problems: (1) lowered dopamine production and (2) blocking acetylcholine.

Dopamine synthesis may be disturbed by Cd, Pb, and Ag in the medulla of adrenal glands, neuron cells, and substantia nigra. Transport of molecules, e.g., dopamine, may be blocked by Pb, Cd, and Ag. Interactions with aldosterone formed in cortex (adrenal glands) are known as an important regulator of Na, K may be disturbed. The high concentration of Cd, Pb, and Ag may interact with the hormone controlled by, e.g., hypothalamus, thalamus, and adrenal glands.

8. Changed metal ion and selenium homeostasis by overloaded Pb, Cd, and Ag in erythrocytes related to receptor functions in Alzheimer's and Parkinson's diseases

Important calcium-dependent receptors were reported in Section 3. Receptors may respond to metal ions and compounds but in a hierarchy to respond correctly. Receptors in the different brain regions may need to be restored; excess Pb, Cd, and Ag may block restoring procedures. Receptor feasibility is dependent on metal ions and organic compounds to maintain hierarchy in selectivity and efficacy. If receptors are exposed to overload of Pb, Cd, and Ag in erythrocytes, receptor activity may be destroyed or renewal not be possible. Patients with Alzheimer's and Parkinson's diseases with changed metal ion homeostasis meet incomplete selenium proteins or not properly adapted proteins [60, 61]. In Parkinson's disease, dopamine synthesis in neuron cells, e.g., substantia nigra and hypothalamus, is decreased. In parkinsonian patient's postmortem substantia nigra, increased concentration of iron was observed [62]. Transport of iron by SLC41 (membrane iron carrier) to the substantia nigra can be disrupted by erythrocytes overloaded with Pb, Cd, and Ag and decrease the synthesis of dopamine. Lowered Ca homeostasis is coupled with selenium deficiency in ER in both Parkinson's and Alzheimer's diseases [26, 63–69]. In Alzheimer's disease increased production of β-amyloid is implicated. Patients with Alzheimer's and Parkinson's diseases may have in common increased Pb, Cd, and Ag in the erythrocytes with possible interactions with selenoproteins and phosphate groups in nuclei, ER, mitochondrial ATP, and IP3 [27]. SelP (selenoprotein P) in the brain with about 10 Se atoms is important to support different brain regions with selenium. As SelP is very reactive, Pb, Cd, and Ag and their protective role may be blocked [70]. A more basic work is necessary to understand how the regulation of metal ion homeostasis in cells is related to selenium homeostasis at the local level.

9. Epigenetic effects on DNA and RNA repair systems after exposure to Cd, Pb, and Ag from erythrocytes

Cells exposed to Cd, Pb, and Ag can disturb the genomic stability which is dependent on Mg [71, 72]. DNA is dependent on efficient repair systems due to as many as 10,000 errors/cell/day [73]. If Cd, Pb, and Ag from erythrocytes are introduced to cells, repair systems will not work properly [74]. Deformed molecules or decreased production of important protective compounds may initiate problems in cell metabolism, e.g., it starts wrong apoptosis signals and Cd, Pb, and Ag may compete with repair systems, e.g., enzymes and ligases of DNA polymerases [75, 76]. Excess Cd, Pb, and Ag can also impair Zn-dependent RNA polymerases by competing with the active center in the binding domain and also create cross-linking of DNA [77–79].

10. Conclusions

ICP-MS may be used for the determination of the element profile of erythrocytes as a biomarker in Alzheimer's and Parkinson's diseases. The increased concentration of Pb, Cd, and Ag in erythrocytes in Alzheimer's and Parkinson's diseases indicates changes in the filter capacity of the kidneys combined with the changes of the adrenal glands. Studying multifactorial problems using element profiles in diseases may help to identify early changes in the pathophysiological process and epigenetic progress. The increase of Pb, Cd, and Ag in the erythrocytes may indicate changes in metal ion homeostasis at the cellular level in other parts of the body, e.g., the brain.

Parkinson's and Alzheimer's diseases are neurodegenerative diseases. A variety of treatment recommendations in the treatment guidelines have been proposed, including physical activity and disease-modifying medication, which should be initiated at the early stage of the disease. The complex synchronistic effects at the cellular level when Cd, Pb, and Ag enter in a noncontrolled way may be approached by using ICP-MS. It is hoped that this knowledge will allow the identification of novel therapeutic targets that will eventually lead to a more efficient treatment, based on the patient's individual genetic predispositions.

Many candidate biomarkers of the neurodegenerative diseases have been proposed in the scientific literature, but in all cases, their variability in cross-sectional studies is considerable, and therefore no single measurement has proven to serve a useful marker, possibly lacking the power of directly predicting disease risk, as the underlying physiological change may per se be harmless and without functional compromise.

This necessitates the development of new effective strategies for the prevention and early diagnosis of such conditions. Contrary to the common perception that personalized medicine is completely based on a genetic approach, clinical subtypes, personality, lifestyle, aging, and comorbidities constitute the true personalized medicine.

Acknowledgements

The authors would like to thank the Crafoord Foundation for providing economic support and Åbo Academy for putting instrumental facilities at our disposal.

Author details

Erland Johansson[1*], Tuomas Westermarck[2], Paul Ek[3], Arno Latvus[4] and Faik Atroshi[5†]

*Address all correspondence to: 101jejohansson@gmail.com

1 EJSelenkonsult AB, Uppsala, Sweden

2 Rinnekoti Research Centre, Espoo, Finland

3 Laboratory of Analytical Chemistry, Åbo Academy, Finland

4 Museokatu 13 B, Helsinki, Finland

5 Pharmacology and Toxicology, University of Helsinki, Finland

†Deceased.

References

[1] Johansson E. Selenium and its protection against the effects of mercury and silver. Journal of Trace Elements and Electrolytes in Health and Disease. 1991;5(4):273-274

[2] Hamburg MA. Paving the way for personalized medicine. USA: FDA; 2013

[3] Johansson E, Westermarck T, Ek P, Atroshi F. Metabolism changes as indicated by the erythrocytes of patients with Alzheimer's disease. In: Atroshi F, editor. Pharmacology and Nutritional Intervention in the Treatment of Disease. Croatia: IntechOpen; 2014. pp. 405-415

[4] Johansson E, Westermarck T, Hasan MY, Nilsson B, et al. Alterations in nickel and cadmium concentrations in erythrocytes and plasma of patients with Parkinson's disease. Trends in Biomedicine in Finland. 2007;XXI 2(4):17-32

[5] Johansson E, Ek P, Holmkvist M, Westermarck T. Erythrocytes as biomarkers of changed metal ion homeostasis in patients with Parkinson's disease. Journal of Trace Elements in Medicine and Biology. 2013;27(S1):45

[6]   Jomova K, Valko M. Advances in metal-induced oxidative stress and human disease. Toxicology. 2011;**283**(2-3):65-87

[7]   Rabinowitz MB. Toxicokinetics of bone lead. Environmental Health Perspectives. 1991;**97**: 33-37

[8]   Lansdown ABG. A pharmacological and toxicological profile of silver as an antimicrobial agent in medical devices. Advances in Pharmacological Sciences. 2010:**16**. Article ID 910686

[9]   Johansson E, Liljefors T. Heavy elements in root tips from teeth with amalgam fillings. In: Momcilovic B, editor. TEMA 7, Zagreb. 1991. pp. 11-18-11-20

[10] Agre P, King LS, Yasui M, Guggino WB, Ottersen CP, Fujoshi Y, et al. Aquaporin water channels—From atomic structure to clinical medicine. The Journal of Physiology. 2002;**542**: 3-16

[11] Tait MJ, Saadoun S, Bell A, Papadopoulos MC. Water movement in the brain: Role of aquaporins. Trends in Neuroscience. 2007;**31**(1):37-43

[12] Schlingman KP, Waldegger S, Konrad M, Chubanov V, Gudermann T. TRPM6 and TPRM7-Gatekeepers of human magnesium metabolism. BBA. 2007;**1772**:813-821

[13] de Rouffignac C, Quamme G. A renal magnesium handling and its hormonal control. Physiological Reviews. 1994;**74**:305-322

[14] Hoenderop JGJ, Bindels RJM. Calciotropic and magnesiotropic TRP channels. Physiology. 2008;**23**:32-40

[15] Herbert SC, Mount DB, Gamba G. Molecular physiology of cation-coupled Cl^- cotransport: SLC 12 family. European Journal of Physiology. 2004;**447**:580-593

[16] He L, Vasilio K, Nebert DW. Analysis and update of human solute carrier (SLC) gene superfamily. Human Genomics. 2009;**3**(2):195-206

[17] Tarling EJ, de Agular Vallim T, Edwards PA. Role of ABC transporters in lipid transport and human disease. Cell. 2013;**24**(7):342-350

[18] Vasilio V, Vasilio K, Nebert DW. Human ATP-binding cassette (ABC) transport family. Human Genomics. 2009;**3**(3):281-290

[19] Valencia CA, Szostak JW, Dong B, Liu R. Scanning the human genome proteome for calmodulin-binding proteins. PNAS. 2005;**102**(12):5969-5974

[20] Ikura M, Ames JB. Genetic polymorphism and protein conformational plasticity in the calmodulin superfamily: Two ways to promote multifunctionality. Proceedings of the National Academy of Sciences of the United States of America. 2005;**103**(5):1159-1164

[21] Young KW, Billups D, Nelson CP, Johnston N, Willets JM, Schell MJ, et al. Muscarinic acetylcholine receptors activation enhances hippocampal neuron excitability and potentiates synaptically evoked Ca^{2+} signals via phosphatidylinositol 4,5-bisphosphate depletion. Molecular and Cellular Neurosciences. 2005;**30**(1):48-57

[22] Surmeier DJ, Guzman JN, Sanchez-Padilla J, Schumacher PT. The role of calcium and mitochondrial oxidant stress in the loss of substantia nigra pars compacta dopaminergic neurons in Parkinson's disease. Neuroscience. 2011;**198**:21-231

[23] Coscum P, Wyrembak J, Schriner SE, Chen H-W, Marciniak C, LaFerla F, et al. A mitochondrial etiology of Alzheimer and Parkinson's disease. BBA. 2012;**1820**:553-564

[24] Jellinger KA. Neuropathological aspects of Alzheimer disease, Parkinson disease and frontotemporal dementia. Neurodegenerative Diseases. 2008;**5**:118-121

[25] Reeves MA, Hoffmann PR. The human selenoproteome: Recent insights into functions and regulation. Cellular and Molecular Life Sciences. 2009;**66**(15):2457-2478

[26] Chen J, Berry J. Selenium and selenoproteins in the brain and brain diseases. Journal of Neurochemistry. 2003;**86**:1-12

[27] Pilial R, Uyshara-Lock JH, Ballinger FP. Selenium and selenoprotein function brain disorders. IUBMB. 2014;**66**(4):220-239

[28] Solito E, Sastre M. Microglia function in Alzheimer's disease. Frontiers in Pharmacology. 2012;**3**(14):1-10

[29] Brugnara C. Erythrocyte membrane transport physiology. Current Opinion in Haematology. 1997;**4**:122-127

[30] O'Brien PM, Legge GJF. Elemental microanalysis of individual blood cells. Biological Trace Element Research. 1987;**13**:159-166

[31] Gambhir KK, Archer JA, Bradley CJ. Characteristics of human erythrocyte insulin receptor. Diabetes. 1978;**27**:701-708

[32] Chiu SL, Chen C-M, Cline HT. Insulin receptor signaling regulates synapse number, dendritic plasticity and circuit function in vivo. Neuron. 2008;**58**:708-719

[33] Clausen T. Clinical and therapeutic significance of the Na^+, K^+ pump. Clinical Science. 1998;**95**:3-17

[34] Gardos G. The function of calcium in the permeability of human erythrocytes. Biochim Biophys Acta. 1958;**30**(3):633-654

[35] Vijverberg HPM, Leinders-Zufall T, van Kleef RGDM. Differential effects of heavy metal ions on Ca^{2+}-dependent K^+-channels. 1994;**14**(6):841-857

[36] Herbert SC, Mount DB, Gamba G. Molecular physiology of cation-coupled Cl^- cotransport: The SLC12 family. Pflügers Archiv: European Journal of Physiology. 2004;**447**: 580-593

[37] Lijnen P, Staessen J, Fagard R, Amery A. Effect of cadmium on transmembrane Na^+ and K^+ transport system in human erythrocytes. British Journal of Industrial Medicine. 1991;**48**:392-398

[38] Shen X, Valencia CA, Szostak JW, Dong B, Liu R. Scanning the human proteome for calmodulin-binding protein. PNAS. 2005;**102**(17):5969-5974

[39] Chao SH, Suzuki Y, Zysk JR, Cheung WY. Activation of calmodulin by various metal cations as a function ionic radius. Molecular Pharmacology. 1984;**26**(1):75-89

[40] Kihara T, Shimohama S. Alzheimer's disease and acetylcholine receptors. Acta Neurobiologiae Experimentalis. 2004;**64**:99-105

[41] Emre M. Dementia associated with Parkinson's disease. The Lancet Neurology. 2003;**2**: 229-237

[42] Marlove M, Errera J, Jacobs J. Increased lead and cadmium burdens among mentally retarded children with borderline intelligence. American Journal of Mental Deficiency. 1983;**87**(5):477-483

[43] Zheng W. Toxicology of choroid plexus: Special reference to metal-induced neurotoxicities. Microscopy Research and Technique. 2001;**52**(1):89-103

[44] Redzic ZB, Preston JE, Duncan JA, Chodobski A, Chodobski S. The choroid plexus-cerebrospinal fluid system: From development to aging. Current Topics in Developmental Biology. 2005;**70**:1-37

[45] Zlokovic BV. The blood-brain barrier in health and chronic neurodegenerative disorders. Neuron. 2008;**57**(2):178-201

[46] Ballab P, Braun A, Nedergaard M. The blood-brain barrier: An overview structure, regulation and clinical implications. Neurobiology of Disease. 2004;**16**:1-13

[47] Oettl K, Stauber RE. Physiological and pathological changes in the redox state of human serum albumin critically influence its binding properties. British Journal of Pharmacology. 2007;**15**(5):580-590

[48] He L, Vasiliou K, Nebert DW. Analysis and update of the human solute carrier (SLC) gene superfamily. Human Genomics. 2009;**3**(2):295-306

[49] Gerozissis K. Brain insulin regulation, mechanisms of action and function. Cellular and Molecular Neurobiology. 2003;**23**(1):1-25

[50] Gerozissis K. Brain insulin energy and disease and glucose homeostasis, genes environment and metabolic pathologies. European Journal of Pharmacology. 2008;**585**:38-49

[51] Kratz J. Albumin as drug carrier: Design of products, drug conjugates and nanoparticles. Journal of Controlled Release. 2008;**132**:171-183

[52] Nicholson JP, Wolmarans MR, Park GR. The role of albumin critical illness. British Journal of Anaesthesia. 2000;**85**:599-610

[53] Fasano M, Curry S, Terreno E, Galliano M, Fanali G, Narciso P, et al. The extraordinary ligand binding properties of human serum albumin. IUBMB Life. 2005;**57**(12):787-796

[54] Zhao X, Liu R, Teng Y, Liu X. The interaction between Ag+ and bovine serum albumin: A spectroscopic investigation. The Science of the Total Environment. 2011;**409**:892-897

[55] Peng M, Shi S, Zhang Y. The influence of Cd^{2+}, Hg^{2+} and Pb^{2+} on taxifolin binding to bovine serum albumin by spectroscopic methods with the viewpoint of toxic ions/drug interference. Environ Tox Pharmacol. 2011;**33**(2):327-333

[56] Wirth EK, Schweitzer U, Köhrle J. Transport of thyroid hormone in brain. Frontiers in Endocrinology. 2014;**5**:1-7

[57] Beckett GJ, Arthur JA. Selenium and endocrine systems. The Journal of Endocrinology. 2005;**184**:455-465

[58] Gunter TE, Buntinas L, Sparagna G, Eliseev R, Gunter K. Mitochondrial calcium transport: Mechanisms and functions. Cell Calcium. 2000;**28**(5/6):285-296

[59] Hollenbeck PJ, Saxton WM. The axonal transport of mitochondria. Journal of Cell Science. 2005;**118**:5411-5419

[60] Zhang S, Rocourt C, Cheng WM. Selenoproteins and the aging brain. Mechanisms of Ageing and Development. 2010;**131**:253-260

[61] Chen L, Na R, Gu M, Richardson A, Ran G. Lipid peroxidation up-regulates BACE1 expression in vivo: Possible early event of amyloid genesis in Alzheimer's disease. Journal of Neurochemistry. 2008;**107**:197-207

[62] Sofie E, Riederer P, Heinsen H, Beckmann H, Reynolds GP, Hebenstreit G, et al. Increased iron(III) and total iron content in post mortem substantia nigra of parkinsonian brain. Journal of Neural Transmission. 1988;**74**:199-205

[63] Cardoso BR, Roberts BR, Bush A, Hare DJ. Selenium, selenoproteins and neurodegenerative diseases. Metallomics. 2015;**7**:1213-1228

[64] Nelson N. Metal ion transporters and homeostasis. The EMBO Journal. 1999;**18**(16): 4361-4371

[65] Yokel RB. A blood-brain barrier flux of aluminium, manganese, iron and other metals suspected to contribute to metal-induced neurodegeneration. Journal of Alzheimer's Disease. 2006;**10**:223-253

[66] Jellinger KA, Seppi K, Wenning GK, Poewe W. Impact of coexistent Alzheimer pathology on the natural history of Parkinson's disease. Journal of Neural Transmission. 2002;**109**(3):309-329

[67] Ericsson MA, Banks WA. Blood-brain barrier dysfunction as a cause and consequence of Alzheimer's disease. Journal of Cerebral Blood Flow & Metabolism. 2013;**33**:1500-1513

[68] Stutzmann GE. Calcium dysregulation IP3 signalling and Alzheimer's disease. The Neuroscientist. 2005;**11**(2):110-115

[69] Hare DJ, Faux NG, Roberts BR, Volitakis J, Marlins RN, Bush AI. Lead and manganese levels in serum and erythrocytes in Alzheimer's disease and mild cognitive impairment: Results from the Australian imaging, biomarkers and lifestyle flagship study of ageing. Metallomics. 2016;8(6):628-632

[70] Andrea S, Takemoto BS, Berry BJ, Bellinger PB. Role of selenoprotein P in Alzheimer's disease. Ethnicity & Disease. 2010;20(1 Suppl 1):S1-92-5

[71] Hartwig A. Role of magnesium in genomic stability. Mutation Research. 2001;475:113-121

[72] Adhikari SA, Toretsky JA, Yuan L, Roy R. Magnesium essential for base excision repair enzymes, inhibits substrate binding of N-methylpurine-DNA glycosylase. The Journal of Biological Chemistry. 2006;281:29525-29532

[73] Lindahl T. Instability and decay of the primary structure of DNA. Nature. 1993;362:709-715

[74] Zhang Y, Baranovsky AG, Tahirov ET, Tahirov TH, Pavlov YI. Divalent ions attenuate DNA synthesis by human DNA polymerase alfa by changing the structure of the template primer or by perturbing the polymerase reaction. DNA Repair. 2016;43:24-33

[75] Sirover MA, Loeb LA. On the fidelity of DNA replication. The Journal of Biological Chemistry. 1977;252:3605-3610

[76] Naryshiskina T, Bruning A, Gadal A, Severinov K. Role of second largest RNA polymerase I subunit Zn binding domain in enzyme activity. Eukaryote Cell. 2003;2(5): 1046-1052

[77] Bertin G, Averbeck D. Cadmium cellular effects, modifications of biomolecules, modulation of DNA repair and genomic consequences (a review). Biochimie. 2006;88:549-5569

[78] Li Q, Zang ZL. Linking DNA replication to heterochromatin silencing and epigenetic inheritance. Acta Biochimica et Biophysica Sinica. 2012;44:3-13

[79] Sancar A, Lindsey-Boltz LA, Unsal-Kacmaz K, Linn S. Molecular mechanisms of mammalian DNA repair and DNA damage checkpoints. Annual Review of Biochemistry. 2004;73:39-85

Chapter 4

Diet, Aging, Microbiome, Social Well-Being, and Health

Mohamed Abdulla

Additional information is available at the end of the chapter

http://dx.doi.org/10.5772/intechopen.91997

Abstract

Over the past few decades, researchers have established that the human body has a complex ecosystem. It is a social network between our own cells and bacteria and other microorganisms. Bacteria cells in the human body outnumber our own cells by 10 to 1. Despite this huge number, they are usually no threat to us. They offer vital help to many of our basic physiological processes. It is becoming increasingly clear that the microbes in our gut play crucial roles in health and disease. It is likely that the bacterial flora in our body may also influence the aging process. Apart from the influence of bacterial flora in our bodies and the diet we consume, there are certain pharmacological substances such as rapamycin, metformin, and resveratrol that are shown to influence longevity in animals and humans. Calorie restriction is known to increase life span in many animal species. Other factors that influence aging include the role of free radicals, gene modifications, chronic inflammation, and certain spices such as curcumin and capsaicin. Modern life style that promotes obesity and social isolation are other factors that contribute to a number of human illnesses. This paper will present some of the latest findings related to gut flora, aging, and social well-being.

Keywords: diet, microbiome, gut flora, social well-being, health

1. Introduction

The relation between our body and the food we eat on a regular basis throughout our lifespan is a very close and intimate one when compared to all other human relationships. Therefore, many researchers in the field of nutrition have often proclaimed "we are what we eat." According to anthropologists, our ancestors cultivated the art of cooking more than a million years ago, and the hot and cooked meals made us what we are today [1]. The oversized

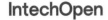

brain, shrunken teeth, guts, and other peculiar traits of our race arose as *Homo sapiens* turned to cooking in order to improve the quality of the food and easy digestion. Unlike our close cousins, the apes, our race cannot survive on raw food in the wild for a long time. On the other hand, the lifespan of our species is much higher than that of the primates. It is often thought that the increased lifespan of humans during the last couple of centuries is due to the advent of antibiotics and other medical advances, the development of modern urban sanitation systems, and the availability of fresh, nutritious vegetables and fruits round the year. This assumption, however, is being challenged by the findings from the study of mummies a few thousand years ago [2, 3]. These studies indicate that the trend in the increase of lifespan actually started much earlier than what was considered a few decades ago. Compelling data from fields as diverse as physical anthropology, primatology, genetics, and medicine indicate another mechanism for the increased life span. The trend toward slower aging and increased life span started when our ancestors developed defense systems that could ward against the threat from pathogens and irritants in the immediate environment [3]. As human ancestors ate more meat, they evolved defenses against its attendant pathogens. These defense systems may also have contributed to an increased life span as well as diseases of old age. Research is going on at present, and if the above theory is proven correct, it may open new avenues for the development of drugs that may prolong the life span as well as fight the old-age diseases. The new abundance of calories and protein helped to fuel brain growth, and at the same time, such nutritional advances also made it unavoidable to the exposure to various pathogens. The risk of exposure to early pathogens and the subsequent development of immunity favored the rise and spread of adaptations that allowed our ancestors to survive attacks by disease-causing organisms such as bacteria, viruses, and other microbes that seek to invade our tissues.

Agriculture was probably developed by humans around the Nile valley, Indus basin, Mesopotamia, and other regions of early civilizations around 10,000–12,000 years ago. It all started when our ancestors noticed that new plants arise from other plant species. In other words, they learned the secret of seeds. This was probably the starting point of agriculture. Before this new era in human history, the diet of our ancestors was composed of fruits, nuts, and tubers. The hunter-gatherer consumed meat whenever they succeeded in hunting. The early *Homo sapiens* kept moving in order to find food and survive. Once they learned the secret of seeds, they quickly learned to domesticate crops, ultimately crossbreeding different plants to create such staples as wheat, rye, and barley. This in turn resulted in a change in the nomadic way of living. They developed a modern way of living by building villages, towns, and cities. Sugarcane was domesticated in New Guinea around 10,000 years ago. It was a kind of food revolution at that time, and according to New Guinean myths, sugar was an elixir that cured almost everything. The domestication of sugarcane spread slowly from island to island and reached the Asian mainland, the Middle East, and Europe. In India, in olden days, sugar was used as a medicine for headaches, gut flutters, and impotence. Finally, Columbus planted sugar cane in Hispaniola. The slave trade in North and South America is a consequence of sugar plantation.

The eating habits of our hunter-gather ancestors changed drastically since they discovered the secrets and potentials of seeds and plants. Along with the advances in technology and

instrumentation, the early practice of agriculture improved tremendously, and our ancestors quickly learned to domesticate crops and animals as mentioned earlier. The percentage
of carbohydrates in the diets of our ancestors after the introduction of agriculture increased
to as much as 40% compared to fats and proteins. With the advance of industrial revolution
about two centuries ago, our dietary habits changed further. The fast-food business became
very lucrative, and currently, it is being introduced even in the remote corners of the globe.
Alcoholic beverages mainly beer and wine were introduced to human diets around 6000 years
ago. The distillation process discovered by the Alchemists in the Middle East several centuries
ago led to the production of strong alcoholic beverages such as whiskey and brandy. The introduction of fertilizers and other chemicals in recent decades to boost the production of crops
has resulted in the contamination of soil and water. The percentage of heavy metals and other
contaminants in the soil and water increased significantly, and this in turn affected plants and
aquatic ecology. The future of agricultural practices is likely to be changed drastically in the
coming years with increasing population burden. How food is going to transform the future
generations is a challenging situation for scientists and politicians. Genetic engineering might
be a partial solution. Genetically modified vegetables and grains are already available in many
food stores. With the current trend in population explosion, it is crucial to find ways to improve
agriculture without destroying the ecology.

For thousands of years, humans shared the planet with Neanderthals, primates, and a large
number of other species which are extinct. Our species were also at a risk of extinction about
74,000 years ago when a super volcanic eruption took place in Indonesia. The human population at that time was only a few thousands. The heroic ascent of man took place around
35,000–50,000 years ago. At around the time of introduction of agriculture, the human population was around one million [4]. During the industrial revolution about 150–200 years ago,
the human population became one billion. After the Second World War, dramatic changes
took place in the history of *Homo sapiens*. This included population expansion, globalization,
mass production, technological and communication revolutions, improved farming methods,
and advances in health sciences. It is predicted that by 2050, the human population would be
increased to 9 billion. It is the age of man: the *Anthropocene* [4].

In this mini-review, I would describe the current knowledge about human aging and the
importance of bacterial flora in our bodies that have profound influence in our health and
social well-being. It will also describe some of the latest advances in order to deal with the
aging populations throughout our globe.

2. Diet, pharmaceuticals, and aging

Any comparative study of diet and aging depends on the availability of accurate criteria for
defining and assessing the aging processes. Currently, a lot of information is available about
human aging. Burnet in 1974 indicated a linear relation between age and logarithmic values for
total death rates in different populations [5]. The exponential increase in mortality rates with
age was first noted by Gompertz in 1825 [6]. Research on aging in the late 1960s in Sweden and

the United States showed similar patterns. Mortality for both countries was higher for men from birth up to the highest ages, whereas the mortality rate at age 10 shows for both men and women the lowest figures of all age groups. At age 20, there is a limited additional increase that is more pronounced in males than in females. It may have a special significance when it is realized that the blood pressure in normal populations exhibits an almost identical plateau at age 20 [7]. These data are consistent with a genetic control hypothesis for aging which is in turn under environmental influence.

During the 1960s and 1970s, tobacco, alcohol, sugar, coffee, and some other constituents have been singled out as factors increasing the risk of developing diseases of the old age including cardiovascular diseases, diabetes, and cancer. Mormons in Utah, USA, and other parts of the world are forbidden to drink alcoholic beverages and coffee and to smoke. It seemed of interest to compare the mortality rates for Mormons and other groups. Studies by Brown and Forbes in 1976 showed that mortality rates of Mormons in Utah (USA) and a control group in Montreal (Canada) showed an identical pattern [8]. The similarity was pronounced after the age of 40 when cancer and cardiovascular diseases are the dominating cause of death [8]. Similar results were found in Sweden. Does this mean that smoking habits and drinking alcoholic beverages and coffee are less important than other factors? Later studies, however, have proven that drinking, smoking, and the consumption of fatty foods have a profound negative influence in the development of diseases of the old age. Studies in Sweden and other countries during the 1970s suggest two separate selection processes: one from conception until the age of 10 and the other from 10 until death. The early selection period may be more susceptible to social and general living conditions than the second. Those surviving the first 20–30 years of age in Australia 100 years ago showed a lower rise in mortality rate with age than the case in the general population today [5, 9]. These findings indicate that aging might be a continuous process [10]. In China arteriosclerosis was not considered to be a clinical problem in the 1930s, but today there is a high incidence of cardiovascular disease in China [11]. The Chinese diet was considered to be "non-atherogenic." The diet at the present time is basically unchanged, but the life expectancy, which 60–70 years ago was 33 years or less, is now 70 years. Some decades ago, chronic alcoholism appeared to protect against cardiovascular diseases until it was found that the low incidence of the diseases related to the shorter life span of alcoholics [12, 13]. Another paradox related to alcohol consumption is the high level of high-density lipoprotein (HDL) found in the blood of alcoholics [12, 13]. HDL is found to have some protective effect against the development of cardiovascular diseases.

It was only during the latter part of the nineteenth century that the mean life expectancy at birth in Sweden and some other European countries reached 50 years. The decreasing infant mortality, which still contributes to a prolonged life expectancy in Sweden and other affluent countries, suggests that the diet consumed by the mothers during the most susceptible phase of life has no obvious inadequacies. With the exception of infections and toxic agents, most environmental factors are assumed to affect human genes only slowly. Can the prevailing causes of death due to cardiovascular diseases and cancer be eliminated? The latest research indicates that they cannot be eliminated, but can be postponed. Hayflick in 1976 estimated the increase in life expectancy when the old-age diseases are eliminated [14]. According to his estimate, a total elimination of cardiovascular diseases would lead to an increase in life expectancy at birth of 10.9 years. The elimination of cancer on the other hand would lead life expectancy by only 2–3 years. Studies by Pearce and Dayton in 1971 showed that populations consuming a diet that is high in polyunsaturated fatty acids died less frequently from cardiovascular diseases than people on normal diets [15].

In order to understand the interaction between the genetic basis and the environmental factors at different age levels, it seemed desirable to develop a "biological age indicator" system. Burnet's hypothesis mentioned earlier indicating a genetic control of aging giving the thymus and the circulating lymphocytes a leading role seems to be in agreement with the findings described above. At the present time, based on a number of studies employing modern technology, it is doubtful whether genes alone are involved in the aging process. Genes alone are unlikely to explain all the secrets of longevity. Genes account for only 25% of longevity. It is the environment too, but that does not explain all factors involved in the aging process either. **Table 1** shows some of the relevant factors associated with aging.

Retardation of growth in experimental animals by calorie restriction was first described by McCay and his co-workers in 1939 [16]. Tannebaum and Silverstone showed that diet restriction retards the appearance of various types of cancer and thus the diet slows down the aging process [17–20]. Ross and his co-workers in 1976 showed that a food intake in grams was negatively correlated with age [21]. They concluded that the conditions in early life seem to govern the life span and to interweave with factors that regulate susceptibility to age-related diseases. So far, nobody has established a particular nutrient such as an amino acid, a mineral, a trace element, a vitamin, or total energy as the limiting factor. Although eating sparingly may have been less a choice than an involuntary circumstance of poverty in a number of places in the world during the nineteenth and twentieth centuries, early research has suggested that

Agent/process	Known mechanism
Calorie restriction	Gene modification
Rapamycin and related compounds	mTOR modification
Metformin	Glycation of proteins
Resveratrol	Antioxidant, acts on sirtuins
Free radicals	Damage DNA and proteins
Gene modification	Acts on regulating genes
Chronic inflammation	Cytokine excretion
Young blood	Restoration of GDF 11
Drugs	Gene/hormone activation
Spices (e.g., curcumin, capsaicin)	Antioxidants, act on sirtuins

Table 1. Factors associated with aging process.

a severely restricted diet is associated with a long life. Recent research, however, has undermined the link between longevity and caloric restriction.

Rapamycin was isolated from the soil of Easter Islands during the late 1960s. The soil contained a bacterium that made a defensive chemical that was shown to prolong the life span of several animal species. This substance has been shown to interfere with the activity of a protein called target of rapamycin (TOR) [22–25]. This protein is a now a subject of intensive research around the world. A number of recent studies have shown that suppressing the activity of the mammalian version of the protein (mTOR) in cells can lower the risk of major age-related diseases, especially neurological disorders such as dementia [19]. Researchers at Harvard University, USA, have found this protein also acts as a nutrient sensor [22–25]. When food is abundant, its activity rises, prompting cells to increase their overall production of proteins and to divide. On the other hand, when food is scarce, it helps to conserve the resources. Thus, inhibiting the functions of mTOR may oppose the aging process. Rapamycin, unfortunately, has many side effects in humans, and a few drug companies are developing molecules like rapamycin that have fewer side effects. The discovery that the aging process, previously thought to be intractably complex, could be dramatically slowed by altering one or several genes (gerontogenes) had helped make gerontology a very exciting and hot topic. It also suggests that aging can be retarded by drugs as mentioned above. Such drugs that slow aging could act as preventive medicines that could postpone or retard the late-life disorders including dementia, osteoporosis, cancer, and cataracts. They can be compared with modern drugs for cardiovascular diseases that have pushed off conditions such as early myocardial infarcts [22–25].

Metformin is a very common drug that is prescribed to patients with diabetes throughout the world. Millions of people have taken it for long periods in order to control blood glucose. Considerable efforts have been made since the 1950s to understand the cellular and molecular mechanisms of the action of metformin. The main effect of this drug from the biguanide family is to decrease hepatic glucose production, mainly through the inhibition of mitochondrial respiratory-chain complex 1. In addition, it activates the AMP-activated protein kinase (AMPK) [26]. Its mechanism of action is not yet absolutely very clear at present. It has, however, been shown that metformin inhibits the TOR pathway. It also activates another aging-related enzyme called AMPK, which is likewise stimulated by calorie restriction. Metformin also has been shown to activate certain genes associated with aging in experimental animals. Recent studies at the university in Cardiff University in Wales, UK, showed that patients with type 2 diabetes who took the drug lived on an average 15% longer than a group of healthy controls [26, 27]. Scientists speculate that metformin interferes with a normal aging process called glycation in which glucose combines with proteins and other molecules gumming up their normal functions. This finding is interesting because people who have diabetes, even if it is well controlled, have somewhat shorter life span than their healthy counterparts. Only time can tell us if metformin can retard aging.

Resveratrol is a molecule that is found in grapes, other berries, and red wine. This molecule has attracted considerable attention in recent years in research concerned with aging process. Researchers have found that this molecule can activate enzymes such as sirtuins that regulate some of the genes that control aging process. In animal models, resveratrol appears to activate one of the sirtuins, STRT1, which switches on multiple chemical pathways that mediate hormetic effects [28]. It also guarded the brain and spinal cord against damaging effects from the cutting off of blood flow that occurs in some types of stroke [28]. Not all of the research is uniformly positive. Scientists are uncertain about the specific pathway that resveratrol may be involved in the death of neurons. Moreover, recent studies in rodents have failed to show an anti-aging effect. It is possible that resveratrol and similar molecules modify genes associated with aging. Further studies are in progress.

Reactive oxygen species (ROS) have attracted considerable attention in scientific circles during the last few decades. Metabolites of dioxygen such as superoxide, hydrogen peroxide, and hydroxyl ions are potentially damaging to biological systems. Univalent reduction of dioxygen produces superoxide which can be converted to hydrogen peroxide and hydroxyl radical. Superoxide dismutase which is a zinc-containing enzyme and other antioxidants may be useful in combating cell damage. A few important trace elements such as zinc, copper, iron, and selenium are important components of enzymes that deactivate the damaging effects of ROS and other free radicals. Although the first paper showing the association between trace elements such as manganese and disorders of the central nervous system appeared more than a century ago, much new information has accumulated in recent years concerning the role of free radicals in the etiology and pathogenesis of several neurological diseases. These include Parkinson's disease, dementia, amyotrophic lateral sclerosis, Down syndrome, and Huntington's disease. The similarities in the histopathological changes and the coexistence of these diseases implicate close relationships among the mechanisms of these illnesses. Age is certainly one of the deciding factors in the appearances of degenerative diseases of the central nervous system. The causes of these, diseases, however, are multifactorial. The reduction in the volume of brain is the most evident abnormality in most of the degenerative diseases mentioned above although the distinction between the changes due to the normal aging of the brain and the pathological changes observed in many degenerative diseases of the brain is arbitrary. The role of ROS and other free radicals in the premature aging process and the subsequent increase in the incidence of a number of degenerative diseases has attracted considerable attention during the last few decades. Oxidant stress caused by free radicals is known to disturb calcium homeostasis by altering the calcium transport across the cell and mitochondrial membranes. Mitochondrial DNA is particularly susceptible to oxidative stress, and there is evidence of age-dependent damage and deterioration of respiratory enzyme activities with normal aging. If free radicals are associated with deterioration of neurons and the aging process, it is probable that high levels of antioxidants may prevent such damage. Fruits, vegetables, and nuts are very rich in many antioxidants, and people who regularly consume a diet rich in antioxidants are known to have healthier brains and to be less likely to suffer from neurodegenerative diseases [29]. On the other hand, supplementations of synthetic antioxidants such as vitamin C, E, and A in experimental animals have failed to prevent or ameliorate diseases. Recent studies by Mattson have shown that the beneficial effect of fruits and vegetables are due to the natural pesticides that plants produce [29]. Plants have developed an elaborate set of chemical defenses to ward off insects. When we consume fruits and vegetables, we are exposed to such chemicals in very low doses. Exposures to these chemicals cause a mild stress reaction that lends resilience to cells in our bodies [29]. Adaptation to these stresses accounts for a number of health benefits, including healthy aging. This is currently a very exciting area of research.

A number of genes that control the body's defenses can dramatically improve health and prolong life. Recent studies indicate that a family of genes involved in an organism's ability to withstand a stressful environment has the power to keep its natural defense and repair systems going strong, regardless of age [29]. Many recently discovered genes have been found to affect stress resistance and life span in many laboratory organisms suggesting that they could be part of a fundamental mechanism for surviving unfavorable environment. Scientists studying groups of people genetically isolated by location or culture have found gene mutations that seem to prevent diseases that most often shorten life. **Table 2** shows some of the most important genes associated with aging.

All the known genes associated with the aging process are not included in the table. Along with the recent advances in gene technology, we are definitely going to find more genes that will influence aging.

Chronic inflammation is another component associated with aging. It is stress-related and associated with anxiety. It is well-known that stress modulates the sympathetic nervous system and results in the secretion of hormones such as epinephrine and cortisol. These hormones signal the immune system to release cytokines. These molecules alert leucocytes and other cells to deal with inflammatory process. When one is chronically stressed, the body is flooded with inflammatory chemicals. The chronic inflammation may lead to the development of cardiovascular diseases, cancer, and brain deterioration. Meditation and mindfulness exercises have recently been shown to have positive effect to combat chronic stress. Regular meditation may also reduce the loss of gray matter in the brain [29, 30].

Gene code	Known function
SIR2 (sirtuin family)	Master regulators of survival
CETP	Reduces risk of dementia and hypertension
APOC-3	Lowers risk of CVD and dementia
GHR	Suppresses insulin-like growth factor
	Lowers fat in the blood
FOXO3a	Lowers the incidence of cancer and heart disease
CAT (catalase)	Detoxification of hydrogen peroxide
AMPK	Metabolism and stress response
KLOTHO	Insulin, IGF 1, and vitamin D regulation
DAF/FOXO proteins	Growth and glucose metabolism
Telomerase genes	Effect on chromosomes

Table 2. Some genes that are currently known to be associated with aging and disease.

A recent discovery in mice shows that young blood contains a protein called GD11 [31]. This protein has been shown to rejuvenate an aging animal by stimulating nerve cell growth and retarding myocardial enlargement. No such studies are done in humans. It is interesting to see if people with long life span have increased levels of GD11 in their blood. It is likely that people with low levels of this protein may be at risk of developing chronic diseases at an early stage and this shortens the life span.

As mentioned earlier, a number of pharmaceutical companies are involved in the development of drugs that may influence the aging process. Molecules similar to rapamycin are of great interest. Novartis has already shown that a molecule called everolimus that is chemically similar to rapamycin may retard the age-related chronic diseases in humans. Side effects and cost are the limiting factors. With current state of knowledge concerned with human aging, it is likely that many new drugs may be available in the future for postponing the aging process. The trend is already visible. Lower calorie intake, regular exercise, eating a variety of fruits and vegetables, and getting proper sleep are probably better than drugs to enjoy a healthy old age.

3. Diet and microbiome

Scientists in the past believed that the human body is capable of regulating the metabolic functions through complex network of enzymes and the immune system. Over the last few years, researchers have found out that the human body has a complex ecosystem. It is a social network between our own cells and bacteria and other microorganisms. Trillions of bacteria inhabit our skin, genital areas, mouth, and intestine. Bacterial cells in the human body outnumber our own cells by 10 to 1. Despite this huge number, they are usually no threat to us. Instead, they offer vital help to many of our basic physiological processes [31]. Employing the latest gene technology, researchers have characterized most prevalent species of microbes in our body. It is becoming increasingly evident that the microbes, mainly bacteria, in our guts play crucial roles in health and diseases. Modern lifestyle has definitely contributed in upsetting the normal flora of our guts, and many diseases such as certain autoimmune disorders, obesity, and gastrointestinal problems are probably due to this imbalance. Compared to many developing and poor countries of our planet, the bacterial flora of the people living in affluent countries is certainly different, especially women. This is especially the case in the microbiota of the genital tract. Urinary tract infections are far more common in the females of industrialized countries than that of women living in poor countries in Asia, Africa, and South America.

Newborns through normal delivery are sterile at the time of birth. While passing through the birth canal, babies pick up some of the bacteria from the mother, and they are gradually exposed to other members in the family including pets and other domesticated animals. During the last few decades, Caesarian deliveries have become very common in both developed and developing countries, and this practice has definitely contributed to the difference in quality and quantity of microbes in infants. By late infancy, our bodies support one of the most complex microbial ecosystems on our planet. As mentioned earlier, modern gene technology has helped to create a catalogue of the entire human microbiome. It has turned out that the bacterial genes outnumber our own genes by a factor of 1–150. The latest studies also reveal that each individual belonging to the human race has his/her own bacterial make-up [32]. Most people associate bacteria with diseases such as respiratory tract and urinary tract infections. It is only during the last few decades that we have learned that we host to a number of friendly microbes as well.

Most bacteria found in the healthy guts of humans are beneficial to us. For example, the gut bacteria help to produce vitamins such as cobalamins and break down indigestible food components so that we can make use of them. Humans need vitamin B12 for cellular energy production, DNA synthesis, and the manufacture of fatty acids. Gut bacteria can also break down starch and fiber. They are normally called as commensals. Our own cells in the gastrointestinal tract cannot handle indigestible food components such as starch. At the same time, it must be pointed out that even the most beneficial bacteria in the gut can cause serious disease if they are translocated to some other parts of the body than where they are supposed to be. I shall describe the influence of the two commensals in order to show their importance in human health and social well-being.

Two bacterial species, namely, *Bacteroides thetaiotaomicron* and *Helicobacter pylori*, play crucial roles in digestion and the regulation of appetite. The first one degrades complex carbohydrates. The human genome lacks most of the genes required to synthesize enzymes that degrade carbohydrates as mentioned earlier. The second one *H. pylori* is notorious in the sense that they cause dyspepsia, a dysfunction discovered already in the 1980s by the Australian physicians Marshall and Warren. This is one of the few bacteria that seem to thrive in the acidic environment of our stomachs. After this discovery, it was common to treat peptic ulcers by antibiotics, and the incidence of bacteria-induced peptic ulcers dropped to 50%. Apart from regulating the acidity in the stomach, this bacterium also regulates appetite. The stomach of our species produces two hormones, namely, ghrelin and leptin, that regulate appetite [32]. Patients who are treated with antibiotics and proton-pump inhibitors to eliminate these bacteria from the stomach usually gain weight gradually, and it has been suggested that the obesity seen even in children in affluent countries like the United States is related to elimination of this bacteria from our stomachs. A recent study in the United States shows that only 6% of children have these bacteria. Repeated prescription of penicillin and other antibiotics for minor respiratory illnesses and ear infections is probably the main reason for this imbalance. Eradication of this bacteria from the stomach by proton-pump inhibitors and antibiotics has become the common practice in most countries at the present time, and with time, it is likely that this beneficial bacteria is totally eradicated. It is uncertain at the moment whether the elimination of these bacteria alone will be one of the major causes of obesity in the future.

So far, I have only described the influence of two commensals in our body. What about the trillions of others? A healthy, mature, immune system depends on the constant intervention of beneficial bacteria in the gastrointestinal tract. *Bacteroides fragilis* and the *Lactobacillus* species are another group of gut bacteria found in a majority of human population [32, 33]. These microbes are known to help to keep the immune system in balance by boosting its anti-inflammatory arm. Because of lifestyle changes, especially after the introduction of fast foods over the last few decades, a number of beneficial bacteria species in our guts are disappearing. The microbiota of Westerners is significantly reduced in comparison to rural individuals living similar lifestyle to our Paleolithic ancestors and other free-living primates [34]. What has happened to modern lifestyle during a short period of time has completely changed our association with the microbial world. The rise in a number of autoimmune disorders and obesity is closely associated with the imbalance in our gut flora. Despite the advances in health sciences during the last century, we are still far away from understanding the role of microbiome in health and disease. Intensive research is taking place throughout the world to learn more about the microbiota and health.

4. Food and social well-being

According to the World Health Organization (WHO), the fundamental cause of obesity and overweight is an energy imbalance between calories consumed and calories expended. Physicians and other health personnel throughout the world have advised their overweight patients to eat less and exercise more. In spite of such efforts, the prevalence of obesity or the accumulation of unhealthy amounts of body fat has climbed to unprecedented levels. Currently, 30% of the US populations are overweight, and the health budget has increased to astronomical levels to treat diseases associated with obesity. Similar trends are noted in other affluent countries. Even in fast-growing countries such as China, India, Brazil, Russia, and South Africa (the so-called BRICS), overweight-associated diseases are on the increase. In the good old days, fat babies were considered to be healthier than the thin ones. Even at the present time, many mothers who attend the child care centers in the Western countries are worried when their kids are underweight according to the current growth charts. In many Asian countries, a round belly is considered to be a sign of opulence. The fast-food revolution mentioned earlier is probably the most dominant cause of overweight in affluent countries. If the current trend continues, obesity will soon surpass smoking in most countries as the biggest contributing factor in the development of chronic diseases and early death. For a species that evolved to consume energy-rich food in the environment where starvation was a constant threat, losing weight and staying trimmer in an affluent world fueled by marketing messages and cheap empty calories is, in fact, very difficult. Recent research findings are yielding new and important insights about social and behavioral factors that influence diet, physical activity, and sedentary life. The general public love to believe and react to neat and cheap fixes, and the mass media oblige by playing up new scientific findings in headline after headline as if they were the solutions. Behavior-focused studies of obesity and diets have identified some basic conditions that seem correlated with greater chance of losing weight and keeping it off. These include initial assessment, self-monitoring, behavior shifts, and support from others with similar problems. Unfortunately, people are getting more and more isolated and live a sedentary life mainly due modern lifestyle.

As mentioned in the earlier section, our body hosts trillions of microorganisms, especially in the gut. Bacteria and other microbes dwelling in our body produce molecules that can interact with our central nervous system in ways that appear to affect our anxiety and stress response. Some of these molecules resemble hormones and neurotransmitters. Gut microbiome appear to alter gene activity, especially in the brain, as mentioned earlier. These molecules may also be involved in memory and learning. The mood changes in an individual are known to relate to the activity of the gut microbiota. This again depends on the type and quantity of diet we consume on an everyday basis. Evidence supporting a connection between gut ecology and human brain is trickling in. It is very likely that the microbes on our skin interact with those in the gut and thereby influence our behavior.

The final question is about the kind of diet that could provide a healthy long life. Apart from healthy aging, an ideal diet should have components that can prevent illnesses such as cardiovascular disease and diabetes. Such a diet should be rich in vegetables, fruits, and whole grains, with moderate amounts of protein and less added sugars and bad fats. It is impossible to point out one single nutrient in certain diets that provides health benefits such as reduced death from cardiovascular diseases, and many experts on human nutrition think that it is the result of various foods in combination that provide the most benefit. The important thing is to cut back on how much we eat overall. Therefore, a diet low in added sugars and bad fats, with moderate protein intake, and high in plants, nuts, and fruit, can currently be considered good for healthy aging and social well-being.

Author details

Mohamed Abdulla

Address all correspondence to: abdulla39@hotmail.com

Primary Care Center, Swedish Medical Board, Älmhult, Sweden

References

[1] Finch CE. Evolution of the human lifespan and disease of aging: Roles of infection, inflammation and nutrition. Proceedings of the National Academy of Sciences, USA. 2010;**107**(Supplement 1):1718-1724

[2] Thompson RC et al. Atherosclerosis across 4000 years of human history. Lancet. 2013;**381**: 1211-1222

[3] Pringle H. Long live the humans. Scientific American. 2013;**309**(4):34-41

[4] Vince G. Adventures in the Anthropocene. A Journey to the Heart of the Planet we Made. London: Chatto & Windus; 2014. pp. 1-14

[5] Burnet M. A genetic interpretation of ageing. Lancet. 1973;**II**:480

[6] Gompertz B. On the nature of the function expressive of the law of human mortality, and on a new mode of determining the value of life contingencies. In a letter to Fransis Baily, ESQ. FRS & c. Philosophical Transaction of the Royal Society of London. 1825:513

[7] Thulin T. Blood pressure in a defined population. Studies of individuals and families [PhD thesis]. Lund, Sweden: Studentliteratur; 1977

[8] Brown KS, Forbes WF. A mathematical model of aging processes. Journals of Gerontology. 1976;**31**:385

[9] Norden Å. Ageing. In: Borgström B, Norden Å, Åkesson B, Abdulla M, Jägerstad M, editors. Nutrition and Old Age. Scandinavian Journal of Gastroenterology. 1979;**14** (supplement 52):15-21

[10] Carlsson LA. Nutrition in Old Age. Symposia of the Swedish Nutrition Foundation. Uppsala: Almqvist & Wiksell; 1972. p. 9

[11] Corday F, Corday SR. Prevention of heart disease by control of risk factors. American Journal of Cardiology. 1975;**35**:330

[12] Barona F, Lieber CS. Hyperlipidemia and ethanol. In: Feldman EB, editor. Nutrition and Cardiovascular Disease. New York: Appleton-Century Crofts; 1976. p. 158

[13] Miller NE et al. The Tromsö heart study. High density lipoprotein and coronary heart disease: A prospective case-control study. Lancet. 1977;**I**:968

[14] Hayflick L. The cell biology of human ageing. New England Journal of Medicine. 1976;**295**:1302

[15] Pearce ML, Dayton S. Incidence of cancer in men on a diet high in polyunsaturated fat. Lancet. 1971;**I**:464

[16] McCay CM et al. Retard growth, life span, ultimate body size and age changes in the albino rat after feeding diets restricted in calories. Journal of Nutrition. 1939;**18**:1

[17] Tannebaum A, Silverstone H. Nutrition in relation to cancer. Advances in Cancer Research. 1959;**I**:451

[18] Abdulla M, Sangeeta S. Dietary aspects in cancer prevention. In: Atroshi F, editor. Pharmacology and Nutritional Intervention in the Treatment of Disease. Rijeka: IntechOpen; 2014. pp. 179-189

[19] Abdulla M, Gruber P. Role of diet modification in cancer prevention. BioFactors. 2000;**12**:45-51

[20] Abdulla M. Inorganic chemical elements in prepared meals [PhD thesis]. Sweden: University of Lund; 1985

[21] Ross MH, Lustbader E, Bras G. Dietary practices and growth response as predictors of longevity. Nature. 1976;**262**:548

[22] Stipp D. A new path to longevity. Scientific American. 2012;**2012**:21-27

[23] Blagosklonny MV, Hall MN. Growth and aging: A common molecular mechanism. Aging. 2009;**1**(4):357-362

[24] Harrison DE et al. Rapamycin fed late in life extends life span in genetically heterogeneous mice. Nature. 2009;**460**:392-395

[25] Sharp ZD. Aging and. TOR: Interwoven in the Fabric of Life in Cellular and Molecular Life Sciences. 2011;**68**(4):587-597

[26] Viollett B et al. Cellular and molecular mechanisms of metformin: An overview. Clinical Science (London, England: 1979). 2012;**122**(6):253-270

[27] Bannister CA et al. Can people with type 2 diabetes live longer than those without? A comparison of mortality in people initiated with metformin or sulphonylurea mono-therapy and matched with non-diabetic controls. Diabetes, Obesity and Metabolism. 2014;**16**:1165-1173

[28] Hayden EC. Anti-aging pill pushed as drug. Nature. 2015;**522**:265-266

[29] Mattson M. What does not kill you. Scientific American. 2015;**313**(1):29-33

[30] Hall SS. This baby will live to be 120. National Geographic. 2013;**223**(5):28-47

[31] Carstenson LL et al. The longevity report. Time. 2015;**185**(6-7):56-81

[32] Acherman J. The ultimate social network. Scientific American. 2012;**306**(6):20-27

[33] Junjie Q et al. A human gut microbial catalogue established by metagenomic sequenc-ing. Nature. 2010;**464**:59-65

[34] Bengmark S. Gut microbiota, immune development and function. Pharmacological Research. 2013;**69**:87-113

Chapter 5

Diet-Related Thalassemia Associated with Iron Overload

Somdet Srichairatanakool,
Pimpisid Koonyosying and Suthat Fucharoen

Additional information is available at the end of the chapter

http://dx.doi.org/10.5772/intechopen.91998

Abstract

Thalassemia is an inherited disease caused by the genetic disorder of α- and β-globin genes, resulting in ineffective erythropoiesis and chronic anemia. Transfusion-dependent β-thalassemia patients require red cell transfusion to maintain their blood hemoglobin level in the normal range, whereas non-transfusion-dependent thalassemia patients increase duodenal absorption of dietary iron in an attempt to accelerate erythropoiesis. These changes give rise to iron overload, oxidative stress, organ dysfunction, and other complications. Effective iron chelators are necessary to achieve negative iron balance and to relieve such complications associated with iron overload. Some pharmaceuticals such as hydroxyurea, N-acetylcysteine, ascorbic acid, vitamin E, and glutathione are also given to thalassemia patients in order to overcome oxidative cell and tissue damage and to generate a better quality of life. Interestingly, functional natural products (such as mango, tea, caffeine, and curcumin), vegetables, and cereal (e.g., rice) are helpful for their health-providing properties by supplementing the endogenous antioxidant defensive power in the body. Natural products exhibit many pharmacological activities, but they are safer if used in the traditional manner.

Keywords: thalassemia, personalized medicine, antioxidant, green tea, functional fruits, iron

1. Introduction

Thailand is one of the countries located in Southeast Asia (SEA) with an ongoing thalassemia endemic and has been affected by this inherited disease for a long time. In 2012, we had an official meeting for reviewing progression in the field to develop a good clinical practice guideline (CPG) for thalassemia management in Thailand.

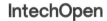

2. Etiology of thalassemia

Thalassemia is an inherited autosomal recessive disorder of hemoglobin molecules (ineffective erythropoiesis) that is characterized by an imbalanced α- and β-globin chain synthesis. The accumulation of unbound α-globin chains in erythroid cells is the major cause of pathology in β-thalassemia. Stimulation of γ-globin chain synthesis can relieve disease severity because it combines with the α-globin chain to form a fetal hemoglobin (Hb F). The disease occurs prevalently from Southeast Asia to the Mediterranean.

2.1. α-Thalassemia

α-Thalassemia is due to an impaired production of α-globin chains from 1, 2, 3, or all 4 of the α-globin genes, leading to a relative excess of β-globin chains. The severity of the disease is based on how many genes are affected. Four clinical conditions of increased severity are recognized: two carrier states, $α^+$-thalassemia caused by the deletion or dysfunction of one of the four α-globin genes, and $α^0$-thalassemia resulting from deletion or dysfunction of two α-globin genes in *cis*. The two clinically relevant forms are Hb Bart's hydrops fetalis syndrome and Hb H disease. Patients with Hb Bart's hydrops fetalis syndrome (homozygous α-thalassemia) have nonfunctioning α-globin genes (genotype α-thal 1/α-thal 1 or − −/− −) and mostly die before birth. Mothers usually suffer hypertension, edema, and toxic pregnancy. Hb H disease patients carry only one functioning α-globin gene (genotype α-thal 1/α-thal 2 or − −/− α, and α-thal 1/ Hb Constant Spring (CS) or −/$α^{CS}$α) and mostly suffer mild-to-severe anemia, jaundice, febrile, and splenomegaly and hepatomegaly. α-Thalassemia is prevalent in tropical and subtropical regions similar to other common globin gene disorders such as β-thalassemia and sickle cell anemia where malaria was and still is an epidemic. As a consequence of massive population migrations, α-thalassemia has become a relatively common clinical problem in North America, Europe, and Australia [1–3].

In northeast Thailand, thalassemia patients suffered with Hb H disease mostly due to the interaction of α-thalassemia 1 (SEA type) with the Hb CS, the deletion of three α-globin genes with the SEA type α-thalassemia 1 and the 3.7- or 4.2-kb deletion of α-thalassemia 2, and the interaction of the SEA α-thalassemia 1 with the Hb Pakse [4]. In Cambodia, α-globin gene mutation was mostly caused by the α-(3.7) (rightward) deletion (frequency 0.098–0.255), α-thal-1 (− −(SEA)) (frequency 0.008–0.011), and α-thal-2 [-alpha(4.2) (leftward deletion)] (frequency 0.003–0.008) [5].

2.2. β-Thalassemia

Human β-thalassemia is characterized by the deficient production of the β-globin chains of adult hemoglobin (Hb A), typically due to mutations of the β-globin gene. Over 200 mutations have been identified in this gene, and the type of mutation can influence the severity of the disease. There are three main types of β-thalassemia, listed in order of decreasing severity: homozygous β-thalassemia major (TM) (genotype $β^0/β^0$) caused by mutations in both alleles, β-thalassemia intermedia (TI) (genotype $β^0/β^+$, $β^+/β^+$, and $β^+/β^E$) caused by diverse mutations, and heterozygous β-thalassemia minor caused by single mutation, including hereditary persistent fetal hemoglobin (HPFH). TI patients usually become mildly anemic (baseline Hb level 7–10 g/dl) and have widely varying severity. Some patients require blood transfusion and chelation to promote their growth in childhood and prevent bone deformities in adults and sometimes get splenectomy due to hypersplenism and mechanical encumbrance. Enhancing Hb F synthesis is useful in some patients, and anti-oxidative compounds were found not to improve blood Hb levels. Stem cell transplantation and gene therapy are possible in well-developed countries but limited in developing countries and in some severe cases. Many complications such as pulmonary hypertension, thrombosis, hypercoagulability, pseudoxanthoma elasticum, and osteoporosis are reported in TI patients and can affect their treatment [6].

β-Thalassemia hemoglobin E (Hb E) (genotype β^0/β^E or β^+/β^E) is most prevalent in SEA countries including Thailand where the carrier frequency is around 50%. The interaction of thalassemia Hb E and β-thalassemia results in a clinical spectrum ranging from a condition indistinguishable from TM to a mild form of TI. Three categories can be identified depending on symptoms as followed: asymptomatic (normal Hb level), mild (baseline Hb level <9.0 g/dl), moderate (baseline Hb level 7–9 g/dl), and severe (baseline Hb level <7.0 g/dl). In transgenic mice, homozygous beta-knockout (BKO) thalassemia shows many clinical features of red blood cells (RBC) indices, in particular mild anemia similar to human TI. The abnormalities include decreased blood Hb concentration, hematocrit (Hct), numbers and osmotic fragility of RBC, and the increase of reticulocyte count. Additionally, Perl's staining and colorimetric assays shows deposition of iron in the spleen, liver, and kidneys but not in the heart [7].

3. Anemia in thalassemia

The accumulation of excess unbound α-globin chains in erythroid cells of β-thalassemia patients can result in RBC hemolysis and anemia; nevertheless, stimulation of γ-globin gene to produce γ-globin chain which can combine with the α-globin to form Hb F is a therapeutic approach. Like cell apoptosis, eryptosis is a programmed cell death or suicidal death of erythrocytes which is characterized by shrinkage, membrane bleb, activation of proteases (e.g., caspase and calpain) after oxidative stress, and phosphatidylserine (PS) exposure at the outer plasma membrane leaflet of the affected RBC. Eryptosis can be triggered by osmotic shock, energy depletion, hyperthermia, curcumin, ceramide, prostaglandin E_2, platelet-activating factor, valinomycin, amyloid peptide, hemolysin, chlorpromazine, cyclosporine, paclitaxel, stressors-induced injury, and iron-induced oxidative stress. In contrast, it is inhibited by erythropoietin (EPO), catecholamines, and nitric oxide (NO). Eryptosis is probably a useful mechanism to get rid of defective RBC and infectious agents. Nonetheless, excessive eryptosis found in iron deficiency, intoxication of metals (such as Al, Cu, Pb, and Hg), xenobiotics, β-thalassemia, sickle cell disease (SCD), glucose-6-phosphate dehydrogenase (G6PD) deficiency, hereditary spherocytosis, paroxysmal nocturnal hemoglobinuria, myelodysplastic syndrome (MDS), phosphate depletion, sepsis, hemolytic uremic syndrome, renal insufficiency, diabetes, pathogenic infection (e.g., malaria, mycoplasma, and hemolysin-producing bacteria), and Wilson's disease can result in short lifespan and microvesicles of the RBC, consequently leading to anemia and impaired microcirculation [8–10]. Synthetic compounds and natural products of interests need to be investigated to elucidate their therapeutic potential of inhibitors of excessive eryptosis in β-thalassemia with chronic anemia.

4. Iron overload in thalassemia

4.1. Pathophysiology and complications

Iron overload in thalassemia is assessed with an increase of plasma iron and transferrin saturation, the presence of redox iron as non-transferrin-bound iron (NTBI) and labile plasma iron (LPI), and a high deposition of tissue iron in the forms of hemosiderin, ferritin, and labile iron pools (LIP). Excessive iron accumulation in the vital organs is the cause of liver diseases (e.g., hepatitis, hepatic fibrosis, and hepatocellular carcinoma), cardiomyopathies (e.g., cardiac arrhythmia and heart failure), and endocrinopathies (e.g., diabetes, growth retardation, defective puberty, hypopituitarism, hypogonadism, and hypoparathyroidism) [11, 12]. Iron overload can be caused by an increase of dietary iron absorption due to chronic anemia and by multiple blood transfusions to maintain normal blood Hb level. Under incomplete or partial synthesis of β-chains of Hb in β-thalassemia patients, the remaining excessive α-globin chains are unstable and eventually precipitate, causing RBC membrane damage [13]. The affected RBCs are prematurely hemolyzed in the bone marrow and spleen, resulting in increased RBC turnover, ineffective erythropoiesis, and severe anemia, so patients require regular blood transfusions to prevent the anemia and ischemia. Though thalassemia patients do not receive transfusions, abnormal iron absorption produces an increase in the body iron burden evaluated at 2–5 g per year [14]. Regular blood transfusions (420 ml/unit of donor blood equivalent to 200 mg of iron) lead to double this iron accumulation. Consequently, iron accumulation introduces progressive damage in the liver, heart, and in endocrine glands. Circulating NTBI as well as LPI is detected whenever the capacity of transferrin to incorporate iron derived from either gastrointestinal tract or reticuloendothelial (RE) cells becomes a limiting factor. Both forms of toxic iron appear primarily in transfused patients where the total iron-binding capacity (TIBC) has been surpassed [15]. Pathologically, the NTBI fraction seems to be translocated across cell membrane irregularly, while the LPI is redox active and susceptible to chelation [16].

4.2. Redox iron catalysis

In enzymatic reactions as shown in **Figure 1**, superoxide ($O_2^{-\bullet}$) which is one of the reactive oxygen species (ROS) is normally produced by NADH:ubiquinone oxidoreductase catalysis at the complex I (I) in oxidative phosphorylation and will be converted to hydrogen peroxide (H_2O_2) by superoxide dismutase (SOD) catalysis (II). Hydrogen peroxide (H_2O_2) which is another ROS is produced by xanthine oxidase (XO) catalysis of hypoxanthine to xanthine (III) and xanthine to uric acid (IV) in purine catabolic pathway. Finally, hydrogen peroxide will be degraded or detoxified by peroxidase (POD) and catalase (CAT) to water and oxygen (V).

In Haber-Weiss/Fenton nonenzymatic reactions, iron can participate in the oxidation-reduction process known to generate ROS including hydrogen peroxide reacts to form hydroxyl radical ($OH^{\bullet}$) and hydroxide anion (OH^-) [17] (**Figure 2**).

ROS can induce cell death through initiating a series of chemical reactions with many significant biomolecules, resulting in DNA oxidation, protein damage, and membrane lipids peroxidation [18, 19]. Among these ROS, hydroxyl radicals might be the most harmful to lipid and

NADH:ubiquinone oxidoreductase

(Complex I)

$$NADH + Ubiquinone + O_2 \longrightarrow NAD^+ + Ubiquinol + O_2^{\bullet -} .. (I)$$

SOD

$$O_2^{\bullet -} + 2 H^+ \longrightarrow H_2O_2 \qquad .. (II)$$

XO

$$Hypoxanthine + O_2 \longrightarrow Xanthine + H_2O_2 \qquad .. (III)$$

XO

$$Xanthine + O_2 \longrightarrow Uric\ acid + H_2O_2 \qquad .. (IV)$$

POD or CAT

$$H_2O_2 \longrightarrow H_2O + \tfrac{1}{2} O_2 \qquad .. (V)$$

Figure 1. Enzymatic production of ROS.

$$Fe^{3+} + O_2^{\bullet -} \rightarrow Fe^{2+} + O_2 \qquad \textbf{\textit{Haber-Weiss reaction}}$$

$$Fe^{2+} + H_2O_2 \rightarrow Fe^{3+} + HO^{\bullet} + HO^- \qquad \textbf{\textit{Fenton reaction}}$$

$$O_2^- + H_2O_2 \rightarrow O_2 + HO^{\bullet} + HO^- \qquad \textbf{\textit{Net reaction}}$$

Figure 2. Iron-catalyzed redox reactions of biological importance.

protein membrane components. The $^{\bullet}OH$-induced membrane damage can be related directly to a membrane-associated Fenton reagent [20]. Oxidative cell damage has been attributed to the emergence of excessive levels of LPI that promote the production of ROS exceeding the cellular defensive capacity [21]. Cellular LIP is a source of chelatable and redox-active iron, which is transitory and serves as a crossroad of cell iron metabolism. The nature of the LIP has been revealed by its capacity to promote ROS generation in its "rise-and-fall" patterns. LIP plays a role as a self-regulatory pool that is sensed by cytosolic iron-regulatory proteins (IRPs) and its feedback regulated by an IRP-dependent expression of iron import and storage. LIP is influenced by a range of biochemical reactions that are capable of overriding the IRP regulatory loops. Excess labile iron can react with unsaturated lipids [22]. Such redox reactions lead to the damage of cells, tissues, and organs as demonstrated as the iron overload associated with β-thalassemia.

4.3. Tissue iron deposition

The spleen contains macrophages that digests hemoglobin and stores the resulting iron in ferritin. The number of blood transfusions in β-TM patients correlates with their splenic hemosiderosis and weight [23]. Hemosiderin deposition was found to be greater in the iron-overloaded livers than in the iron-overloaded spleens. Ferritin and hemosiderin increased in hepatocytes and splenic RE cells [24]. Splenectomy is one of the clinical complications of hypertransfused TM patients to reduce hyperactivity of RE macrophage; nevertheless, it may increase the iron overload.

The liver is one of the main storage organs for iron. Iron overload is considered when the ferritin level consistently exceeds 1,000 ng/ml (normal range 20–200 ng/ml). Excess free radicals can cause progressive tissue injury and eventually cirrhosis or hepatocellular carcinoma in iron overload patients whose iron is sequestrated predominantly in ferritin or hemosiderin [25]. When plasma transferrin becomes highly saturated, NTBI is detectable and rapidly transported across the hepatocyte membrane via a specific pathway. Likely, ferroportin 1 is the only protein that mediates the transport of iron out of hepatocytes and is then oxidized by ceruloplasmin and bound to transferrin [26]. Iron deposition affects hepatic parenchymal cells (hepatocytes and bile duct cells) and mesenchymal cells (endothelial cells, macrophage, and Kupffer cells) and often distributes differently from one area to another [27].

The heart is one of the most mitochondrial-rich tissues in the body, making the iron of particular importance to cardiac function. Iron as iron-sulfur cluster and cytochromes plays a key role for oxidative phosphorylation and superoxide production in the mitochondria. Iron deposition in the heart cells can lead to cellular oxidative stress and damage and an alteration of myocardial function. Heart failure is the leading cause of death among hemosiderosis β-thalassemia patients, of whom around 60% die from cardiac failure. Harmful effects of iron overload on the heart of TM patients can be monitored efficiently by using noninvasive techniques as described below, whereas invasive techniques such as Perl's stained in biopsied heart tissue are rather impossible. Treatment with effective iron chelators can protect these patients from iron-loaded cardiomyopathy [28, 29].

Bone marrow iron deposition (186 μg/g wet weight) increases in proportion to the total body iron store in dietary iron overload of African Bantu people and Caucasian idiopathic hemochromatosis patients [30]. MDS patients who are a heterogeneous group of clonal hematopoietic stem cell malignancies show bone marrow hemosiderosis and may develop systemic iron overload.

Though hematological care is improved in homozygous transfusion-dependent β-thalassemia (TDT) patients, multi-endocrine dysfunction is still a common complication. Thyroid dysfunction is defined as overt hypothyroidism, subclinical hypothyroidism, and an exaggerated thyroid-stimulating hormone response was reported in β-thalassemia patients [31]. Possibly, growth retardation, secondary hypogonadotropic hypogonadism and hypothyroidism are originated from pituitary damage primarily caused by iron overload and oxidative stress [32, 33]. Approximately half of patients' pituitary gland dysfunction associated with iron overload is irreversible [34].

The redox irons in TDT patients with TM and TE are catalytically harmful to adrenal glands and can cause adrenal insufficiency [35]. Though all TM patients were nondiabetic, some of them decreased in the oral glucose tolerance test. They showed normal response of cortisol to insulin and adrenocorticotropic hormone stimulation. Moreover, the β-cell pancreatic function and adrenal cortical function were depressed in the severely iron-loaded. Recently, Koonyosying and colleagues have demonstrated green tea extract could reduce cellular the levels of iron and ROS and increase insulin secretion in concentration-dependent manner in iron-loaded pancreatic cell line (RINm5F), indicating the amelioration of oxidative stress and endocrinal improvement of pancreatic β-cells [36]. They also found that eltrombopag, which is a thrombopoietin receptor agonist and potent metal ion-chelating agent, efficiently decreased cellular levels of iron and ROS from cultured HuH7, H9C2, and RINm5F cells and restored insulin secretion from iron-loaded RINm5F cells [37].

4.4. Assessment of tissue iron content

Serum ferritin level has been used as a surrogate biochemical marker to correlate closely with liver iron concentration for a long time and would be a valuable alternative to assess visceral iron overload in heavily iron-loaded TM patients [38]. Sophisticated noninvasive magnetic resonance imaging, magnetic iron detector susceptometry, superconducting quantum interference device, and nuclear resonance scattering techniques can also be used to assess iron status in tissues. Alternatively, invasive tissue biopsied needle aspiration associated with ferrozine colorimetry or graphite-furnace atomic absorption spectrometry is routinely quantitated for nonheme iron in tissues (e.g., myocardium, liver, pancreas, adrenal glands, anterior pituitary gland, and skin) [39–41]. These methods are all valuable when evaluating iron load in the tissues and monitoring the response of different organs to chelation therapy.

5. Thrombotic events in thalassemia

Heart failure and arrhythmia are the main causes of death in TM patients with cardiac siderosis, pulmonary hypertension, and thrombosis and also the major cardiovascular complications in TI patients possibly due to pro-atherogenic biochemical factors (e.g., iron status and lipid profile) [42, 43]. Hypercoagulable pulmonary microthromboembolism in Thai pediatric TE patient was previously investigated [44]. After splenectomy TI patients mostly had thrombosis, thrombocytosis, and lower levels of anticoagulation inhibitors (e.g., protein S, protein C, and antithrombin III) [45]. Splenectomy promotes portal vein thrombosis in TM patients [46]. Ineffective erythropoiesis, chronic anemia, iron overload, and polycythemia by erythrocytosis and thrombosis are coincidently occurring in β-thalassemia patients. Signs of cerebrovascular accident (brain ischemia, hemorrhage, and infarct) and heart disease (congestive heart failure and atrial fibrillation) were described in chronically hypercoagulable thromboembolic thalassemia patients, so anticoagulant and/or antiplatelet therapy is recommended. Hypoxia and iron overload are the two major mechanisms of ROS overproduction [47]. The levels of plasma hemostatic and thrombotic markers were significantly higher in splenectomized TE patients than non-splenectomized ones, implying splenectomy increases platelet hyperactivity, blood hypercoagulability, and risk of thrombosis. ROS-induced activation of vascular endothelial cells can cause vasculitis and thrombosis, showing increased levels of many soluble adhesion molecules and von Willebrand factor (vWF) in thalassemia blood [48]. Procoagulant activity of circulating RBC microvesicles or microparticles (MPs) may contribute to thrombotic events in thalassemia hypercoagulability [49]. Carotid artery thrombus is usually associated with severe cardiovascular diseases (CVD), iron deficiency anemia, and thrombocytosis. Thromboembolic complications are documented in thalassemia patients, possibly due to aggregation of abnormal RBC and high amounts of RBC membrane-derived MPs [50]. Antioxidant treatment of β-thalassemia HbE patients can improve oxidative stress and hypercoagulable state [51]. Iron overload, in particular NTBI level, would be one of the risk factors in pulmonary thrombosis and hypertension in splenectomized non-transfusion-dependent thalassemia (NTDT) patients [52]. Iron chelators are useful and effective in the amelioration of iron overload and oxidative stress in thalassemia mice, possibly in the prevention of pulmonary thrombosis [53]. Nitric oxide (NO•) synthesized from L-arginine by catalysis of nitric oxide synthase (NOS) species is a free-radical, physiologic vasodilator, and potent inhibitor of platelet function. Excessive iron-liberated heme degradation contributes to hypercoagulability [54]. Low arginine bio-availability in β-thalassemia patients can cause pulmonary hypertension and cardiopulmonary dysfunctions [55]. Splenectomy, thrombocytosis, RBC, and platelet MPs may be residual hypercoagulable/thrombotic risks in TDT patients [56, 57]. Liver inflammation and cirrhosis can involve in hypercoagulability, thrombosis, and reduced fibrinolysis [58, 59].

6. Treatment and implements

Strategy and approach have been suggested for the treatment and support of thalassemia patients to have better quality of life and well-being [60]. These approaches include occasional/regular blood transfusions, iron chelation therapy, antioxidant supplement, Hb F switching agents, anti-allergic drugs, antibiotics (such as antibacterial, antiviral, antifungal, and antimalarial drugs), splenectomy (in the past), dental care, and hemopoietic stem cell transplantation.

6.1. Iron chelation therapy

Iron chelation therapy aims to prevent the accumulation of toxic iron and eliminate the excess iron in TDT patients. Effective chelation and good management of the patients have been correlated with a decline in early deaths and complications [61]. Reduction of plasma and cellular chelatable iron such as NTBI, LPI, and LIP is a slow process and requires aggressive chelation therapy. The chelation will maintain the iron balance at safe levels to prevent high iron accumulation and oxidative tissue injury. Such non-iron and iron-overloaded models as RBC, cell cultures (e.g., hepatocytes, HepG2 cells, and cardiomyocytes), animals (e.g., mice, gerbils, rats, and transgenic BKO mice), and even human thalassemia patients are experimentally investigated and clinically tested to assess the safety and efficacy of iron chelators. At present, three standard iron chelators including desferrioxamine (DFO), deferiprone (DFP), and deferasirox (DFX) are widely used for the treatment of β-thalassemia patients with iron overload to prevent oxidative stress-induced organ dysfunctions and such complications (**Figure 3**). Combined DFO/DFP and DFP/DFX treatments can reverse endocrine complications by improving glucose intolerance and gonadal dysfunction in TDT patients [62].

Under continuous chelation therapy, many TDT patients with moderate-to-severe pituitary iron overload had normal volume and function of the pituitary gland, representing a potential therapeutic window, while some hypogonadal patients preserved their pituitary volumes

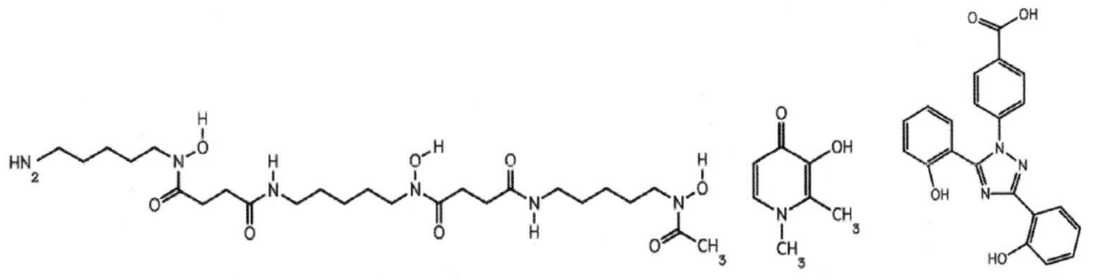

DFO   **DFP**   **DFX**

Figure 3. Chemical structures of DFO, DFP, and DFX.

and functions. Thai clinicians have reported that DFO chelation therapy for 1.5 years largely decreased serum ferritin level and improved secretion of prolactin (PRL) and growth hormone (GH) but not other pituitary hormones [63].

6.2. Supplementation of antioxidants

Compounds such as vitamins A, C, E, β-carotene, reduced glutathione (GSH), and N-acetylcysteine (NAC) and enzymes such as SOD, CAT, glutathione peroxidase (GPx), and glutathione reductase (GR) can remove free radicals by enzymatic and nonenzymatic antioxidant systems in the body (**Figure 4**). Since β-thalassemia patients have a higher oxidative stress level than normal people, effective antioxidants would be a complementary treatment of choice in these patients. Ideas for using drug antioxidants to eliminate oxidative tissue damage and empower antioxidant systems in thalassemia patients have been applicable for a long time [64]. Commercially available compounds included vitamin C, vitamin E, NAC, coenzyme Q_{10}, and hydroxyurea (HU) which were used for the treatment, with vitamin E being the most popular [65–79]. Importantly, treatment with vitamin E significantly lowered the levels of plasma lipid peroxidation products and adenosine diphosphate (ADP)-challenged platelet activity in non-splenectomized and splenectomized HbE/β-thalassemia patients [80]. Regarding other anti-oxidative natural products, silymarin restored glutathione level in thalassemia patients [81]. Fermented papaya preparation (FPP) increased glutathione levels in blood cells and platelets and decreased membrane lipid peroxidation products in β-thalassemia patients [82]. Treatment with a cocktail of DFP, NAC, vitamin E, and curcumin for 1 year improved antioxidant capacity in HbE/β-thalassemia patients [80, 83]. The levels of serum vitamins A and E, Zn, Se, and Cu were lower in young thalassemia patients than in controls, whereas serum ferritin and iron levels were inversely correlated with

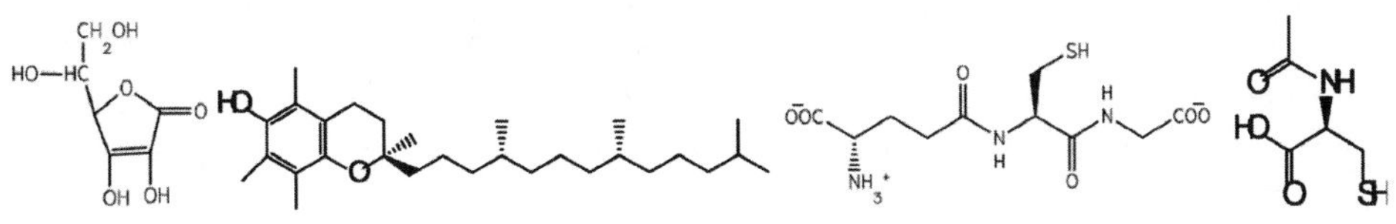

Vitamin C   **Vitamin E**   **Glutathione**   **NAC**

Figure 4. Structures of antioxidants.

serum retinol and selenium levels ($p < 0.05$). Interestingly, vitamin E and polyphenols can abolish increased oxidative stress in thalassemia patients; if given along with iron chelators, then they may provide a substantial improvement in chronic anemia and complications [84].

6.3. Vitamin C

Ascorbic acid or vitamin C is a simple water-soluble vitamin which cannot be enzymatically synthesized in the human body. The substance normally functions as a cofactor of proline and lysine hydroxylase in collagen synthesis. The levels of leukocyte and urinary AA are decreased in idiopathic hemochromatosis patients, TDT patients, and Bantu people [85]. Platelet vitamin C level is lower in thalassemia patients with iron overload than normal people [86]. When TM patients are treated with vitamin C, their levels of serum iron, transferrin saturation, and ferritin are increased [87]; possibly vitamin C would be involved in the mobilization of storage iron from tissues and increase oxidative damage in the patients. However, vitamin C plus vitamin E supplementation for β-thalassemia patients has benefits more than vitamin E alone in promoting their antioxidant activity [66].

6.4. Vitamin E

Vitamin E (α-tocopherol) is considered to be the most important lipid-soluble exogenous antioxidant in humans. Low serum level of vitamin E is found in homozygous TM and TE patients. Oral administration of high doses of vitamin E effectively decreased plasma lipid peroxidation in β-thalassemia patients and prolonged RBC survival in some patients [71, 88]. A therapeutic trial with vitamin E was carried out in TM and TI patients with 750–1000 IU/day for an average period of 16 months. The treated patients showed fourfold increase in both serum and RBC vitamin E levels and a reduced level of malonyldialdehyde (MDA) when compared with the untreated group [89]. Daily vitamin E supplementation for 3 months significantly increased plasma α-tocopherol levels and reduced plasma oxidant levels in splenectomized TE patients [80].

6.5. Glutathione

Glutathione (γ-glutamylcysteinylglycine) is a tripeptide synthesized by the catalysis of γ-glutamyl cysteine synthetase and glutathione synthetase in cells and indicated as a very important endogenous free-radical scavenger due to the presence of cysteine sulfhydryl group in the molecule. In addition, GR, GPx, and glutathione-S-transferase (GST) work as antioxidants to get rid of harmful free radicals mostly in the cells. Physiologically, GR together with reduced nicotinamide adenine dinucleotide phosphate functions to recycle oxidized glutathione (GSSG) back to GSH to scavenge ROS, and GPx converts hydrogen peroxide to water and oxygen. GSH is approximately 80% present in the liver. GR activity was slightly decreased in TDT patients, whereas GPx activity was not different when compared with healthy persons [90]. Blood GSH levels of α-, β-, and HbE/β-thalassemia patients with iron overload were significantly lower than those of the healthy controls [91–95]. Importantly, treatment with flavonoid silymarin restored a decreased GSH content in T cells of β-thalassemia major patients [81]. Though endogenous GSH content is unable to be filled up with direct consumption due to digestive peptidase activity, oral administration of some antioxidants such as vitamin E (10 mg/kg/day), commercially available FFP, silymarin tablet (140 mg three times a day), HU (10–20 mg/kg/day), NAC (2,400 mg/day), and curcumin (500 mg/day)/vitamin E cocktail can increase/restore intracellular GSH content in thalassemia patients instead.

6.6. Hydroxyurea

HU (alternatively hydroxycarbamide) is a drug of choice used for enhancing γ-globin gene expression and modifying γ-globin chain production, as a consequence of Hb F production in SCD and β-thalassemia patients. In controversy, the compound is toxic and suspected to the pathogenesis of colonic ulcerative [96]. Indeed, HU effectively increases Hb F production in patients with SCD, SCD with α-thalassemia, and TI and results in a decrease in the number of blood transfusions required [97–99]. A current clinical study in TI patients has shown HU decreased serum ferritin (50 vs. 33%), LIP (20 vs. 13%), apoptotic event (62 vs. 15%), and ROS (60 vs. 50%) levels and increased GSH level (66 vs. 25%) in the responders compared to the nonresponders [100]. In addition to the increase in Hb F synthesis, treatment with HU (30 mg/day) in β-thalassemia patients with Hb E for 3 months decreased SOD activity and MDA concentration of the RBC, probably due to inhibition of cytosolic superoxide radical and membrane lipid peroxidation [101, 102].

6.7. *N*-acetylcysteine (NAC)

NAC, an anti-oxidative thiol-containing compound, is able to trap ROS and reactive nitrogen species (RNS) and therefore protect cells from such free-radical-mediated damage. After crossing the cell membrane, the compound will be hydrolyzed to cysteine used for the synthesis of GSH. Importantly, NAC can protect the RBC of SCD patients and of normal subjects from oxidative stress condition [65, 103]. In vitro treatment of blood cells including RBC, platelets (PLT), and polymorphonuclear leukocytes of β-thalassemia patients with *N*-acetylcysteine amide increased GSH content and reduced ROS level in these cells, possibly resulting in a significant reduction in the sensitivity of thalassemia RBC to hemolysis and phagocytosis by macrophages [65]. They also showed that the intraperitoneal injection of AD4 to β-thalassemia mice (150 mg/kg) significantly reduced all parameters of oxidative stress. One β-thalassemia with hemoglobin sickle (Hb S) who received NAC (2400 mg/day) for 6 weeks showed an increase in whole-blood GSH levels and a decrease in the RBC membrane PS exposure [104]. Consistently, TDT patients who received NAC (10 mg/kg/day) for 3 months showed a decrease in total oxidative stress and total oxidative stress index and an increase in total antioxidant capacity and blood Hb level [105]. Our group has reported that treatment of β-thalassemia HbE with a cocktail of DFP, NAC, and either vitamin E or cucumin for 12 months significantly decreased levels of iron overload (e.g., NTBI, LPI, erythrocyte membrane nonheme iron) and oxidative stress (e.g., MDA and erythrocyte ROS) parameters and increased levels of blood Hb and antioxidant indicators (e.g., CAT, SOD, and GSH), suggesting an effective antioxidant property [51].

7. Supplementation of functional food

7.1. Curcuminoids

Curcumin (diferuloylmethane) is one of the major phytochemicals (70–80%, w/w) from the golden spice turmeric *Curcuma longa* Linn (family Zingiberaceae). The three main constituents of curcuminoids are curcumin, demethoxycurcumin, and *bis*-demethoxycurcumin, of which the important molecular structure for biological activity is diketone moiety (**Figure 5**).

Apparently, curcumin and its metabolites including di-, tetra-, and hexa-hydrocurcumin exhibit strong antioxidant, free-radical scavenging, anti-lipid peroxidative, antithrombotic, and anti-inflammatory activities. Many clinical investigations have addressed pharmacokinetics, safety (maximum dose 12 g/day over 3 months), and efficacy of this attractive nutraceutical against several human diseases including β-thalassemia. Many formulations of curcumin including nanoparticles, liposomal encapsulation, emulsions, capsules, tablets, and powder are available for a single and adjunctive treatment [106]. Curcumin is claimed to be a potential hexadentate iron chelator and found to remove NTBI in thalassemia serum and also suppress the ROS generation and lipid peroxidation in thalassemia RBC [83, 107–111]. Curcuminoids (particularly *bis*-demethoxycurcumin) and its metabolite (hexahydrobisdemethoxycurcumin) potentially enhanced the upregulation of γ-globin gene and synthesis of Hb F in human erythroid leukemia (K562) and primary erythroid precursor cells [112]. Curcumin is reported one of the triggers of eryptosis to allow defective RBC to escape hemolysis [8]. The oxidative stress condition in circulating RBC of TE patients is reduced after treatment with a curcumin cocktail, leading to improvement in their quality of life [83]. Curcumin markedly decreased iron deposition and lipid peroxidation product as MDA in the liver and spleen and the liver of iron-loaded rats [113].

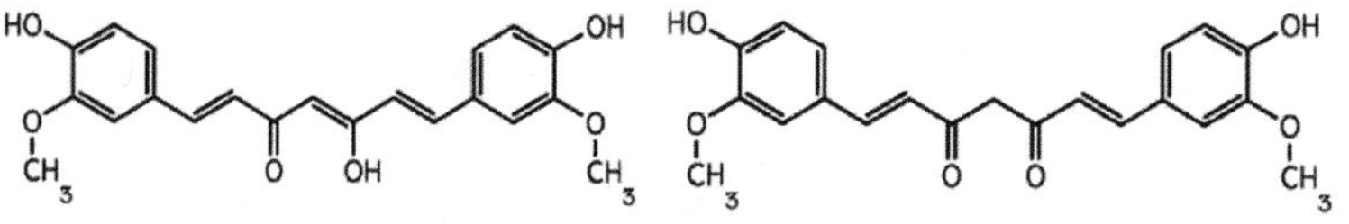

enol form   *keto form*

Curcumin

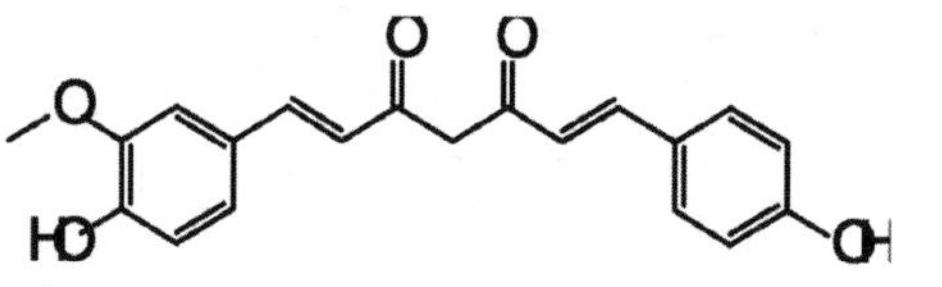

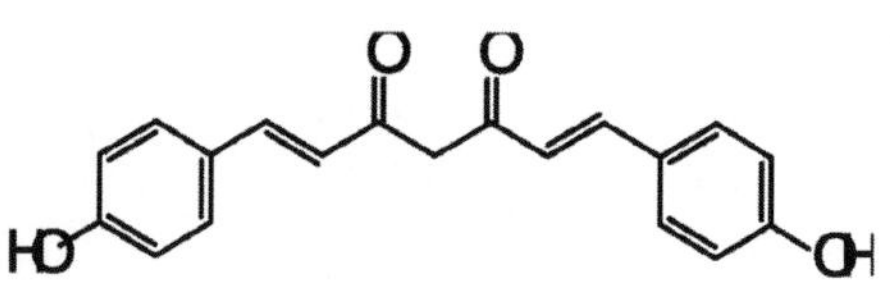

Demethoxycurcumin   ***bis*-Demethoxycurcumin**

Figure 5. Structures of ingredients in curcuminoids.

7.2. Green tea

Tea (*Camellia sinensis* L., Theaceae family) is one of the most popular beverages in the world in which the products, depending on duration of fermentation, can be classified into green tea (GT), oolong tea, white tea, yellow tea, black tea, pu-erh tea, and Miang tea. GT (*C. sinensis* L. var japonica) is produced without any fermentation (oxidation), so the major persisting catechins are not destroyed by naturally occurring polyphenol oxidase (PPO) in fresh tea leaves. Oolong tea (*C. sinensis* var sinensis) is processed from tea leaves under semi-fermentation, in which β-glycosidic aroma precursors including 8-hydroxygeranyl β-D-primeveroside, *trans*- and *cis*-linalool 3,6-oxide 6-O-β-D-xylopyranosyl-β-D-glucopyranosides, and (2R,3S,4S,4aS,11bS)-3,4,11-trihydroxy-2-(hydroxymethyl)-8-(4-hydroxyphenyl)-3,4,4α, 11β-tetrahydro-2H,10H-pyrano[2′,3′:4,5]furo[3,2-g]chromen-10-one are the main volatile constituents besides the catechin derivatives. Black tea (long fermentation) and Miang tea (*C. sinensis* L. kuntze var assamica) require very long fermentation times depending on the manufacturing process. Miang (a northern Thai word) is a chewing tea and commonly used for gum chewing in elderly people, relief of skin burn and inflammation, and as an antidiarrheal remedy.

In industry, GT is produced from steaming or roasting fresh tea leaves at high temperatures, consequentially drying and inactivating the PPO enzymes and leaving polyphenols known as flavonols or catechins at 30–40% by weight of dry tea leaves. It contains at least four major catechin derivatives including (−)-epigallocatechin-3-gallate (EGCG), (−)-epigallocatechin (EGC), (−)-epicatechin-3-gallate (ECG), and (−)-epicatechin (EC), of which the lipophilic permeable EGCG exhibits anti-oxidative and iron-chelating activities (**Figure 6**) [114]. Additionally, other phenolic acids including chlorogenic acid (CGA), caffeic acid (CA), and gallic acid (GA) and flavonols including kaempferol, myricetin, and quercetin are present in green tea [115]. Green tea extract (GTE) and EGCG, which show iron-chelating and antioxidant properties [116, 117] decrease labile iron (e.g., NTBI and LPI) level and consequently deplete lipid peroxidation as well as oxidative stress in both iron-loaded rats and thalassemia mice [118, 119]. The compounds were effective in the inhibition of RBC hemolysis, resulting in a prolonged RBC lifespan and decreased iron deposition and oxidative damage in the liver [119].

TI showed higher intestinal nonheme iron absorption than TM, while tea produced 41–90% inhibition of iron absorption in these patients, suggesting that tea consumption would be

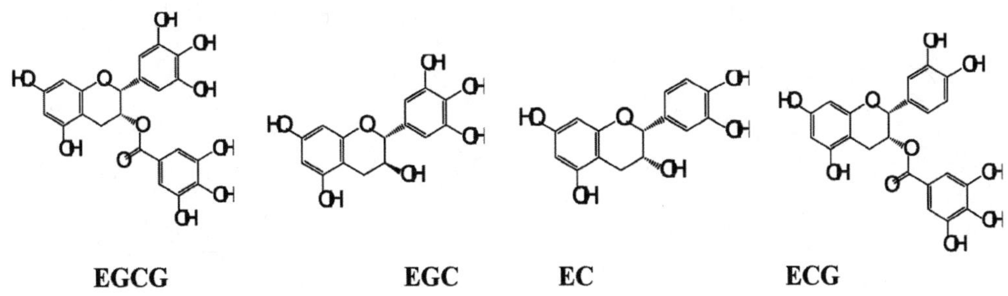

EGCG   **EGC**   **EC**   **ECG**

Figure 6. Structures of catechins in green tea.

recommended to thalassemia patients, particularly TI patients [120]. Logically, anti-oxidative GTE interferes duodenal absorption of dietary iron and iron-chelating properties in vitro and in vivo [116–119]. The preparation also showed inhibitory effect on catecholamine secretion from isolated rabbit adrenal glands, possibly by blocking L-type calcium channels in the adrenal medullary glands [121]. Therefore, GTE might be helpful to decrease iron deposition, reduce ROS levels, and ameliorate functions of targeted endocrine glands (e.g., pancreas and adrenal cortex) in β-thalassemia models. In controversy, a study reports development of thrombotic thrombocytopenic purpura in a person after consuming a weight-loss product containing green tea [122]. Most importantly, green tea showed antithrombosis ex vivo and inhibition of cyclooxygenase 1 activity [123, 124].

In our recent study, we have produced a functional GT-CUR concentrate (**Figure 7**) for investigating its effects in Thai adult TDT patents. We found that the drink did not affect white blood cell and platelet numbers, Hb, and Hct but increased RBC numbers following daily consumption for 2 months. The levels of blood urea, serum alanine aminotransferase, aspartate aminotransferase, and alkaline phosphatase activity tended to decrease but neither significantly nor dose dependently. In month 1 and 2 of the treatments, there were a decrease of serum MDA (-0.07 ± 2.95 and -0.87 ± 1.68 μM, respectively), NTBI (-1.20 ± 8.03 and -3.93 ± 3.83 μM, respectively), and LPI (1.91 ± 4.99 and -1.10 ± 2.94 μM, respectively) and increase of serum antioxidant activity (5.08 ± 8.86 and 0.28 ± 13.39 mg trolox equivalent/ml, respectively). These findings suggest GT-CUR drink would increase erythropoiesis, improve liver and kidney function, and diminish oxidative stress and iron overload in thalassemia patients [125]. Surprisingly, we demonstrate that treatment of GTE (1–10 μM EGCG equivalent) decreased cellular iron approximately 45% and ROS level in a concentration-dependent manner in iron-loaded pancreatic cell line (RINm5F) when compared with control cells. Secretory insulin level was nearly 2.5-fold times the highest safe concentration of the GTE [36]. The results imply that catechin-rich GT would indeed be an effective drink to remove iron, decrease ROS, and improve pancreatic cell function thereby increasing insulin production, leading to the amelioration of diabetic complications in thalassemia patients with iron overload.

Evidently, green tea is abundant with phytonutrient and enriched with active phytochemicals that exhibit many biological and pharmacological activities and it can be utilized for a functional

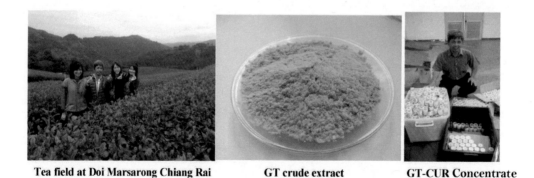

Tea field at Doi Marsarong Chiang Rai   **GT crude extract**   **GT-CUR Concentrate**

Figure 7. GT-CUR concentration: from field to nutraceutical product.

drink and health benefits. Up to now, many green tea products are being marketed worldwide for many purposes in different population ages. We are eager to use our multifunctional cocktail containing green tea extract, DFP, and vitamin E to examine if the product could diminish hypercoagulability and excessive platelet activity in thalassemia patients and thrombosis-related diseases, besides iron chelation.

7.3. Coffee

Coffee is also one of the most widely consumed beverages in the world because they contain many active ingredients that are a benefit for human health. Coffee (*Coffea arabica* L., *Coffea canephora* L. family Rubiaceae) is an original crop that will be further processed to roast coffee, coffee powder, coffee brew, coffee biscuit, and coffee candy for commercial purposes. Coffee is widely naturalized in many parts of the world including Africa, Latin America, the Pacific and Caribbean Ocean, Southeast Asia, and China. In Thailand, coffee is usually cultivated on the highlands at Doi Chang and Huay Nam Khun of Chiang Rai, Doi Saket District of Chiang Mai, and Kraburi District of Ranong (**Figure 8**).

Caffeine (1,3,7-trimethylxanthine) is a predominant ingredient persisting in tea and coffee, which is the most widely used pharmacologic substance showing prooxidant and antioxidant and hydroxyl radical scavenger [126–128]. Coffee contains many kinds of monosaccharide including sucrose, polysaccharides, D-arabinose, D-mannose, D-glucose, D-galactose, D-rhamnose, and D-xylose in nearly equal amounts. The amounts of caffeine and CGA are slightly higher in raw arabica coffee (0.9–1.2% and 1.6–2.4% w/w, respectively) than in raw robusta coffee (5.5–8.0% and 7.0–10.0% w/w, respectively) [129]. Interestingly, only arginine and cysteine are much more abundant in the green coffee (3.61% and 2.89% for arabica 2.28% and 3.87% for robusta) when compared with the roast coffee (0% and 0.76% for arabica 0% and 0.14% for robusta). Phenolic compounds including mono- and di-caffeoylquinic acids, CA, ferulic acid, *p*-coumaric acid, sinapic acid, 4-hydroxybenzoic acid, and CGA were detected in spent coffee by-product [130, 131] (**Figure 9**). Phenolic compounds, in particular CGA in coffee was able to chelate metal ion such as Zn [132]. In controversy for CVD incidence, one

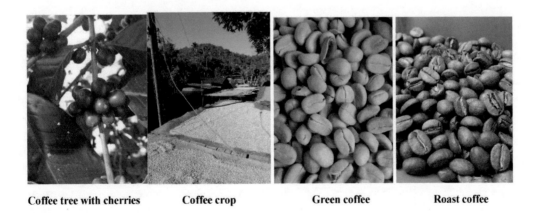

Coffee tree with cherries   **Coffee crop**   **Green coffee**   **Roast coffee**

Figure 8. Coffee crop in Thailand.

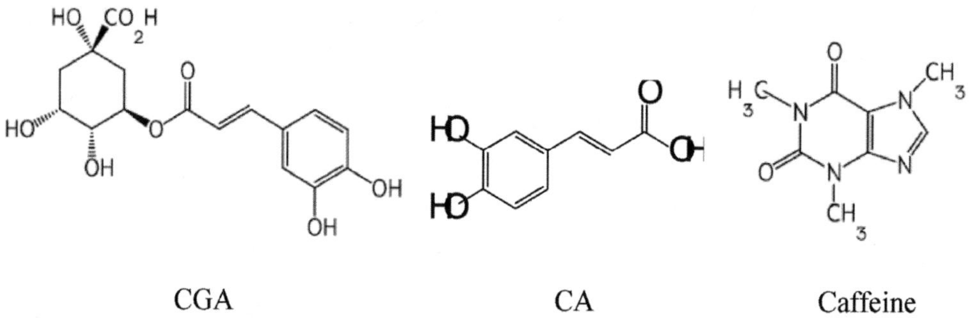

Figure 9. Some major constituents in coffee.

report supports the administration of caffeine augments endothelium-dependent vasodilation in young healthy volunteers through an increase in NO production [133]. Approximately one third of CGA and almost all of the CA are absorbed in the small intestine of humans, so the two antioxidants might have preventive effect of CVD [134]. The 10-kDa or less fractions but no other common components (e.g., CGA, CA, caffeine, quinic acid, trigonelline hydrochloride, and 5-(hydroxymethyl)-2-furfural) in hot-water extract of coffee had antithrombin and antiplatelet activity [135]. CGA protected oxidative damage and dose dependently increased the production of NO of human aortic endothelial cells [136].

Caffeine increases intracellular calcium-stimulating endothelial NOS to accelerate the production of NO which will be diffused to vascular smooth muscle cell to produce vasodilation [137]. Tocopherols are found in coffee bean oil [138]. Caffeine (300 mg, equivalent to two to three cups) is metabolized in the human body to theophylline (170 ng/ml plasma) 7 hours post-administration [139]. Tea and coffee dose dependently inhibited absorption of nonheme iron of either animal or plant food [140]. Dihydrocaffeic acid, a metabolite of CA detected in human plasma following coffee ingestion, was able to decrease ROS and increase NOS activity in human-derived EA.hy926 endothelial cells [141]. Ingestion of green coffee extract for 4 months led to the decrease in plasma level of homocysteine and improvement of human vessel reactivity [142]. Coffee ground residual has higher phenolic contents than roast coffee bean and shows inhibitory effects on the production of NO and pro-inflammatory cytokines in the macrophage [143]. Surprisingly, healthy volunteers who consumed coffee for 2 months (420 and 780 mg CGA equivalent/day) showed increase of plasma total antioxidant capacity [144]. A recent study has demonstrated coffee would counteract cerebral arterial constriction via endothelial NOS induction and smooth muscle dilation [145]. Two catechols, particularly CGA and CA which is abundant in coffee, could potentially scavenge free radicals and subsequently inhibit the production of pro-inflammatory cytokines as interleukin-8 in intestinal epithelial cells [146]. Consistent with our previous study, healthy adults consuming CGA-enriched coffee showed a significant increase of plasma antioxidant capacity when compared with the control group [144, 147]. Additionally, CGA-enriched green and roast coffee can protect oxidative damage of biomolecules in human consumers [148].

Nowadays, there are varieties of coffee products including green coffee powder, green coffee capsules, green coffee extracts, green coffee cleans detox, roast coffee, roast coffee, coffee brew, and herbal coffee that are commercially available for all-level consumers. In socioeconomics, the coffee beverage business is very popular and a growing industry in Thailand. We are applying the wonderful properties of coffee for health benefits in thalassemia patients regarding anti-oxidation, metal chelation, and antithrombosis.

8. Fruits and vegetables

Epicarp extracts of bergamot (*Citrus bergamia* Risso) containing "citropten" and "bergapten" powerfully induced the expression and differentiation of γ-globin gene in human erythroid cells (K562) and consequently the production of Hb F, suggesting a potential therapy application in β-thalassemia and sickle cell anemia [149]. Fermented papaya preparation (FPP) increased the glutathione levels in blood cells and platelets and also decreased erythrocyte ROS level and membrane lipid peroxidation product levels such as MDA and phosphatidylserine in β-thalassemia patients [82, 150]. Mango (*Mangifera indica* L., family Anacardiaceae) is a tropical edible fruit cultivated globally and is annually produced from March to May. The seasonal fruit gives a high yield in Thailand and can be consumed in the forms of green and yellow fruits. It was found that aqueous extracts of the stem barks and peel from Vimang mango displayed potent antioxidant, free-radical scavenging and divalent metal ion-chelating properties due to the presence of a major polyphenol "mangiferin" [151]. Consistently, our group demonstrated that aqueous and ethanolic extracts of Thai mango (*M. indica* var Mahachanok and *M. indica* var Kaew) lowered plasma levels of glucose and triglyceride in streptozotocin-induced rats. Obviously, the extract showed analgesic, anti-gastric ulcerative, and chemical-induced hepatoprotective effects in rats. In addition, the extracts increased plasma antioxidant capacity in rats and humans [152]. The results suggest fresh and fermented mangoes would be a potential functional and therapeutic food against the deleterious action of ROS generated during iron overload (e.g., β-thalassemia, Friedreich's ataxia, hemochromatosis, and inflammation).

Rice (*Oryza sativa* L.) is the chief economic crop cultivated in every region of Thailand. One study demonstrated that consumption of wheatgrass juice and tablets decreased the requirement of RBC transfusions in Indian β-thalassemia patients by 25% or more [153, 154]. It was possible that pheophytin compound in the wheatgrass would increase hemoglobin synthesis. In controversy, another study showed that the juice therapy did not affect the production of hemoglobin [155]. Pancytopenia such as leukocytopenia and thrombocytopenia is observed in the chelation treatment of thalassemia; however, herbs like wheatgrass, papaya leaves, and garlic would be effective in treating single lineage cytopenias [156]. We found that ethanol extract of neem (*Azadirachta indica* var siamensis Valeton) leaves displayed free-radical scavenging and iron-binding activities in vitro, and the study of the extract will be extended to β-thalassemia mice with iron overload [157].

9. Conclusions

Regular iron chelation therapy with high dietary intake of antioxidants effectively lowers the harmfulness of iron overload-mediated oxidative tissue damage and organ dysfunctions in thalassemia patients. The supplementation with single nutrients, like antioxidants, is generally not effective in ameliorating such iron overload conditions or in slowing the progression of the disease. It is recommended that these nutrients should be consumed as part of a healthy diet/functional fruits in daily meals. Nutritional and herbal strategies for modifying the pathological and clinical courses of thalassemia disease should consider the major active ingredients, nutraceuticals, biological activities, and hematological efficacy. Moreover, pre-implant/prenatal detections of thalassemia in the fetus using sensitive and specific molecular-biological and ultrasonic techniques could block new cases and problematic carriers of hemoglobinopathies. Understanding the genetics underlying the heritable subphenotypes of thalassemia would be prognostically useful and inform us further about personalized therapeutics as well as help the discovery and development of new pharmacogenomics. An effective medical regime, adjunctive supplementation of synthetic and natural antioxidants, and caregiver education could also be important factors to prevent or treat symptoms/complications in thalassemia. Selected protocols using single or combined chelators could be designed for personalized iron chelation therapy in TDT and NTDT patients, which would effectively and safely remove all the excess toxic iron (e.g., NTBI, LPI, and LIP) and prevent cardiac, liver, and other organ damage. Finally, a reliable approach based on genomics and proteomics may be effective to build a rational personalized medicine framework that can be applied in the preclinical, clinical, and therapeutic settings of hypercoagulability in thalassemia.

Acknowledgements

We appreciate the Global Society for Nutrition, Environment and Health (GSNEH) for their support. We thank Emeritus Professor Robert C. Hider, PhD., King's College London, and Mr. Michael Creswell from the University of Manchester, Manchester, UK, for English proofreading.

Symbols and abbreviations

α	alpha
β	beta
γ	gamma
ADP	adenosine diphosphate
BKO	beta-knockout
CA	caffeic acid
CAT	catalase
CGA	chlorogenic acid
CS	Constant Spring
CVD	cardiovascular diseases

DFO	desferrioxamine
DFP	deferiprone
DFX	deferasirox
EC	(−)-epicatechin
ECG	(−)-epicatechin-3-gallate
EGC	(−)-epigallocatechin
EGCG	(−)-epigallocatechin-3-gallate
EPO	erythropoietin
FPP	fermented papaya preparation
G6PD	glucose-6-phosphate dehydrogenase
GA	gallic acid
GPx	glutathione peroxidase
GR	glutathione reductase
GSH	reduced glutathione
GST	glutathione-S-transferase
GT	green tea
GTE	green tea extract
Hb	hemoglobin
Hb A	adult hemoglobin
Hb E	hemoglobin E
Hb F	fetal hemoglobin
Hb S	hemoglobin sickle
Hct	hematocrit
HPFH	hereditary persistent fetal hemoglobin
HU	hydroxyurea
IRPs	iron-regulatory proteins
LIP	labile iron pools
LPI	labile plasma iron
MDA	malonyldialdehyde
MDS	myelodysplastic syndrome

MPs	microparticles
NAC	N-acetylcysteine
NO	nitric oxide
NOS	nitric oxide synthase
NTBI	non-transferrin-bound iron
NTDT	non-transfusion-dependent thalassemia
POD	peroxidase
PPO	polyphenol oxidase
PS	phosphatidylserine
RBC	red blood cells
RE	reticuloendothelial
ROS	reactive oxygen species
SAE	Southeast Asia
SCD	sickle cell disease
SOD	superoxide dismutase
TDT	transfusion-dependent β-thalassemia
thal	thalassemia
TI	β-thalassemia intermedia
TIBC	total iron-binding capacity
TM	β-thalassemia major
vWF	von Willebrand factor
XO	xanthine oxidase

Author details

Somdet Srichairatanakool[1], Pimpisid Koonyosying[1] and Suthat Fucharoen[2]*

*Address all correspondence to: suthat.fuc@mahidol.ac.th

1 Department of Biochemistry, Faculty of Medicine, Chiang Mai University, Chiang Mai, Thailand

2 Thalassemia Research Centre, Institute of Molecular Biosciences, Mahidol University Salaya Campus, Nakornpathom, Thailand

References

[1] Fucharoen G, Fucharoen S, Wanhakit C, Srithong W. Molecular basis of alpha (0)-thalassemia in northeast of Thailand. The Southeast Asian Journal of Tropical Medicine and Public Health. 1995;**26**(Suppl 1):249-251

[2] Fucharoen S, Viprakasit V. Hb H disease: Clinical course and disease modifiers. Hematology-American Society of Hematology Education Program. 2009;**2009**(1):26-34

[3] Fucharoen S, Winichagoon P, Siritanaratkul N, Chowthaworn J, Pootrakul P. Alpha- and beta-thalassemia in Thailand. Annals of the New York Academy of Sciences. 1998;**850**: 412-414

[4] Boonsa S, Sanchaisuriya K, Fucharoen G, Wiangnon S, Jetsrisuparb A, Fucharoen S. The diverse molecular basis and hematological features of Hb H and AE Bart's diseases in Northeast Thailand. Acta Haematologica. 2004;**111**:149-154

[5] Munkongdee T, Tanakulmas J, Butthep P, Winichagoon P, Main B, Yiannakis M, et al. Molecular epidemiology of hemoglobinopathies in Cambodia. Hemoglobin. 2016;**40**: 163-167

[6] Borgna-Pignatti C. Modern treatment of thalassaemia intermedia. British Journal of Haematology. 2007;**138**:291-304

[7] Garrick LM, Strano-Paul LA, Hoke JE, Kirdani-Ryan LA, Alberico RA, Everett MM, et al. Tissue iron deposition in untransfused beta-thalassemic mice. Experimental Hematology. 1989;**17**:423-428

[8] Foller M, Huber SM, Lang F. Erythrocyte programmed cell death. IUBMB Life. 2008;**60**:661-668

[9] Lang F, Abed M, Lang E, Foller M. Oxidative stress and suicidal erythrocyte death. Antioxidants & Redox Signaling. 2013;**21**:138-153

[10] Lang F, Qadri SM. Mechanisms and significance of eryptosis, the suicidal death of erythrocytes. Blood Purification. 2012;**33**:125-130

[11] Kushner JP, Porter JP, Olivieri NF. Secondary iron overload. Hematology-American Society of Hematology Education Program. 2001;**2001**(1):47-61

[12] Weatherall DJ. Pathophysiology of thalassaemia. Baillière's Clinical Haematology. 1998;**11**:127-146

[13] Weatherall DJ, Pressley L, Wood WG, Higgs DR, Clegg JB. Molecular basis for mild forms of homozygous beta-thalassaemia. Lancet. 1981;**1**:527-529

[14] Hershko C, Konijn AM, Link G. Iron chelators for thalassaemia. British Journal of Haematology. 1998;**101**:399-406

[15] Breuer W, Hershko C, Cabantchik ZI. The importance of non-transferrin bound iron in disorders of iron metabolism. Transfusion Science. 2000;**23**:185-192

[16] Esposito BP, Breuer W, Sirankapracha P, Pootrakul P, Hershko C, Cabantchik ZI. Labile plasma iron in iron overload: Redox activity and susceptibility to chelation. Blood. 2003;**102**:2670-2677

[17] Jomova K, Valko M. Importance of iron chelation in free radical-induced oxidative stress and human disease. Current Pharmaceutical Design. 2011;**17**:3460-3473

[18] Cairo G, Recalcati S, Pietrangelo A, Minotti G. The iron regulatory proteins: Targets and modulators of free radical reactions and oxidative damage. Free Radical Biology & Medicine. 2002;**32**:1237-1243

[19] Yurkova I, Kisel M, Arnhold J, Shadyro O. Iron-mediated free-radical formation of signaling lipids in a model system. Chemistry and Physics of Lipids. 2005;**137**:29-37

[20] Hebbel RP. Auto-oxidation and a membrane-associated 'Fenton reagent': A possible explanation for development of membrane lesions in sickle erythrocytes. Clinics in Haematology. 1985;**14**:129-140

[21] Hershko CM, Link GM, Konijn AM, Cabantchik ZI. Iron chelation therapy. Current Hematology Reports. 2005;**4**:110-116

[22] Schafer FQ, Qian SY, Buettner GR. Iron and free radical oxidations in cell membranes. Cellular and Molecular Biology (Noisy-le-Grand, France). 2000;**46**:657-662

[23] Okon E, Levij IS, Rachmilewitz EA. Splenectomy, iron overload and liver cirrhosis in beta-thalassemia major. Acta Haematologica. 1976;**56**:142-150

[24] Matsuno T, Mori M, Awai M. Distribution of ferritin and hemosiderin in the liver, spleen and bone marrow of normal, phlebotomized and iron overloaded rats. Acta Medica Okayama. 1985;**39**:347-360

[25] Jensen PD. Evaluation of iron overload. British Journal of Haematology. 2004;**124**:697-711

[26] Andrews NC. Disorders of iron metabolism. The New England Journal of Medicine. 1999;**341**:1986-1995

[27] Deugnier Y, Turlin B. Pathology of hepatic iron overload. Seminars in Liver Disease. 2011;**31**:260-271

[28] Freeman AP, Giles RW, Berdoukas VA, Talley PA, Murray IP. Sustained normalization of cardiac function by chelation therapy in thalassaemia major. Clinical and Laboratory Haematology. 1989;**11**:299-307

[29] Wolfe L, Olivieri N, Sallan D, Colan S, Rose V, Propper R, et al. Prevention of cardiac disease by subcutaneous deferoxamine in patients with thalassemia major. The New England Journal of Medicine. 1985;**312**:1600-1603

[30] Brink B, Disler P, Lynch S, Jacobs P, Charlton R, Bothwell T. Patterns of iron storage in dietary iron overload and idiopathic hemochromatosis. The Journal of Laboratory and Clinical Medicine. 1976;**88**:725-731

[31] Zervas A, Katopodi A, Protonotariou A, Livadas S, Karagiorga M, Politis C, et al. Assessment of thyroid function in two hundred patients with beta-thalassemia major. Thyroid. 2002;**12**:151-154

[32] Soliman AT, elZalabany MM, Mazloum Y, Bedair SM, Ragab MS, Rogol AD, et al. Spontaneous and provoked growth hormone (GH) secretion and insulin-like growth factor I (IGF-I) concentration in patients with beta thalassaemia and delayed growth. Journal of Tropical Pediatrics. 1999;**45**:327-337

[33] Tato L, Lahlou N, Zamboni G, De Sanctis V, De Luca F, Arrigo T, et al. Impaired response of free alpha-subunits after luteinizing hormone-releasing hormone and thyrotropin-releasing hormone stimulations in beta-thalassemia major. Hormone Research. 1993;**39**:213-217

[34] Wood JC, Noetzl L, Hyderi A, Joukar M, Coates T, Mittelman S. Predicting pituitary iron and endocrine dysfunction. Annals of the New York Academy of Sciences. 2010;**1202**:123-128

[35] Nakavachara P, Viprakasit V. Adrenal insufficiency is prevalent in HbE/beta-thalassaemia paediatric patients irrespective of their clinical severity and transfusion requirement. Clinical Endocrinology. 2013;**79**:776-783

[36] Koonyosying P, Uthaipibull C, Fucharoen S, Koumoutsea EV, Porter JB, Srichairatanakool S. Decrement in cellular iron and reactive oxygen species, and improvement of insulin secretion in a pancreatic cell line using green tea extract. Pancreas. 2019;**48**(5):636-643

[37] Vlachodimitropoulou E, Chen YL, Garbowski M, Koonyosying P, Psaila B, Sola-Visner M, et al. Eltrombopag: A powerful chelator of cellular or extracellular iron(III) alone or combined with a second chelator. Blood. 2017;**130**:1923-1933

[38] Letsky EA, Miller F, Worwood M, Flynn DM. Serum ferritin in children with thalassaemia regularly transfused. Journal of Clinical Pathology. 1974;**27**:652-655

[39] Butensky E, Fischer R, Hudes M, Schumacher L, Williams R, Moyer TP, et al. Variability in hepatic iron concentration in percutaneous needle biopsy specimens from patients with transfusional hemosiderosis. American Journal of Clinical Pathology. 2005;**123**: 146-152

[40] Mavrogeni SI, Markussis V, Kaklamanis L, Tsiapras D, Paraskevaidis I, Karavolias G, et al. A comparison of magnetic resonance imaging and cardiac biopsy in the evaluation of heart iron overload in patients with beta-thalassemia major. European Journal of Haematology. 2005;**75**:241-247

[41] Youssry I, Mohsen NA, Shaker OG, El-Hennawy A, Fawzy R, Abu-Zeid NM, et al. Skin iron concentration: A simple, highly sensitive method for iron stores evaluation in thalassemia patients. Hemoglobin. 2007;**31**:357-365

[42] Cohen AR, Galanello R, Pennell DJ, Cunningham MJ, Vichinsky E. Thalassemia. Hematology-American Society of Hematology Education Program. 2004;**2004**(1):14-34

[43] Sirachainan N. Thalassemia and the hypercoagulable state. Thrombosis Research. 2013; **132**:637-641

[44] Chuansumrit A, Hathirat P, Isarangkura P, Pintadit P, Mahaphan W. Thrombotic risk of children with thalassemia. Journal of the Medical Association of Thailand. 1993;**76** (Suppl 2):80-84

[45] Bhattacharyya M, Kannan M, Chaudhry VP, Mahapatra M, Pati H, Saxena R. Hypercoagulable state in five thalassemia intermedia patients. Clinical and Applied Thrombosis/Hemostasis. 2007;**13**:422-427

[46] Al-Hawsawi ZM, Haouimi AS, Hassan RA, Tarawah AM. Portal vein thrombosis after splenectomy for beta-thalassemia major. Saudi Medical Journal. 2004;**25**:225-228

[47] Tyan PI, Radwan AH, Eid A, Haddad AG, Wehbe D, Taher AT. Novel approach to reactive oxygen species in nontransfusion-dependent thalassemia. BioMed Research International. 2014;**2014**:350432

[48] Butthep P, Bunyaratvej A, Funahara Y, Kitaguchi H, Fucharoen S, Sato S, et al. Possible evidence of endothelial cell activation and disturbance in thalassemia: An in vitro study. The Southeast Asian Journal of Tropical Medicine and Public Health. 1997;**28**(Suppl 3): 141-148A

[49] Cappellini MD, Grespi E, Cassinerio E, Bignamini D, Fiorelli G. Coagulation and splenectomy: An overview. Annals of the New York Academy of Sciences. 2005;**1054**:317-324

[50] Pattanapanyasat K, Gonwong S, Chaichompoo P, Noulsri E, Lerdwana S, Sukapirom K, et al. Activated platelet-derived microparticles in thalassaemia. British Journal of Haematology. 2007;**136**:462-471

[51] Yanpanitch OU, Hatairaktham S, Charoensakdi R, Panichkul N, Fucharoen S, Srichairatanakool S, et al. Treatment of beta-thalassemia/hemoglobin E with antioxidant cocktails results in decreased oxidative stress, increased hemoglobin concentration, and improvement of the hypercoagulable state. Oxidative Medicine and Cellular Longevity. 2015;**2015**:537954

[52] Inthawong K, Charoenkwan P, Silvilairat S, Tantiworawit A, Phrommintikul A, Choeyprasert W, et al. Pulmonary hypertension in non-transfusion-dependent thalassemia: Correlation with clinical parameters, liver iron concentration, and non-transferrin-bound iron. Hematology. 2015;**20**:610-617

[53] Yatmark P, Morales NP, Chaisri U, Wichaiyo S, Hemstapat W, Srichairatanakool S, et al. Effects of iron chelators on pulmonary iron overload and oxidative stress in beta-thalassemic mice. Pharmacology. 2015;**96**:192-199

[54] Nielsen VG, Pretorius E. Iron and carbon monoxide enhance coagulation and attenuate fibrinolysis by different mechanisms. Blood Coagulation & Fibrinolysis. 2014;**25**:695-702

[55] Morris CR, Kim HY, Klings ES, Wood J, Porter JB, Trachtenberg F, et al. Dysregulated arginine metabolism and cardiopulmonary dysfunction in patients with thalassaemia. British Journal of Haematology. 2015;**169**:887-898

[56] Cappellini MD, Musallam KM, Poggiali E, Taher AT. Hypercoagulability in non-transfusion-dependent thalassemia. Blood Reviews. 2012;**26**(Suppl 1):S20-S23

[57] Musallam KM, Taher AT, Karimi M, Rachmilewitz EA. Cerebral infarction in beta-thalassemia intermedia: Breaking the silence. Thrombosis Research. 2012;**130**:695-702

[58] Gonzalez-Reimers E, Quintero-Platt G, Martin-Gonzalez C, Perez-Hernandez O, Romero-Acevedo L, Santolaria-Fernandez F. Thrombin activation and liver inflammation in advanced hepatitis C virus infection. World Journal of Gastroenterology. 2016;**22**:4427-4437

[59] Kell DB, Pretorius E. Serum ferritin is an important inflammatory disease marker, as it is mainly a leakage product from damaged cells. Metallomics. 2014;**6**:748-773

[60] Fucharoen S, Weatherall DJ. Progress toward the control and management of the thalassemias. Hematology/Oncology Clinics of North America. 2016;**30**:359-371

[61] Porter JB. Optimizing iron chelation strategies in beta-thalassaemia major. Blood Reviews. 2009;**23**(Suppl 1):S3-S7

[62] Farmaki K, Tzoumari I, Pappa C. Oral chelators in transfusion-dependent thalassemia major patients may prevent or reverse iron overload complications. Blood Cells, Molecules & Diseases. 2011;**47**:33-40

[63] Vannasaeng S, Fucharoen S, Pootrakul P, Ploybutr S, Yansukon P. Pituitary function in thalassemic patients and the effect of chelation therapy. Acta Endocrinologica. 1991;**124**:23-30

[64] Halliwell B. Drug antioxidant effects. A basis for drug selection? Drugs. 1991;**42**:569-605

[65] Amer J, Atlas D, Fibach E. N-acetylcysteine amide (AD4) attenuates oxidative stress in beta-thalassemia blood cells. Biochimica et Biophysica Acta. 2008;**1780**:249-255

[66] Dissayabutra T, Tosukhowong P, Seksan P. The benefits of vitamin C and vitamin E in children with beta-thalassemia with high oxidative stress. Journal of the Medical Association of Thailand. 2005;**88**(Suppl 4):S317-S321

[67] Giardini O, Cantani A, Donfrancesco A. Vitamin E therapy in homozygous beta-thalassemia. The New England Journal of Medicine. 1981;**305**:644

[68] Giardini O, Cantani A, Donfrancesco A, Martino F, Mannarino O, D'Eufemia P, et al. Biochemical and clinical effects of vitamin E administration in homozygous beta-thalassemia. Acta Vitaminologica et Enzymologica. 1985;**7**:55-60

[69] Hyman CB, Landing B, Alfin-Slater R, Kozak L, Weitzman J, Ortega JA. Dl-alpha-tocopherol, iron, and lipofuscin in thalassemia. Annals of the New York Academy of Sciences. 1974;**232**:211-220

[70] Kalpravidh RW, Wichit A, Siritanaratkul N, Fucharoen S. Effect of coenzyme Q_{10} as an antioxidant in beta-thalassemia/Hb E patients. BioFactors. 2005;**25**:225-234

[71] Miniero R, Canducci E, Ghigo D, Saracco P, Vullo C. Vitamin E in beta-thalassemia. Acta Vitaminologica et Enzymologica. 1982;**4**:21-25

[72] Miniero R, David O, Ghigo D, Luzzatto L, Ramenghi U, Saracco P, et al. Administration of vitamin E in heterozygous beta-thalassaemia: The effect on red blood cell survival. Panminerva Medica. 1984;**26**:283-286

[73] Miniero R, Piga A, Luzzatto L, Gabutti V. Vitamin E and beta-thalassaemia. Haematologica. 1983;**68**:562-563

[74] O'Brien RT. Ascorbic acid enhancement of desferrioxamine-induced urinary iron excretion in thalassemia major. Annals of the New York Academy of Sciences. 1974;**232**:221-225

[75] Ozsoylu S, Gurgey A. Vitamin E treatment in triplicated alpha-globin gene-heterozygous beta-thalassemia. American Journal of Hematology. 1991;**38**:335-336

[76] Palasuwan A, Soogarun S, Wiwanitkit V, Luechapudiporn R, Pradniwat P, Lertlum T. Preliminary study of the effect of vitamin E supplementation on the antioxidant status of hemoglobin-E carriers. The Southeast Asian Journal of Tropical Medicine and Public Health. 2006;**37**(Suppl 3):184-189

[77] Pfeifer WP, Degasperi GR, Almeida MT, Vercesi AE, Costa FF, Saad ST. Vitamin E supplementation reduces oxidative stress in beta thalassaemia intermedia. Acta Haematologica. 2008;**120**:225-231

[78] Tesoriere L, D'Arpa D, Butera D, Allegra M, Renda D, Maggio A, et al. Oral supplements of vitamin E improve measures of oxidative stress in plasma and reduce oxidative damage to LDL and erythrocytes in beta-thalassemia intermedia patients. Free Radical Research. 2001;**34**:529-540

[79] Vatanavicharn S, Yenchitsomanus P, Siddhikol C. Vitamin E in beta-thalassaemia and alpha-thalassaemia (HbH) diseases. Acta Haematologica. 1985;**73**:183

[80] Unchern S, Laoharuangpanya N, Phumala N, Sipankapracha P, Pootrakul P, Fucharoen S, et al. The effects of vitamin E on platelet activity in beta-thalassaemia patients. British Journal of Haematology. 2003;**123**:738-744

[81] Alidoost F, Gharagozloo M, Bagherpour B, Jafarian A, Sajjadi SE, Hourfar H, et al. Effects of silymarin on the proliferation and glutathione levels of peripheral blood mononuclear cells from beta-thalassemia major patients. International Immunopharmacology. 2006;**6**:1305-1310

[82] Amer J, Goldfarb A, Rachmilewitz EA, Fibach E. Fermented papaya preparation as redox regulator in blood cells of beta-thalassemic mice and patients. Phytotherapy Research. 2008;**22**:820-828

[83] Kalpravidh RW, Siritanaratkul N, Insain P, Charoensakdi R, Panichkul N, Hatairaktham S, et al. Improvement in oxidative stress and antioxidant parameters in beta-thalassemia/Hb E patients treated with curcuminoids. Clinical Biochemistry. 2009;**43**:424-429

[84] Fibach E, Rachmilewitz EA. The role of antioxidants and iron chelators in the treatment of oxidative stress in thalassemia. Annals of the New York Academy of Sciences. 2010;**1202**:10-16

[85] Wapnick AA, Lynch SR, Krawitz P, Seftel HC, Charlton RW, Bothwell TH. Effects of iron overload on ascorbic acid metabolism. British Medical Journal. 1968;**3**:704-707

[86] Chatterjea B, Maitra A, Banerjee DK, Basu AK. Status of ascorbic acid in iron deficiency anaemia and thalassaemia. Acta Haematologica. 1980;**64**:271-275

[87] Chapman RW, Hussain MA, Gorman A, Laulicht M, Politis D, Flynn DM, et al. Effect of ascorbic acid deficiency on serum ferritin concentration in patients with beta-thalassaemia major and iron overload. Journal of Clinical Pathology. 1982;**35**:487-491

[88] Livrea MA, Tesoriere L, Pintaudi AM, Calabrese A, Maggio A, Freisleben HJ, et al. Oxidative stress and antioxidant status in beta-thalassemia major: Iron overload and depletion of lipid-soluble antioxidants. Blood. 1996;**88**:3608-3614

[89] Vatanavicharn S, Anuwatanakulchai M, Yenchitsomanus P, Siddhikol C. Relationship of serum vitamin E, erythrocyte nonheme iron, and malonyldialdehyde (lipid membrane peroxidation product) in thalassemia. Birth Defects Original Article Series. 1987;**23**:207-211

[90] Selden C, Seymour CA, Peters TJ. Activities of some free-radical scavenging enzymes and glutathione concentrations in human and rat liver and their relationship to the pathogenesis of tissue damage in iron overload. Clinical Science (London, England). 1980;**58**:211-219

[91] Amer J, Fibach E. Oxidative status of platelets in normal and thalassemic blood. Thrombosis and Haemostasis. 2004;**92**:1052-1059

[92] Aphinives C, Kukongviriyapan U, Jetsrisuparb A, Kukongviriyapan V, Somparn N. Impaired endothelial function in pediatric hemoglobin E/beta-thalassemia patients with iron overload. The Southeast Asian Journal of Tropical Medicine and Public Health. 2015;**45**:1454-1463

[93] Chakraborty D, Bhattacharyya M. Antioxidant defense status of red blood cells of patients with beta-thalassemia and E/beta-thalassemia. Clinica Chimica Acta. 2001;**305**:123-129

[94] Cheng ML, Ho HY, Tseng HC, Lee CH, Shih LY, Chiu DT. Antioxidant deficit and enhanced susceptibility to oxidative damage in individuals with different forms of alpha-thalassaemia. British Journal of Haematology. 2005;**128**:119-127

[95] Chiou SS, Tsao CJ, Tsai SM, Wu YR, Liao YM, Lin PC, et al. Metabolic pathways related to oxidative stress in patients with hemoglobin H disease and iron overload. Journal of Clinical Laboratory Analysis. 2014;**28**:261-268

[96] Boonyawat K, Wongwaisayawan S, Nitiyanant P, Atichartakarn V. Hydroxyurea and colonic ulcers: A case report. BMC Gastroenterology. 2014;**14**:134

[97] Bradai M, Abad MT, Pissard S, Lamraoui F, Skopinski L, de Montalembert M. Hydroxyurea can eliminate transfusion requirements in children with severe beta-thalassemia. Blood. 2003;**102**:1529-1530

[98] Bradai M, Pissard S, Abad MT, Dechartres A, Ribeil JA, Landais P, et al. Decreased transfusion needs associated with hydroxyurea therapy in Algerian patients with thalassemia major or intermedia. Transfusion. 2007;**47**:1830-1836

[99] Darbari DS, Nouraie M, Taylor JG, Brugnara C, Castro O, Ballas SK. Alpha-thalassaemia and response to hydroxyurea in sickle cell anaemia. European Journal of Haematology. 2013;**92**:341-345

[100] Italia K, Chandrakala S, Ghosh K, Colah R. Can hydroxyurea serve as a free radical scavenger and reduce iron overload in beta-thalassemia patients? Free Radical Research. 2016;**50**:959-965

[101] Ajanta H, Chakraborty S, Madhusnata D, Bhattacharya DK, Manisha D. The activity of superoxide dismutase in hydroxyurea-treated E beta thalassemia. The Journal of the Association of Physicians of India. 2002;**50**:1034-1035

[102] De M, Banerjee N, Talukdar G, Bhattacharya DK. Lipid peroxidation and spectrin of RBC membrane in hydroxyurea treated E/beta thalassaemia. Indian Journal of Clinical Biochemistry. 2000;**15**:56-59

[103] Udupi V, Rice-Evans C. Thiol compounds as protective agents in erythrocytes under oxidative stress. Free Radical Research Communications. 1992;**16**:315-323

[104] Nur E, Brandjes DP, Teerlink T, Otten HM, Oude Elferink RP, Muskiet F, et al. N-acetylcysteine reduces oxidative stress in sickle cell patients. Annals of Hematology. 2012;**91**:1097-1105

[105] Ozdemir ZC, Koc A, Aycicek A, Kocyigit A. N-Acetylcysteine supplementation reduces oxidative stress and DNA damage in children with beta-thalassemia. Hemoglobin. 2014;**38**:359-364

[106] Gupta SC, Patchva S, Aggarwal BB. Therapeutic roles of curcumin: Lessons learned from clinical trials. The AAPS Journal. 2012;**15**:195-218

[107] Iqbal M, Okazaki Y, Okada S. In vitro curcumin modulates ferric nitrilotriacetate (Fe-NTA) and hydrogen peroxide (H_2O_2)-induced peroxidation of microsomal membrane lipids and DNA damage. Teratogenesis Carcinogenesis and Mutagenesis. 2003; **Suppl 1**:151-160

[108] Sharma OP. Antioxidant activity of curcumin and related compounds. Biochemical Pharmacology. 1976;**25**:1811-1812

[109] Srichairatanakool S, Thephinlap C, Phisalaphong C, Porter JB, Fucharoen S. Curcumin contributes to in vitro removal of non-transferrin bound iron by deferiprone and desferrioxamine in thalassemic plasma. Medicinal Chemistry. 2007;**3**:469-474

[110] Thephinlap C, Phisalaphong C, Fucharoen S, Porter JB, Srichairatanakool S. Efficacy of curcuminoids in alleviation of iron overload and lipid peroxidation in thalassemic mice. Medicinal Chemistry. 2009;**5**:474-482

[111] Thephinlap C, Phisalaphong C, Lailerd N, Chattipakorn N, Winichagoon P, Vadolas J, et al. Reversal of cardiac iron loading and dysfunction in thalassemic mice by curcuminoids. Medicinal Chemistry. 2011;**7**:62-69

[112] Chaneiam N, Changtam C, Mungkongdee T, Suthatvoravut U, Winichagoon P, Vadolas J, et al. A reduced curcuminoid analog as a novel inducer of fetal hemoglobin. Annals of Hematology. 2012;**92**:379-386

[113] Badria FA, Ibrahim AS, Badria AF, Elmarakby AA. Curcumin attenuates iron accumu-lation and oxidative stress in the liver and spleen of chronic iron-overloaded rats. PLoS ONE. 2015;**10**:e0134156

[114] McKay DL, Blumberg JB. The role of tea in human health: An update. Journal of the American College of Nutrition. 2002;**21**:1-13

[115] Cabrera C, Artacho R, Gimenez R. Beneficial effects of green tea—A review. Journal of the American College of Nutrition. 2006;**25**:79-99

[116] Srichairatanakool S, Ounjaijean S, Thephinlap C, Khansuwan U, Phisalpong C, Fucharoen S. Iron-chelating and free-radical scavenging activities of microwave-pro-cessed green tea in iron overload. Hemoglobin. 2006;**30**:311-327

[117] Thephinlap C, Ounjaijean S, Khansuwan U, Fucharoen S, Porter JB, Srichairatanakool S. Epigallocatechin-3-gallate and epicatechin-3-gallate from green tea decrease plasma non-transferrin bound iron and erythrocyte oxidative stress. Medicinal Chemistry. 2007;**3**:289-296

[118] Ounjaijean S, Thephinlap C, Khansuwan U, Phisalapong C, Fucharoen S, Porter JB, et al. Effect of green tea on iron status and oxidative stress in iron-loaded rats. Medicinal Chemistry. 2008;**4**:365-370

[119] Saewong T, Ounjaijean S, Mundee Y, Pattanapanyasat K, Fucharoen S, Porter JB, et al. Effects of green tea on iron accumulation and oxidative stress in livers of iron-chal-lenged thalassemic mice. Medicinal Chemistry. 2010;**6**:57-64

[120] de Alarcon PA, Donovan ME, Forbes GB, Landaw SA, Stockman JA 3rd. Iron absorp-tion in the thalassemia syndromes and its inhibition by tea. The New England Journal of Medicine. 1979;**300**:5-8

[121] Lim DY. Comparison of green tea extract and epigallocatechin gallate on secretion of catecholamines from the rabbit adrenal medulla. Archives of Pharmacal Research. 2005;**28**:914-922

[122] Liatsos GD, Moulakakis A, Ketikoglou I, Klonari S. Possible green tea-induced throm-botic thrombocytopenic purpura. American Journal of Health-System Pharmacy. 2010;**67**:531-534

[123] Kang WS, Lim IH, Yuk DY, Chung KH, Park JB, Yoo HS, et al. Antithrombotic activi-ties of green tea catechins and (−)-epigallocatechin gallate. Thrombosis Research. 1999;**96**:229-237

[124] Lee DH, Kim YJ, Kim HH, Cho HJ, Ryu JH, Rhee MH, et al. Inhibitory effects of epigal-locatechin-3-gallate on microsomal cyclooxygenase-1 activity in platelets. Biomolecules & Therapeutics. 2013;**21**:54-59

[125] Koonyosying P, Tantiworawit A, Hantrakool S, Utama-Ang, N, Cresswell M, Fucharoen S, et al. Consumption of a green tea extract-curcumin drink decreases blood urea nitrogen and redox iron in β-thalassemia patients. Food & Functions. 2020;**11**(1):932-943

[126] Devasagayam TP, Kamat JP, Mohan H, Kesavan PC. Caffeine as an antioxidant: Inhibition of lipid peroxidation induced by reactive oxygen species. Biochimica et Biophysica Acta. 1996;**1282**:63-70

[127] Shi X, Dalal NS, Jain AC. Antioxidant behaviour of caffeine: Efficient scavenging of hydroxyl radicals. Food and Chemical Toxicology. 1991;**29**:1-6

[128] Stadler RH, Turesky RJ, Muller O, Markovic J, Leong-Morgenthaler PM. The inhibitory effects of coffee on radical-mediated oxidation and mutagenicity. Mutation Research. 1994;**308**:177-190

[129] Chu YF, Farah A. Coffee constituents. In: Coffee. New Jersey, USA: John Wiley & Sons Inc. and the Institute of Food Technologists; 2012. pp. 22-58 (Chapter 2)

[130] Monente C, Ludwig IA, Irigoyen A, De Pena MP, Cid C. Assessment of total (free and bound) phenolic compounds in spent coffee extracts. Journal of Agricultural and Food Chemistry. 2015;**63**:4327-4334

[131] Monente C, Ludwig IA, Stalmach A, de Pena MP, Cid C, Crozier A. In vitro studies on the stability in the proximal gastrointestinal tract and bioaccessibility in Caco-2 cells of chlorogenic acids from spent coffee grounds. International Journal of Food Sciences and Nutrition. 2015;**66**:657-664

[132] Takenaka M, Sato N, Asakawa H, Wen X, Murata M, Homma S. Characterization of a metal-chelating substance in coffee. Bioscience, Biotechnology, and Biochemistry. 2005;**69**: 26-30

[133] Umemura T, Ueda K, Nishioka K, Hidaka T, Takemoto H, Nakamura S, et al. Effects of acute administration of caffeine on vascular function. The American Journal of Cardiology. 2006;**98**:1538-1541

[134] Olthof MR, Hollman PC, Katan MB. Chlorogenic acid and caffeic acid are absorbed in humans. The Journal of Nutrition. 2001;**131**:66-71

[135] Naito S, Yatagai C, Maruyama M, Sumi H. Effect of coffee extracts on plasma fibrinolysis and platelet aggregation. Nihon Arukōru Yakubutsu Igakkai Zasshi. 2011;**46**:260-269

[136] Jiang R, Hodgson JM, Mas E, Croft KD, Ward NC. Chlorogenic acid improves ex vivo vessel function and protects endothelial cells against HOCl-induced oxidative damage, via increased production of nitric oxide and induction of Hmox-1. The Journal of Nutritional Biochemistry. 2015;**27**:53-60

[137] Echeverri D, Montes FR, Cabrera M, Galan A, Prieto A. Caffeine's vascular mechanisms of action. International Journal of Vascular Medicine. 2010;**2010**:834060

[138] Folstar P, van der Plas HC, Pilnik W, de Heus JG. Tocopherols in the unsaponifiable matter of coffee bean oil. Journal of Agricultural and Food Chemistry. 1977;**25**:283-285

[139] Sved S, Hossie RD, McGilveray IJ. The human metabolism of caffeine to theophylline. Research Communications in Chemical Pathology and Pharmacology. 1976;**13**:185-192

[140] Morris ER. An overview of current information on bioavailability of dietary iron to humans. Federation Proceedings. 1983;**42**:1716-1720

[141] Huang J, de Paulis T, May JM. Antioxidant effects of dihydrocaffeic acid in human EA.hy926 endothelial cells. The Journal of Nutritional Biochemistry. 2004;**15**:722-729

[142] Ochiai R, Jokura H, Suzuki A, Tokimitsu I, Ohishi M, Komai N, et al. Green coffee bean extract improves human vasoreactivity. Hypertension Research. 2004;**27**:731-737

[143] Lopez-Barrera DM, Vazquez-Sanchez K, Loarca-Pina MG, Campos-Vega R. Spent coffee grounds, an innovative source of colonic fermentable compounds, inhibit inflammatory mediators in vitro. Food Chemistry. 2016;**212**:282-290

[144] Agudelo-Ochoa GM, Pulgarin-Zapata IC, Velasquez-Rodriguez CM, Duque-Ramirez M, Naranjo-Cano M, Quintero-Ortiz MM, et al. Coffee consumption increases the antioxidant capacity of plasma and has no effect on the lipid profile or vascular function in healthy adults in a randomized controlled trial. The Journal of Nutrition. 2016;**146**:524-531

[145] Chang J, Fedinec AL, Kuntamallappanavar G, Leffler CW, Bukiya AN, Dopico AM. Endothelial nitric oxide mediates caffeine antagonism of alcohol-induced cerebral artery constriction. The Journal of Pharmacology and Experimental Therapeutics. 2015;**356**:106-115

[146] Shin HS, Satsu H, Bae MJ, Totsuka M, Shimizu M. Catechol groups enable reactive oxygen species scavenging-mediated suppression of PKD-NF kappaB-IL-8 signaling pathway by chlorogenic and caffeic acids in human intestinal cells. Nutrients. 2017;**9**:E165. DOI: 10.3390/nu9020165

[147] Bakuradze T, Boehm N, Janzowski C, Lang R, Hofmann T, Stockis JP, et al. Antioxidant-rich coffee reduces DNA damage, elevates glutathione status and contributes to weight control: Results from an intervention study. Molecular Nutrition & Food Research. 2011;**55**:793-797

[148] Hoelzl C, Knasmuller S, Wagner KH, Elbling L, Huber W, Kager N, et al. Instant coffee with high chlorogenic acid levels protects humans against oxidative damage of macromolecules. Molecular Nutrition & Food Research. 2010;**54**:1722-1733

[149] Guerrini A, Lampronti I, Bianchi N, Zuccato C, Breveglieri G, Salvatori F, et al. Bergamot (*Citrus bergamia* Risso) fruit extracts as gamma-globin gene expression inducers: Phytochemical and functional perspectives. Journal of Agricultural and Food Chemistry. 2009;**57**:4103-4111

[150] Fibach E, Tan ES, Jamuar S, Ng I, Amer J, Rachmilewitz EA. Amelioration of oxidative stress in red blood cells from patients with beta-thalassemia major and intermedia and E-beta-thalassemia following administration of a fermented papaya preparation. Phytotherapy Research. 2010;**24**:1334-1338

[151] Pardo-Andreu GL, Sanchez-Baldoquin C, Avila-Gonzalez R, Yamamoto ET, Revilla A, Uyemura SA, et al. Interaction of Vimang (*Mangifera indica* L. extract) with Fe(III)

improves its antioxidant and cytoprotecting activity. Pharmacological Research. 2006;**54**:389-395

[152] Srichairatanakool S et al. Nutritional values and pharmacological activities of Mangifera indica Linn. cv Mahachanok. In: A Final Report of Thailand Research Fund. 2013

[153] Marawaha RK, Bansal D, Kaur S, Trehan A. Wheat grass juice reduces transfusion requirement in patients with thalassemia major: A pilot study. Indian Pediatrics. 2004;**41**:716-720

[154] Singh K, Pannu MS, Singh P, Singh J. Effect of wheat grass tablets on the frequency of blood transfusions in thalassemia major. Indian Journal of Pediatrics. 2010;**77**:90-91

[155] Choudhary DR, Naithani R, Panigrahi I, Kumar R, Mahapatra M, Pati HP, et al. Effect of wheat grass therapy on transfusion requirement in beta-thalassemia major. Indian Journal of Pediatrics. 2009;**76**:375-376

[156] Bagwe SM, Kale PP, Bhatt LK, Prabhavalkar KS. Herbal approach in the treatment of pancytopenia. Journal of Complementary and Integrative Medicine. 2017;**14**(1):1-11

[157] Pangjit K, Tantiphaipunwong P, Sajjapong W, Srichairatanakool S. Iron-chelating, free radical scavenging and anti-proliferative activities of *Azadirachta indica*. Journal of the Medical Association of Thailand. 2014;**97**(Suppl 4):S36-S43

Free Radicals and Antioxidants: Opportunities for Enhancing Treatment of Epilepsy with Personalized Medicine

Jerzy Majkowski, Tuomas Westermarck and Faik Atroshi

Additional information is available at the end of the chapter

http://dx.doi.org/10.5772/intechopen.91999

Abstract

Introduction: Epileptic seizures and antiepileptic drugs (AEDs) are a source of oxygen stress. Oxygen stress can have negative effects. These effects which can be prevented are largely unknown in clinical epileptology. Objective: The objective of the study is to discuss (a) homeostatic oxidant, antioxidant imbalance due to epileptic seizures and AEDs, (b) the protective factors that help prevent oxygen stress (OS), and personalized medicine based on pharmacogenomics and diet as therapeutic challenges in epilepsy. Discussion: Experimental models of epileptic seizures evoked by various means suggest that seizures can cause neuronal destruction. This is accompanied by an increased activity of free radicals and a reduction of total antioxidant capacity (in red blood cells, blood serum, and cerebrospinal fluid). A number of antioxidants have been found to attenuate the negative effects of OS and act neuroprotectively if they are administered prior to seizure occurrence: vitamins (C, E), trace elements (Se, Zn), melatonin, erdosteine, or natural herbal extracts. New AEDs (GBP, LEV, LTG, and TGB) cause no, or very little, OS as opposed to other drugs (CBZ, PHT, PB, VPA, TPM, or OXC), which have pronounced albeit heterogeneous and dose-dependent effects. It is suggested that AEDs should be administered together with free radical sweepers (vitamins, trace elements, electrolytes, melatonin) and other anti-oxidizing substances. Conclusions: (1) Epileptic seizures and AEDs cause OS. The effects vary greatly depending, among other things, on the daily drug dose. (2) The findings of research using a variety of seizure models are more unequivocal than the findings of research on patients with epilepsy. This suggests that the relations among seizures, AEDs, OS etiology, and OS consequences are complex. (3) Since existing AEDs cause OS, it is necessary to develop a new approach to AED treatment. (4) It is important to know the patient's specific characteristics, including previous history, lifestyle, age, gender, weight, diet, environment, etc. They can be valuable tools to improve the quality of life of a person suffering from epilepsy. This concept of managing the patient health is called targeted medicine or personalized medicine.

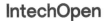

Keywords: epileptic seizures, epilepsy, oxygen stress, antioxidants, personalized medicine

1. Introduction

Within the last three decades, interest in oxygen stress and its role in the development of organ pathology has increased considerably, and the importance of this phenomenon has been increasingly recognized. Oxygen stress means that the production of free radicals and reactive forms of oxygen (RFO) has exceeded the antioxidant defense mechanism capacity [1, 2]. Bartosz [3] thinks that RFO research may be the key to a better understanding of certain biochemical, physiological, and pathological aspects of living organisms and suggests that such understanding could be applied to clinical practice. Free radicals, the product of oxygen stress, may play an important role as physiological markers that control cell process signals. However, when produced in excess, or when the antioxidant defense system is weak, they may lead to cell injury.

Excessive free radical production is related to various physiological and pathological states such as aging, epileptic seizures, or the use of xenobiotics, including fat-soluble drugs [4, 5]; this also applies to antiepileptic drugs (AEDs) [6–8]. A number of nonspecific factors [9] as well as dietary habits affect the state of antioxidants in the healthy elderly [10]. This suggests that oxidation and anti-oxidation processes are rather ubiquitous and hence nonspecific.

As far as epilepsy is concerned, when the number of free radicals in the neuron increases, this interferes with the respiratory chain in the mitochondria, destabilizes the lysosomal membranes, and lowers the convulsion threshold [11–13]. Peroxydation of the neuronal membranes modifies their electrophysiological properties and leads to an abnormal bioelectric discharge in the neurons.

Epilepsy is frequent in diseases involving dysfunction in the mitochondrial structures. It is a sign of energetic anomalies in the ATP synthesis due to ADP phosphorylation [14]. The mitochondria have vital functions such as energy production, cellular harm control, neurotransmitter synthesis, and free radical production. It is not clear yet which of these functions are affected in epileptic seizures [15]. Liang and Patel found an increase in spontaneous and evoked epileptic attacks in a subgroup of mice with a partial inherent mitochondrial SOD deficit. This effect correlated with chronic mitochondrial oxygen stress (aconitase enzyme deactivation) and reduced oxygen use. They think that oxygen stress caused by free radical peroxides increases seizure susceptibility in this subgroup of mice. This susceptibility increases with age and also with increased environmental stimulation and the use of stimulants. Oxygen stress and mitochondrial dysfunction may both cause and be caused by epileptic attacks [16]. According to Dubenko and Litovchenko [17], the application of energy metabolism activators improves the clinical and electroencephalographic course of epilepsy. This has been demonstrated experimentally by positive histological changes. According to these writers, this treatment prevents neuronal harm and the development of encephalopathy.

Research on various seizure models, in animals and humans, has shown that not only epileptic seizures but also EEG discharges themselves may cause complex metabolic neural lesions and oxidation-antioxidant disequilibrium [18–21].

On the other hand, a number of experimental studies have shown that AEDs can also produce free radicals and significantly increase the peroxydation of neuronal membrane lipids and reduce the protective effects of antioxidants. These changes may lead to increased seizure and idiosyncratic drug effect frequency [7, 22–25]. PHT initiates an oxidation damage to proteins and fats in the maternal and embryonic liver tissue organelle in murine rodents [1].

A group of researchers have also found that oxidation stress and resistance to AEDs trigger adaptive mechanisms, i.e., production of endogenous antioxidant sweepers, which prevent the harmful effects of oxidation [26]. These researchers studied nitrogen oxide and endogenous antioxidant GSH sweepers, GSH-Px, complete (T) and superoxide dismutase (T-SOD), Mn-SOD, and catalase in the cerebrospinal fluid of children with various neurological diseases. All the antioxidant parameters were the highest in the children with bacterial meningitis compared with the other groups. In the epilepsy group, nitrogen oxide, GSH, and GSH-Px were higher than in the aseptic meningitis and control group [26]. The authors think that oxygen stress may be related to seizure pathology and that its reduction may lead to a better prognosis for the course of epilepsy.

Akarsu et al. [27] came to similar conclusions. They studied the state of oxidation in 21 children with febrile seizures and 21 children without febrile seizures. They assessed the level of arginase and catalase in the red blood cells, malondialdehyde—an indicator of lipid peroxidation (MDA)—and nitrogen oxide in the plasma and cerebrospinal fluid. The control group consisted of 41 children divided into three subgroups: (1) with fever, (2) without convulsions, and (3) without fever and without convulsions. Both fever and convulsions had a significant effect on the oxidation mechanism. Febrile and afebrile convulsions differed in their generation of oxygen stress. According to the authors, higher levels of oxygen stress may be a factor that protects against neuronal lesion during convulsions in afebrile convulsions.

Not only can oxygen stress initiate epileptogenesis, it can also worsen the course of epilepsy. Consistently with these conclusions, using antioxidants in conventional epilepsy therapy and hence attenuating oxygen stress could have a positive effect on the course of epilepsy [28]. Many researchers share this opinion, but few of them are clinical epileptologists. Earlier, a review was published of research on the possible role of oxygen stress in the early stages of epileptogenesis, both in animal models and humans [29]. There has also been discussion of attempts to use exogenous antioxidants which, according to many writers, have antiepileptogenic properties (which AEDs do not).

It has been reported that refractory epileptic patients may benefit from pharmacogenetic testing for variations in the genes encoding drug-metabolizing enzymes and drug transporters of AEDs [30]. Since the treatment options are limited, the use of personal medication, which could have beneficial effects in epilepsy treatment, is indicated [31]. The aim of personalized medication is to maximize the likelihood of therapeutic efficacy and to minimize the risk of drug toxicity. Specific genes have been linked to adverse drug reactions in the form of a severe rash in Stevens-Johnson syndrome [32, 33].

2. Preventing oxidation stress due to epileptic seizures

Experimental research with animal models and clinical observation have shown that epileptic seizures lead to a number of harmful activities in the brain: disturbed blood circulation, increased cerebrospinal fluid pressure, brain edema, and hypoxia, all of which lead to a sudden reduction of energy carriers (ADP, ATP, phosphocreatine) and pH neuron reduction. During seizures, arachidic acid is released in the postsynaptic membranes. This has an activating effect on presynaptic neuronal endings and leads to increased glutamate release. Arachidic acid also increases the production of free oxygen radicals, leading to increased lipid peroxidation. These in turn may activate phospholipase C and then lead to the release of arachidic acid from cellular membranes, setting a vicious circle in motion [3].

2.1. The metrazol seizure model (PTZ)

Intraperitoneally induced seizures in rats by means of PTZ rupture the blood-brain barrier. This has been demonstrated with Evans dye, used to mark the permeability of this barrier [34]. Research suggests that free radicals are involved in the permeability of the blood-brain barrier; this permeability leads to albumin extravasation to the thalamic nuclei, brain stem, frontal cortex, and occipital cortex. The animals that have been given vitamin E or selenium (Se) prior to the seizure induction had less extravasation in these structures. It has also been demonstrated that in young rats in normothermic conditions, the barrier permeability was greater in males ($p < 0.05$) [35].

In this convulsion model in mice, prior administration of erdosteine (mucoliticum), which acts as an antioxidant, leads to much weaker oxygen stress and much longer latency time from pentylenetetrazol (PTZ) administration to convulsion onset ($p < 0.05$) [36]. On the other hand, compared with the control group, the experimental group had lower levels of MDA and xanthine oxidase (oxidizers) and a higher level of SOD ($p < 0.001$). These studies show that administration of erdosteine reduces convulsion-induced oxygen stress and therefore protects the neurons.

In mice, *Nigella sativa* oil (NSO), a powerful antioxidant that has been in used in folk medicine and the kitchen for thousands of years, prevented epileptic seizures induced by PTZ kindling much more effectively than valproic acid (VPA) [20].

2.2. The kainic acid model

Kainic acid (KA) is used as a model substance in the assessment of neurotoxicity. It leads to excessive RFT production due to reduced antioxidant activity. When KA was administered to rats, lipid peroxidation of the neuronal membrane increased in proportion to seizure progression [37]. In the same model, SOD and catalase activity increased significantly on day 5 following KA administration and returned to the base level 3 weeks later; GGH-PX activity also increased significantly on day 5 but was still high 3 weeks later [38]. Lipid and protein peroxidation, assessed by MDA concentration, increased significantly 8 and 16 h later then decreased on day 2 and day 5 following KA injection. The authors attribute the rapid increase in MDA and protein peroxidation to free radicals produced in this phase of the pathological KA effect; they think that the changes in the enzymatic scavenger activity and the reduced MDA concentration may have been caused by glia proliferation due to neuronal death.

In the KA model in mice, prior or simultaneous administration of melatonin (a powerful hydroxyl radical scavenger) (20 mg/kg i.p.) had an anti-oxidizing effect and prevented lipid peroxidation, cerebral mitochondria DNA injury, and seizures [39].

In the KA model, prior administration of vineatrol significantly reduced the MDA level in rats' brains but had no effect on the glutation level [40]. Doses exceeding 20 and 40 mg/kg lengthened the latency time to that of the first seizures. Additional administration of vineatrol 30 and 60 min after KA administration significantly reduced seizure incidence. The authors suggest that vineatrol could potentially be administered in the epileptic state.

Sok et al. [21] studied the anticonvulsive effects of *Petasites japonicum* (BMP), a plant grown in East Asia and used for both culinary purposes and in folk medicine. Its root extracts are still used for headaches and asthma. Prolonged administration of BMP, prior to KA administration, reduced mortality in mice by one half, and administration of the BMP-I subfraction reduced convulsive seizures and also significantly reduced neuronal loss in parts CA_1 and CA_3 of the hippocampus. The authors suggest that BMP-I is the factor responsible for prevention of oxidization lesion in the mouse brain.

Hsieh et al. [41] tested a traditional Chinese herb (*Gastrodia elata* B1—GE) administered to treat epilepsy in a controlled study using the KA seizure model in rats. They found that prior administration of GE significantly reduced in vitro lipid peroxydation in the rats' brains, an effect analogous to the effect of phenytoin (PHT—20 mg/kg). The authors think that GE has an antiepileptic effect and is a free radical scavenger. This antiepileptic effect may be at least partly attributable to the GE's vanilla component [42].

2.3. The pilocarpine model

Pilocarpine, an imidazole alkaloid extracted from the leaves of the *Pilocarpus jaborandi* shrub, is a parasympathomimetic, cholinergic antagonist that acts similarly to acetylcholine. It is often used to evoke epileptic convulsions and epileptic states in animal models. The mechanisms leading to seizures or status epilepticus are unknown. It is thought that oxygen stress plays an important role, but we still do not know which brain structures are more sensitive. Studies of the activity of catalase, a free radical scavenger, have found different effects of the epileptic state on the catalase level in different brain structures [19]. The highest elevation was found in the hippocampus (36%), striatum (31%), and frontal cortex (15%); no changes in the level of catalase activity were found in the cerebellum. The authors think that the endogenous increase in the catalase activity, responsible for removal of free oxygen radicals produced during convulsions, may be a compensatory defense mechanism that counteracts the negative effects of oxygen stress in the status epilepticus. Other researchers have come to similar conclusions [26, 43]. Tejada et al. [43] evoked a pilocarpine epileptic state and found that MDA increased significantly (64%), suggesting oxygen injury. They found a simultaneous increase in the anti-oxidizing activity of catalase enzymes (28%), GSH-Px (28%) and SOD

(21%). On the other hand, vitamin E concentration in the cerebral cortex was reduced (15%) due to increased lipid peroxydation following pilocarpine administration.

Barros et al. [18] applied the same model and found that administration of vitamin E (200 mg/g i.p.) 30 min prior to the administration of pilocarpine (400 mg/kg s.c.) led to increased (214%) catalase activity in the hippocampus compared with rats given only pilocarpine (67%) or physiological saline. The authors think that increased catalase activity may be responsible for the regulation of free radicals evoked by the status epilepticus.

In this same model in rats, prior administration of vitamin C (250 mg/kg i.p.) reduced the negative effects of oxygen stress and neuronal lesion [44]. The latency time to convulsion onset following pilocarpine administration was longer, and mortality in the status epilepticus was reduced compared with the group which did not receive vitamin C or received physiological saline. This study also demonstrated that in the group receiving only vitamin C, the level of lipid peroxidation was lower than in the group that received (a) pilocarpine and (b) pilocarpine and vitamin C. In all the experimental groups, catalase activity in the hippocampus increased compared with the control group which only received physiological saline. The authors think that the neuroprotective function of vitamin C in adult rats may be due to reduced lipid peroxidation and increased catalase activity following convulsions and status epilepticus [44].

2.4. The audiogenic seizure model

Prolonged melatonin administration to rats congenitally predisposed to audiogenic convulsions (the Krushinsky-Molodkina model) had no effect on seizures evoked by a 20 times more powerful auditory stimulus [45]. VPA administration significantly reduced convulsions, but VPA and melatonin combination had a significantly larger anti-seizure effect—it lengthened the latency time and reduced seizure severity. However, the rats receiving the combined treatment displayed a much more rapid onset of myclonia than the rats receiving either VPA or melatonin [45].

3. Counteracting AED-evoked oxygen stress

3.1. AEDs in animal models of epileptic seizures

Researchers using animal models have found a variety of effects of AEDs, administered in various doses, on oxidant and antioxidant processes in an astrocyte culture in rats [46]. Here is a selected list of studied variables: LDH and GS levels, RFT production, lipid peroxidation, and DNA fragmentation. Drugs such as CBZ, TPM, and OXC caused oxygen stress whatever their dose. GBP, LEV, LTG, and TGB, on the other hand, caused no significant metabolic changes whether given in large or small doses. Cortical astrocytes seem to tolerate this latter group of AEDs better than the former group.

In a similar model of rat cortical cell culture, VPA was found to protect against the negative effects of oxygen stress [47]. Administration of VPA for 7 days prevented lipid and protein oxidization anomalies. The authors think that by preventing the accumulation of free radicals, VPA affects one or more of the neuroprotective processes.

VPA is a relatively safe drug, but it can sometimes be related to allergic idiosyncratic hepatopathy, a rare condition but more frequent in children less than 2 years of age taking more than one type of AED. The mechanism of toxic hepatopathy is unknown, but it has been suggested that it is caused by oxygen stress which leads to excessive RFT production and reduction of total antioxidant capacity [48, 49]. Therefore, therapeutic strategies or specific medicines that reduce oxygen stress may protect against toxic hepatopathy in patients taking VPA. Sabayan et al. [49] have hypothesized that garlic (allium) preparations may prevent this liver damage by removing free radicals and preventing the reduction of glutathione activity which accompanies the treatment with VPA.

TPM with its many mechanisms of action has undoubted effectiveness in the treatment of epilepsy in children. However, TPM administered in rat stomachs for 3 months may lead to such adverse effects as toxic liver dysfunction [50]. In a study of young rats, it was found that small doses of TPM (40 mg/kg a day) might reduce total antioxidant capacity in the organism and lead to a minor liver pathology. Large doses of TPM (80 mg/kg a day) or a combination of TPM (40 mg/kg) and VPA (300 mg/kg a day) significantly increased the risk of such adverse effects. Glutathione levels in the liver were significantly lower in the rats given large doses of TPM and in the rats on the TPM + VPA regime than that in the rats taking small doses of TPM and the controls given only distilled water. Histopathological examination also revealed disseminated punctual necrosis as well as lipid and degenerative changes in some hepatocytes.

In this same model, TPM (40 and 80 mg/kg i.p.) had no effect either on rats' status epilepticus or mortality, but larger doses significantly reduced KA-evoked lipid peroxidation [51].

LEV (2000 mg/kg i.p.) administered prior to pilocarpine administration (400 mg/kg s.c.) in mice prevented peroxidation increase in the hippocampus (but did not increase the nitrate level or reduce catalase activity in the hippocampus or cortical glutation) [52]. Perhaps the anti-oxidizing, neuroprotective effect of LEV and the consequent reduction of oxygen stress can be attributed to a different mechanism than the one which is active in the case of other AEDs.

In the KA convulsion model in rats, pre-convulsion administration of zonisamide led to an increased antioxidant level in the hippocampus [53]. The authors think that zonisamide has neuroprotective properties against free radicals.

LTG does not lead to detectable increases in lipid peroxydation in rats in vivo [54]. The antiepileptic effectiveness of LTG in the partial complex epilepsy model (stimulation of the dentate gyrus) in rats was in reverse proportion to the level of activity of nitrogen oxide [55].

3.2. AEDs in human epilepsy

When used in human epilepsy, AEDs have various but equivocal effects on the oxidization processes [7, 22]. The authors studied the effects of epilepsy and prolonged AED treatment (CBZ, PHT, and VPA) on the levels of trace elements, electrolytes, and oxidization and anti-oxidization activity in the blood serum in 70 patients with epilepsy and 14 untreated patients with epilepsy (controls) [7, 22]. They found increased Zn, Ca, Na, MDA, and GSH-Px and reduced copper, ceruloplasmin, and total antioxidant capacity in the treated patients (especially in those treated with VPA); treatment had no effect on the levels of Se, Mg, and K. In the untreated patients with epilepsy, uric acid (a powerful free oxygen radical scavenger) was elevated but the total antioxidant capacity in the serum was reduced, suggesting that different antioxidants had different activities in this epileptic group.

According to these authors, some nutrients may have a positive effect on the reduction of seizure frequency (vitamin B_6, vitamin E, Mg, Mn, taurine, glycine, omega-3 fatty acids; vitamin B_1 may improve cognitive functioning in patients with epilepsy).

In order to prevent the negative effects of LPP, prophylactic or therapeutic replenishment of folic acid, vitamin B_6, vitamin D, and L-carnitine may be advisable. Vitamin K is recommended toward the end of pregnancy in women taking AEDs. In some cases melatonin may reduce seizure frequency. However, supplementation can very seldom substitute AEDs completely [56].

Mahle and Dasgupta [1] found that PHT monotherapy significantly increased lipid hydroperoxidase in blood serum concentration compared with the control group. The total blood serum antioxidant capacity was lower in patients than in healthy controls. These researchers found a weak correlation between lipid hydroperoxidase concentrations, trygliceridemia, and cholesterol level in the serum of patients with epilepsy.

The negative consequences of oxygen stress in the serum were significantly larger in women with epilepsy treated with PHT monotherapy than in healthy women and women with untreated epilepsy [57]. According to the authors, as an addition to glutathione to PHT treatment, modification of the activity of CuZn-SOD enzymes and reduction of copper absorption during pregnancy may prevent the incidence of the aforementioned, albeit somewhat controversial, fetal phenytoin syndrome [58]. PHT is very rarely administered to patients with epilepsy in Poland (1–2%) and probably only exceptionally to epileptic women in reproductive (childbearing) age.

Comparative studies of the effects of PHT and CBZ monotherapies found a significant increase in the blood serum level of MDA and CuZn-SOD and a significant reduction of glutathione in patients treated with PHT compared with a healthy control group and a group with untreated epilepsy [59]. No differences were found for CBZ except for a slight increase in CuZn-SOD activity. All in all compared with PTH, CBZ caused fewer interferences with antioxidant activity, lipid peroxidation, and level of trace elements (Cu, Zn).

VPA used in monotherapy for 60 days in 50 children with epilepsy (mean age 8.5 ± 3.6 years) led to liver dysfunction, free radical production, and DNA oxidation injury in the liver cells and neurons. The general oxidation state, measured by the level of 8-hydroxy-2-deoxyguanosine (8-OHdG), depended on the drug dose [60]. A linear relation was found between the VPA serum level and the lipid peroxidation magnitude. In a group of children with a VPA concentration 114 ± 9.7 µg/ml, peroxidation was significantly higher than in a control group of children with a VPA concentration 81.0 ± 8 µg/ml. Free radicals caused DNA oxygen injury due to a significant increase in the serum level of 8-OHdG, which may be a good biological indicator of increased risk of VPA-evoked degeneration.

Other researchers have also found a linear relation between lipid peroxidation and the VPA level in the plasmas of patients with epilepsy [4]. They measured lipid peroxidation spectrofluorometrically, before and after Fenton reaction evocation, in 75 patients and 4 healthy controls. Interestingly, lipid peroxidation was higher in patients with partial epilepsy than in patients with generalized epilepsy and higher in women than men. Gender differences in oxygen stress effects have also been found in PHT-treated patients with epilepsy [57], PTZ rat models [35], and hippocampal sections in patients [61].

A comparative study of the effect of 2-year VPA and CBZ monotherapies on changes in the antioxidant system in children with epilepsy found significant differences in the effects of both AEDs [62]. The researchers measured the level of glutation, GSH-Px, red blood cell SOD, and serum lipid peroxidation. They studied two groups: (1) 25 healthy children and (2) 27 children with epilepsy untreated prior to the study onset, 14 of whom were treated with VPA and 13 with CBZ. The treatment lasted 2 years. Laboratory tests were conducted in treatment months 13 and 24. The antioxidant systems in the children taking VPA for 2 years were more altered than the antioxidant systems of the children taking CBZ.

Another comparative study of the effects of CBZ and VPA on epileptic children found no differences in the serum concentrations of Cu, Zn, Mn, Se, and Mg [24]. The only difference was found for the GSH-Px activity which was significantly higher in the VPA group. There were no differences in the SOD levels.

A more recent comparative study of the effect of VPA, CBZ, and PB monotherapies on the oxidation and anti-oxidation systems in children with epilepsy yielded slightly different results [6]. The control groups consisted of children with untreated epilepsy and healthy children. The researchers found that the level of total antioxidant capacity in the serum was significantly reduced in the group with untreated epilepsy compared with the healthy group. The level of peroxidation was significantly elevated in both the untreated group with epilepsy and the CBZ treatment group compared with the healthy controls. The pattern of results was similar for the children treated with PB and for the control group. According to the authors, children with epilepsy are at risk of oxygen stress due to seizures and AEDs. Their oxidation and anti-oxidation processes are unbalanced. VPA restores this balance more effectively than CBZ or PB.

Bolayir et al. [63] studied the effect of OXC on anti-oxidation processes in 13 adult patients with epilepsy prior to monotherapy and after 1 year of monotherapy. They also studied 15 healthy controls. They measured lipid peroxidation activity, SOD, GSH-Px, and catalase in the red blood cells. The patients had significant differences in the levels of GSH-Px and SOD after 1 year of treatment compared with the pre-treatment levels. The MDA level was also significantly different from the level of the control group and from that assessed before the treatment. These findings suggest that the anti-oxidation systems in patients treated with OXC are negatively affected after 1 year of treatment.

3.3. Dietary management in epilepsy

The idea that a specific way of eating can affect epilepsy was (recognized) first postulated by Hippocrates, who noticed that fasting could prevent convulsions [64]. All forms of dietary therapy that can be used for epilepsy involve ketogenic [65–68] medium-chain triglyceride, modified Atkins, and low-glycemic index diets that restrict carbohydrates and increase fat in the diet. However, most of these metabolic treatments for epilepsy can cause some side effects and nutritional deficiencies such as diarrhea, constipation, nausea, vomiting, and increased acid reflux. There is growing interest in ketogenic diet and it is available in many countries. The reasons why ketogenic diet prevents seizure are not fully understood. One hypothesis is that the ketones produced by the diet are able to enter the brain and reduce the levels of reactive oxygen species and make the brain use energy more efficiently, resulting in fewer seizures [69, 70]. It has been shown that ketogenic diet can produce a significant reduction in seizure frequency in the elderly as well [66, 71, 72].

3.4. Vitamins and minerals

Long-term use of antiepileptic drugs can affect the vitamin and mineral status in epilepsy patients. Antiepileptic drugs have been shown to decrease the levels of the B group vitamins such as folate and vitamins B_6 and B_{12} [73, 74], which are important for controlling the metabolism. For example, the low folate levels caused by AEDs lead to high levels of homocysteine, a risk factor for heart disease [74–76]. Epileptic patients have reduced folic acid levels due to the use of AEDs [77]. It has been reported that epileptic patient using AEDs should be supplemented with B vitamins, especially with the metabolically active form of folic acid, L-methylfolate, to reduce the homocysteine levels [78].

Significantly lower levels of vitamin D are found in the blood of patients taking antiepileptic drugs. The explanation is that the use of AEDs increases the liver enzyme activity of cytochrome P450, which is involved in breaking down of vitamin D [79–83]. Therefore, patients who are taking AEDs may need to take vitamin D and calcium supplements [84].

Pyridoxine-dependent epilepsy is a rare autosomal recessive disorder characterized by a combination of various seizure types that usually occurs during the first hours of life and is unresponsive to standard anticonvulsants, responding only to immediate administration of pyridoxine hydrochloride (vitamin B_6) [85–87]. However, not all types of seizures can be treated with pyridoxine, but a potentially effective option is the biologically active form of vitamin B_6 (pyridoxal-5-phosphate) [88–90].

Other antioxidants that have been reported to have the capacity to mitigate mitochondrial oxidative stress in the brain and lower seizure frequency in epilepsy include vitamin E, vitamin C, and selenium [91–97]. Vitamin E is shown to prevent several types of seizures in animal models [98, 99]. Epileptics are also more likely to have low vitamin E levels, though this may be a result of taking antiepileptic drugs [100].

Magnesium is essential for enzyme function including ATP-generating reactions [101]. It stimulates the production of prostacyclin and nitric oxide [102], supports mitochondrial integrity, and modulates ion transport [103, 104]. Magnesium has been shown to be associated with many health conditions; for example, it is essential for brain function and development [105, 106]. Epileptics have significantly lowered serum magnesium levels, and the seizure activity correlates with the level of hypomagnesemia [107–109].

3.5. Melatonin

Numerous studies on melatonin conducted over the last 30 years have confirmed that this neurohormone is susceptible to circadian rhythms, has antioxidant properties, and modulates immunological activity [110]. Melatonin affects the blood platelets and prolongs their life. It is transported by platelets to all body tissues. Thanks to its lipophilic function, it crosses the cell membranes easily, regulates blood-tissue exchange, and interacts with the endothelial cells. Platelets can behave like mobile and wandering serotonergic and/or melatonergic elements, comparable with cerebral neurotransmitter release [111].

Melatonin was found to be a potent free radical scavenger, and therefore it reduces oxygen stress and prevents excessive arousal from injured neurons as demonstrated with various animal models and humans.

The neuroprotective effect of melatonin was confirmed in a randomized, double-blind trial with epileptic children receiving VPA monotherapy [112]. The researchers administered VPA + melatonin to 15 children and VPA + placebo to 14 children for 14 days. The posttest GSS-R level was significantly higher (p = 0.05) in the VPA + melatonin group, and the percentile difference in the value of this enzyme was also significant (p = 0.005).

Gupta et al. [113] found that CBZ and VPA administered in monotherapy to 22 children with epilepsy had differential effects on the blood serum levels of melatonin. In both groups the researchers measured endogenous and exogenous melatonin 30 min after administration. The serum level of melatonin was higher in the CBZ group (165 pg/ml ± 50–350) than in the VPA group (78 pg/ml ± 13–260). The authors think that these differences in the level of melatonin can be attributed to different effects of these two AEDs, additional epilepsy and CBZ-dependent RFT increase, or differences in melatonin kinetics in conditions of oxygen stress. In a study by the present author [29], adding melatonin to the patients' regular AED for several weeks did not affect seizure frequency in cases in which the course of the epilepsy was severe.

3.6. Selenium

The neuroprotective effect of selenium, one of the trace elements, is related to selenoproteins which are antioxidants [114]. Selenium insufficiency has been found in young children with severe mental retardation and drug-resistant epilepsy [115]. Oral administration of selenium (3–5 µg/kg m.c.) reduced seizure frequency, improved EEG recordings, and normalized liver activity. In another study, the serum level of selenium in 30 patients with intractable epilepsy was also lower (66.88 ng/ml ± 17.58) than in healthy controls matched for age, socioeconomic status, and place of residence (85.93 ng/ml ± 13.93) (p < 0.05) [116]. However, the low selenium level in the blood serum did not correlate with the measured risk factors for drug-resistant epilepsy: age of onset, infant seizures, neurological disorder, or etiology of epilepsy.

The clinical implications of these results, and those quoted above, should be interpreted carefully because epilepsy is such a complex and heterogeneous disease, as suggested by the findings reviewed in this article.

3.7. Drug-resistant epilepsy: polytherapy

Drug-resistant seizures force the physician to use polytherapy with various AEDs. Polytherapy increases the production of free radicals and disturbs mineral balance to a greater extent than monotherapy, leading to increased oxygen stress. Both increased free radical production and inhibition of the enzymes that remove scavengers lead to adverse states and aggravation of the morbid process [22, 117].

Patients with epilepsy and on long-term AED therapy are at greater risk of atherosclerotic changes in the arteries [118]. Metabolic dysfunctions in these patients have been attributed to altered homocysteine, lipid and lipoprotein metabolism, and uric acid. According to the authors, these dysfunctions are indications for routine antioxidant multivitamin supplementation (folic acid, B_{12}, B_6, C and E, and beta-carotene). The protective, anti-atheromatic effect of vitamins is based on their antioxidant and anti-inflammatory properties. However, in the other research quoted above, increased lipid hydroperoxidase concentration had only weak correlations with the risk factors for vascular changes (triglyceridemia, cholesterolemia) [1].

Tupeev et al. [119] found a positive effect of prolonged vitamin E treatment (600 mg/day) in patients with generalized seizures: seizure frequency was reduced, EEG improved, and antioxidant activity increased.

Assuming that AEDs can trigger free radical production and lipid peroxydation, Hung-Ming et al. [23] studied the effects of TW970, a modified version of the Chinese herbal specific *chaihu-longu-muli-tang* which has antiepileptic and antioxidant properties. They administered it for 4 months to 3 groups of patients: (1) 20 patients with drug-resistant epilepsy (at least 4 attacks a month), (2) 20 patients with mild epilepsy (fewer than 4 attacks a month), and (3) a control group of 20 healthy adults matched for age. The patients were tested prior to the introduction of TW970 and 4 months after the introduction. In the resistant group, seizure frequency dropped from 13.4 ± 3.4 to 10.7 ± 2.5 a month, but the difference was not significant (p = 0.084). Prior to the TW970 introduction, the resistant epilepsy group had significantly higher lipid peroxidation and increased MDA and CuZn-SOD activity, including reduced glutathione, compared with the healthy control group. After 4 months of TW970 treatment, the levels of MDA and CuZn-SOD normalized in the resistant epilepsy group, whereas no significant changes in the parameters were found in the mild epilepsy group, either prior to or following TW970 therapy. The authors suggest that TW970 may reduce seizure frequency in resistant epilepsy and that antioxidants may be responsible for this effect.

Many Native American plants are valued by local medical practitioners for their positive effects on health and a number of diseases, including epilepsy: *Celastrus paniculatus* L. (CP), *Picrorhiza kurroa* (PK), and *Withania somnifera* L. (WS). It has been found that extracts of these plants are dose-dependent free radical scavengers and that they prevent DNA injury due to oxygen stress. PK extract had a more powerful effect than CP or WS. These favorable biological properties have been attributed to anti-stress, immune-modulating, anti-inflammatory, and antiaging effects [120].

3.8. The effects of surgery on AED-resistant temporal lobe epilepsy

López et al. [121] studied the activity of antioxidant enzymes (SOD, catalase, and GSH-Px) and markers of oxygen stress-induced molecular neuronal injury (MDA and RFT) before and at various moments after epileptic focus resection in 9 patients and a control group of 32 healthy individuals. All the studied variables normalized postoperatively except the SOD activity. Several other interesting observations seem to be somewhat related to these findings. Turkdogan et al. [122] found that increased lipid peroxidation in the plasma may be causally related to the presence of abnormal structural changes of the brain, as assessed by magnetic resonance (MR) rather than to the treatment of epilepsy, focal or generalized epileptic discharges in the EEG, duration of epilepsy, or to seizure frequency (more or fewer than 1 seizure a month). The authors found an increase in serum lipid peroxidation in 52 children with epilepsy, treated with one or more AEDs and with an abnormal brain MR, compared with 16 healthy children (the difference was significant, $p < 0.05$). No significant differences in antioxidant enzymes were found in either group. The children with well-controlled seizures and the ones with drug-resistant seizures but normal MRs had higher SOD activity than the children in the control group ($p < 0.05$). GSH-Px (an antioxidant) activity was not significantly different among the children with epilepsy and the control group [123]. This interesting and heterogeneous picture of enzymatic activity in children with epilepsy and control children suggests that the relations between various laboratory tests and numerous variables associated with the heterogeneity and treatment of epilepsy are very complex. Although the authors took seizure frequency into consideration, they did not specify when the blood tests were taken relative to the experienced or imminent seizure nor did they report EEG recording of epileptic activity prior to the blood test. This makes it very difficult to interpret the causal relations among the results of the various tests and their epileptic correlates.

4. Conclusions

Epilepsy is a brain disease that has been linked with abnormal brain oxidation processes. Despite a vast spectrum of anticonvulsant therapies toward halting abnormal electrical activity in the brain, it may be suggested that antioxidants can perhaps in the future play a role in controlling seizures. Therefore, further study is necessary, in order to display whether widely accessible antioxidants such as vitamin C or vitamin E in fact possess the ability to synergistically act with anticonvulsant medications and whether this combination can result in improved control of epilepsy.

1. Research on animal models and patients with epilepsy suggests that both epileptic seizures and AEDs (especially polytherapy), as well as other factors evoking oxygen stress, have a negative effect on the oxidation-anti-oxidation balance.

2. AEDs and drug dosage have a differential effect on oxygen stress. The research findings are equivocal or even contradictory, however, with respect to the different AEDs. New AEDs usually have a more favorable effect on the oxidation and anti-oxidation enzyme balance and trace element and electrolytic homeostasis.

3. Neuroprotectors (trace elements, vitamins, and other antioxidants) help to reduce seizure-induced oxygen stress, and therefore it is suggested that they should be used to supplement AED treatment.

4. The fact that AEDs can lead to oxidation-anti-oxidation imbalance suggests that we need to adopt a new approach to the treatment of epilepsy and AED synthesis. We need to take the negative effects of oxygen stress into consideration.

5. No drug is completely safe and effective, and considering the complex and heterogeneous nature of epilepsy, it is evident that the optimal treatment of each individual case requires a carefully performed diagnosis and the application of research-based therapy, which includes the use of personalized medicine as well as drugs. Genes are influenced by the environment and therapy. The value of food as medicine was acknowledged several centuries ago. Therefore, monitoring genomic information, pharmacogenomics, and the food-drug interactions is important as it helps to personalize the treatment to meet the patient's needs.

6. It is important to know the patient's specific characteristics including previous history, lifestyle, age, gender, weight, diet, environment, etc. They can be valuable tools to improve the quality of life of the epileptic. Targeted medicine/personalized medicine is the concept of managing the patients' health. It is believed that Hippocrates (c. 460 BC–c. 370 BC) was the one who applied this idea to medicine. He is best remembered today for his famous Oath "It's far more important to know what person the disease has than what disease the person has."

Author details

Jerzy Majkowski[1]*, Tuomas Westermarck[2] and Faik Atroshi[3]†

*Address all correspondence to: fundacja@epilepsy.pl

1 Epilepsy Diagnostic and Treatment Centre, Foundation of Epileptology, Warsaw, Poland

2 Rinnekoti Research Centre, Espoo, Finland

3 Department of Pharmacology and Toxicology, University of Helsinki, Finland

†Deceased.

References

[1] Mahle C, Dasgupta A. Decreased total antioxidant capacity and elevated lipid hydroperoxide concentrations in sera of epileptic patients receiving phenytoin. Life Sciences. 1997;**61**:437-443

[2] Sies H. Oxidative Stress. New York: Academic Press; 1985

[3] Bartosz G. Druga twarz tlenu. Warszawa: Wyd. Nauk. PWN, wyd. III; 2006

[4] Martinez-Bellesteros C, Pita-Calandre E, Sanchez-Gonzalez Y. Lipid peroxidation in adult epileptic patients treated with valproic acid. Revista de Neurología. 2004;**38**:101-106

[5] Niketic V, Ristic S, Saicic ZS. Activities of antioxidant enzymes and formation of the glutathione adduct of hemoglobin (Hb ASSG) in epileptic patients with long-term anti-epileptic therapy. Farmaco. 1995;**50**:811-813

[6] Avcicek A, Iscan A. The effects of carbamazepine, valproic acid and phenobarbital on the oxidative balance in epileptic children. European Neurology. 2007;**57**:65-69

[7] Hamed SA, Abdellah MM. Trace elements and electrolytes homeostasis and their relation to antioxidant enzyme cavity in brain hyperexcitability of epileptic patients. Journal of Pharmacological Sciences. 2004;**96**:349-359

[8] Sobaniec W, Sołowiej E, Kułak W. Evaluation of the influence of antiepileptic therapy on antioxidant enzyme activity and lipid peroxidation in erythrocytes of children with epilepsy. Journal of Child Neurology. 2006;**21**:558-562

[9] Wilson JX. Antioxidant defense of the brain: A role for astrocytes. Canadian Journal of Physiology and Pharmacology. 1997;**75**:1149-1163

[10] Anlasik T, Sies H, Griffiths HR. Dietary habits are major determinants of the plasma antioxidant status in healthy elderly subject. British Journal of Nutrition. 2005;**94**:639-642

[11] Frantseva MV, Perez Velazquez JL, Carlen PL. Changes in membrane and synaptic properties of thalamocortical circuitry caused by hydrogen peroxide. Journal of Neurophysiology. 1998;**80**:1317-1326

[12] Frantseva MV, Perez Velazquez JL, Tsoraklidis G. Oxidative stress is involved in seizure-induced neurodegeneration in the kindling model of epilepsy. Neuroscience. 2000;**97**:431-435

[13] Tayarani I, Chaudiere J, Lefauconnier JM, Bourre JM. Enzymatic protection against peroxidative damage in isolated brain capillaries. Journal of Neurochemistry. 1987;**48**:1399-1402

[14] Patel MN. Oxidative stress, mitochondrial dysfunction, and epilepsy. Free Radical Research. 2002;**36**:1139-1146

[15] Liang LP, Patel M. Mitochondrial oxidative stress and increased seizure susceptibility in SOD2 (-/+) mice. Free Radical Biology & Medicine. 2004;**36**:542-554

[16] Patel M. Mitochondrial dysfunction and oxidative stress: Cause and consequence of epileptic seizures. Free Radical Biology & Medicine. 2004;**37**:1951-1962

[17] Dubenko AE, Litovchenko TA. The concept of pathogenic therapy of epilepsy with medications restoring energy metabolism. Zhurnal Nevrologii i Psikhiatrii Imeni S.S. Korsakova. 2002;**102**:25-31

[18] Barros DO, Xavier SM, Barbosa CO. Effects of the vitamin E in catalase activities in hippocampus after status epilepticus induced by pilocarpine in Wistar rats. Neuroscience Letters. 2007;**416**:227-230

[19] Freitas RM, Nascimento VS, Vasconcelos SM. Catalase activity in cerebellum, hippocampus, frontal cortex and striatum after status epilepticus induced by pilocarpine in Wistar rats. Neuroscience Letters. 2004;**365**:102-105

[20] Ilhan A, Aladog MA, Kocer A. Erdosteine ameliorates PTZ-induced oxidative stress in mice seizure model. Brain Research Bulletin. 2005;**65**:495-499

[21] Sok DE, Oh SH, Kim YB. Neuroprotection by extract of *Petasites japonicus* leaves, a traditional vegetable, against oxidative stress in brain of mice challenged with kainic acid. European Journal of Nutrition. 2006;**45**:61-69

[22] Hamed SA, Abdellah MM, El-Melegu N. Blood levels of trace elements, electrolytes, and oxidative stress/antioxidant systems in epileptic patients. Journal of Pharmacological Sciences. 2004;**96**:465-473

[23] Hung-Ming W, Liu CS, Tsai JJ. Antioxidant and anticonvulsant effect of a modified formula of chaihu-longu-muli-tang. American Journal of Chinese Medicine. 2002;**30**:339-346

[24] Kurekci AE, Alpay F, Tanindi S. Plasma trace element, plasma glutathione peroxidase, and superoxide dismutase levels in epileptic children receiving antiepileptic drug therapy. Epilepsia. 1995;**36**:600-604

[25] Sudha K, Rao AV, Rao A. Oxidative stress and antioxidants in epilepsy. Clinica Chimica Acta. 2001;**303**:19-24

[26] Kawakami Y, Monobe M, Kuwabara K. A comparative study of nitric oxide, glutathione, and glutathione peroxidase activities in cerebrospinal fluid from children with convulsive diseases/children with aseptic meningitis. Brain & Development. 2006;**28**:243-246

[27] Akarsu S, Yilmaz S, Ozan S. Effects of febrile seizures on oxidant state in children. Pediatric Neurology. 2007;**36**:307-311

[28] Costello DJ, Delanty N. Oxidative injury in epilepsy: Potential for antioxidant therapy. Expert Review of Neurotherapeutics. 2004;**4**:541-553

[29] Majkowski J. Epileptogenesis—The role of oxygen stress. Epileptologia. 2007;**15**:225-240

[30] Depondt C, Godard P, Espel RS, Da Cruz AL, Lienard P, Pandolfo M. A candidate gene study of antiepileptic drug tolerability and efficacy identifies an association of CYP2C9 variants with phenytoin toxicity. European Journal of Neurology. 2011;**18**(9):1159-1164. DOI: 10.1111/j.1468-1331.2011.03361.x. Epub 2011 Feb 22

[31] Walker LE, Mirza N, Yip VL, Marson AG, Pirmohamed M. Personalized medicine approaches in epilepsy. Journal of Internal Medicine. 2015;**277**(2):218-234. DOI: 10.1111/joim.12322. Review

[32] Ackers R, Murray ML, Besag F, et al. Prioritizing children's medicines for research: A pharmacoepidemiological study of antiepileptic drugs. British Journal of Clinical Pharmacology. 2007;**63**:689-697

[33] Egunsola O, Choonara I, Sammons HM. Safety of lamotrigine in paediatrics: A systematic review. BMJ Open. 2015;**5**(6):e007711. DOI: 10.1136/bmjopen-2015-00771

[34] Oztas B, Kilic S, Dural E, Ispir T. Influence of antioxidants on the blood-brain barrier permeability during epileptic seizures. Journal of Neuroscience Research. 2001;**66**:674-678

[35] Oztas B, Akgul S, Seker FB. Gender difference in the influence of antioxidants on the blood-brain barrier permeability during pentylenetetrazol-induced seizures in hyperthermic rat pups. Biological Trace Element Research. 2007;**118**:77-83

[36] Ilhan A, Gurel A, Armatcu F. Antiepileptogenic and antioxidant effects of Nigella sativa oil against pentylenetetrazol-induced kindling in mice. Neuropharmacology. 2005;**49**:456-464

[37] Ueda Y, Yokoyama H, Niwa R. Generation of lipid radicals in the hippocampal extracellular space during kainic acid-induced seizures in rats. Epilepsy Research. 1997;**26**:329-333

[38] Bruce AJ, Baudry M. Oxygen free radicals in rat limbic structures after kainate-induced seizures. Free Radical Biology & Medicine. 1995;**18**:993-1002

[39] Mohanan PV, Yamamoto HA. Preventive, effect of melatonin against brain mitochondria DNA damage, lipid peroxidation and seizures induced by kainic acid. Toxicology Letters. 2002;**129**:99-105

[40] Gupta YK, Briyal S. Protective effect of vineatrol against kainic acid induced seizures, oxidative stress and on the expression of heat shock proteins in rats. European Neuropsychopharmacology. 2006;**16**:85-91

[41] Hsieh CL, Chiang SY, Cheng KS. Anticonvulsive and free radical scavenging activities of Gastrodia elata Bl. In kainic acid-treated rats. American Journal of Chinese Medicine. 2001;**29**:331-341

[42] Hsieh CL, Chang CH, Chiang SY. Anticonvulsive and free radical scavenging activities of vanillyl alcohol in ferric chloride-induced epileptic seizures in Sprague-Dawley rats. Life Sciences. 2000;**67**:1185-1195

[43] Tejada S, Sureda A, Roca C. Antioxidant response and oxidative damage in brain cortex after high dose of pilocarpine. Brain Research Bulletin. 2007;**71**:372-375

[44] Santos LF, Freitas RL, Xavier SM. Neuroprotective actions of vitamin C related to decreased lipid peroxidation and increased catalase activity in adult rats after pilocarpine-induced seizures. Pharmacology Biochemistry & Behavior. 2008;**89**:1-5

[45] Savina TA, Balashova OA, Shchipakina TG. Effect of chronic consumption of sodium valproate and melatonin on seizure activity in Krushinskii-Molodkina rats. Bulletin of Experimental Biology and Medicine. 2006;**142**:601-604

[46] Pavone A, Cardile V. An in vitro study of new antiepileptic drugs and astrocytes. Epilepsia. 2003;**44**(suppl 10):34-39

[47] Wang JF, Azzam JE, Young LT. Valproate inhibits oxidative damage to lipid and protein in primary cultured rat cerebrocortical cells. Neuroscience. 2003;**116**:485-489

[48] Chang TK, Abbott FS. Oxidative stress as a mechanism of valproic acid-associated hepatoxicity. Drug Metabolism Reviews. 2006;**38**:627-639

[49] Sabayan B, Foroughina F, Chohedry A. A postulated role of garlic organosulfur compounds in prevention of valproic acid hepatotoxicity. Medical Hypotheses. 2007;**68**: 512-514

[50] Huang J, Ren RN, Chen CM, Ye LY. An experimental study on hepatotoxicity of topiramate in young rats. Zhongguo Dang Dai Er Ke Za Zhi. 2007;**9**:54-58

[51] Kubera M, Budziszewska B, Jaworska-Feil L. Effect of topiramate on the kainate-induced status epilepticus, lipid peroxidation and immunoreactivity of rats. Polish Journal of Pharmacology. 2004;**56**:553-561

[52] Oliveira AA, Almeida JP, Freitas RM. Effects of levetiracetam in lipid peroxidation level, nitrite-nitrate formation and antioxidant enzymatic activity in mice brain after pilocarpine-induced seizures. Cellular and Molecular Neurobiology. 2007;**27**:395-406

[53] Ueda Y, Doi T, Tokumaru J. In vivo evaluation of the effect of zonisamide on the hippocampal redox state during kainic acid-induced seizure status in rats. Neurochemical Research. 2005;**30**:1117-1121

[54] Lu W, Uetrecht JP. Possible bioactivation pathways of lamotrigine. Drug Metabolism and Disposition. 2007;**35**:1050-1056

[55] Sardo P, Ferraro G. Modulatory effects of nitric oxide-active drugs on the anticonvulsant activity of lamotrigine in an experimental model of partial complex epilepsy in the rat. BMC Neuroscience. 2007;**3**:8-47

[56] Gaby AR. Natural approaches to epilepsy. Alternative Medicine Review. 2007;**12**(1):9-24

[57] Liu CS, Wu HM, Kao SH, Wei YH. Phenytoin-mediated oxidative stress in serum of female epileptics: A possible pathogenesis in the fetal hydantoin syndrome. Human & Experimental Toxicology. 1997;**16**:177-181

[58] Hanson JW, Smith DW. The fetal hydantoin syndrome. The Journal of Pediatrics. 1975;**87**:285-290

[59] Liu CS, Wu HM, Kao SH, Wei YH. Serum trace elements, glutathione, cooper/zinc superoxide dismutase, and lipid peroxidation in epileptic patients with phenytoin or carbamazepine monotherapy. Clinical Neuropharmacology. 1998;**21**:62-64

[60] Schulpis KH, Lazaropoulou C, Regoutas S. Valproic acid monotherapy induces DNA oxidative damage. Toxicology. 2006;**217**:228-232

[61] Li H, Pin S, Zeng Z. Sex differences in cell death. Annals of Neurology. 2005;**58**:317-321

[62] Yuksel A, Cengiz M, Seven M, Ulutin T. Changes in the antioxidant system in epileptic children receiving antiepileptic drugs: Two-year prospective studies. Journal of Child Neurology. 2001;**16**:603-606

[63] Bolayir E, Celik K, Tas A. The effects of oxcarbazepine on oxidative stress in epileptic patients. Methods and Findings in Experimental and Clinical Pharmacology. 2004;**26**:345-348

[64] Kelley SA, Hartman AL. Metabolic treatments for intractable epilepsy. Seminars in Pediatric Neurology. 2011;**18**:179-185

[65] Francois LL, Manel V, et al. Ketogenic regime as anti-epileptic treatment: Its use in 29 epileptic children. Archives de Pédiatrie. 2003;**10**(4):300-306

[66] Mady MA, Kossoff EH, et al. The ketogenic diet: Adolescents can do it, too. Epilepsia. 2003;**44**(6):847-851

[67] Sheth RD, Stafstrom CE. Intractable pediatric epilepsy: Vagal nerve stimulation and the ketogenic diet. Neurologic Clinics. 2002;**20**(4):1183-1194

[68] Stafstrom CE, Bough KJ. The ketogenic diet for the treatment of epilepsy: A challenge for nutritional neuroscientists. Nutritional Neuroscience. 2003;**6**(2):67-79

[69] Bough KJ, Rho JM. Anticonvulsant mechanisms of the ketogenic diet. Epilepsia. 2007;**48**(1):43-58

[70] Kosoff EH, Zupec-Kania BA, et al. Optimal clinical management of children receiving the ketogenic diet: Recommendations of the International Ketogenic Diet Study Group. Epilepsia. 2009;**50**(2):304-317

[71] Klein P, Janousek J, et al. Ketogenic diet treatment in adults with refractory epilepsy. Epilepsy and Behavior. 2010;**19**:575-579

[72] Mosek A, Natour H, et al. Ketogenic diet in adults with refractory epilepsy: A prospective pilot study. Seizure. 2009;**18**:30-33

[73] Linnebank M, Moskau S, et al. Antiepileptic drugs interfere with folate and vitamin B12 serum levels. Annals of Neurology. 2011;**69**:352-359

[74] Sener U, Zorlu Y, et al. Effects of common anti-epileptic drug monotherapy on serum levels of homocysteine, Vitamin B12, folic acid and Vitamin B6. Seizure. 2006;**15**:79-85

[75] Apeland T, Mansoor MA, et al. Antiepileptic drugs as independent predictors of plasma total homocysteine levels. Epilepsy Research. 2001;**47**:27-36

[76] Kurul S, Unalp A, et al. Homocysteine levels in epileptic children receiving antiepileptic drugs. Journal of Child Neurology. 2007;**22**(12):1389-1392

[77] Asadi-Pooya AA, Minzer S, Sperling M. Nutritional supplements, foods, and epilepsy: Is there a relationship? Epilepsia. 2008;**49**(11):1819-1827

[78] Morrell MJ. Folic acid and epilepsy. Epilepsy Currents. 2002;2(2):31-34

[79] Menon B, Harinarayan CV. The effect of anti-epileptic drug therapy on serum 25-hydroxyvitamin D and parameters of calcium and bone metabolism—A longitudinal study. Seizure. 2010;19:153-158

[80] Mintzer S, Boppana P, et al. Vitamin D levels and bone turnover in epilepsy patients taking carbamazepine or oxcarbazepine. Epilepsia. 2006;47(3):510-515

[81] Pack AM, Morell MJ. Epilepsy and bone health in adults. Epilepsy and Behavior. 2004;5:S024-S029

[82] Shellhaas RA, Joshi SM. Vitamin D and bone health among children with epilepsy. Pediatric Neurology. 2010;42:385-393

[83] Valsamis HA, Arora SK, et al. Antiepileptic drugs and bone metabolism. Nutrition and Metabolism. 2006;3(36)

[84] Fong CY, Mallick AA, Burren CP, et al. Evaluation and management of bone health in children with epilepsy on long-term antiepileptic drugs: United Kingdom survey of pae-diatric neurologists. European Journal of Pediatric Neurology. 2011;15(5):417-423

[85] Hunt A, Stokes J, McCrory W, Stroud H. Pyridoxine dependency: Report of a case of intractable convulsions in an infant controlled by pyridoxine. Pediatrics. 1954;13:140-143

[86] Nabbout R, Soufflet C, Plouin P, Dulac O. Pyridoxine dependent-epilepsy: A suggestive electroclinical pattern. Archives of Disease in Childhood—Fetal and Neonatal Edition. 1999;81:F125-FF12

[87] Waldinger C, Berg RB. Signs of pyridoxine dependency manifest at birth in siblings. Pediatrics. 1963;32:161-168

[88] Jiao FY, Gao DY, Takuma Y, et al. Randomized, controlled trial of high-dose intrave-nous pyridoxine in the treatment of recurrent seizures in children. Pediatric Neurology. 1997;17:54-57

[89] Tamura T, Aiso K, Johnston KE, et al. Homocysteine, folate, vitamin B-12 and vitamin B-6 in patients receiving antiepileptic drug monotherapy. Epilepsy Research. 2000;40:7-15

[90] Wang HS, Kuo MF, Chou ML, et al. Pyridoxal phosphate is better than pyridoxine for controlling idiopathic intractable epilepsy. Archives of Disease in Childhood. 2005;90:512-515

[91] Ogunmekan AO, Hwang PA. A randomized, double-blind, placebo-controlled, clinical trial of D-alpha-tocopheryl acetate (vitamin E), as add-on therapy, for epilepsy in chil-dren. Epilepsia. 1989;30(1):84-89

[92] Ogunmekan AO. Plasma vitamin E (alpha tocopherol) levels in normal children and in epileptic children with and without anticonvulsant drug therapy. Tropical and Geographical Medicine. 1985;37(2):175-177

[93]   Ogunmekan AO. Vitamin E deficiency and seizures in animals and man. The Canadian Journal of Neurological Sciences. 1979;**6**:43-45

[94]   Savaskan NE, Brauer AU, et al. Selenium deficiency increases susceptibility to glutamate-induced excitotoxicity. The FASEB Journal. 2003;**17**(1):112-114

[95]   Tamai H, Wakamiya E, Mino M, Iwakoshi M. Alphatocopherol and fatty acid levels in red blood cells in patients treated with antiepileptic drugs. Journal of Nutritional Science and Vitaminology (Tokyo). 1988;**34**:627-631

[96]   Yamamoto N, Kabuto H, et al. Alpha-tocopheryl-l-ascorbate-2-O-phosphate diester, a hydroxyl radical scavenger, prevents the occurrence of epileptic foci in a rat model of post-traumatic epilepsy. Pathophysiology. 2002;**8**(3):205-214

[97]   Zaidi SM, Banu N. Antioxidant potential of vitamins A, E and C in modulating oxidative stress in rat brain. Clinica Chimica Acta. 2004;**340**(1-2):229-233

[98]   Levy SL et al. The anticonvulsant effects of vitamin E: A further evaluation. The Canadian Journal of Neurological Sciences. 1992;**19**(2):201-203

[99]   Levy SL, Burnham WM, et al. An evaluation of the anticonvulsant effects of vitamin E. Epilepsy Research. 1990;**6**:12-17

[100] Higashi A, Tamari H, et al. Serum vitamin E concentration in patients with severe multiple handicaps treated with anticonvulsants. Pediatric Pharmacology. 1980;**1**:129-134

[101] Barbagallo M, Dominguez LJ, Galioto A, Ferlisi A, Cani C, Malfa L, et al. Role of magnesium in insulin action, diabetes and cardio-metabolic syndrome X. Molecular Aspects of Medicine. 2003;**24**:39-52

[102] Sontia B, Touyz RM. Role of magnesium in hypertension. Archives of Biochemistry and Biophysics. 2007;**458**:33-39

[103] Romani AMP. Cellular magnesium homeostasis. Archives of Biochemistry and Biophysics. 2011;**512**(1):1-23

[104] Swaminathan R. Magnesium metabolism and its disorders. Clinical Biochemist Reviews. 2003;**24**(2):47-66

[105] Abumaria N, Yin B, et al. Effects of elevation of brain magnesium on fear conditioning, fear extinction, and synaptic plasticity in the infralimbic prefrontal cortex and lateral amygdala. Journal of Neuroscience. 2011;**31**(42):14871-14881

[106] Jin J, Wu LJ, Jun J, Cheng X, Xu H, et al. The channel kinase, TRPM7, is required for early embryonic development. Proceedings of the National Academy of Sciences of the United States of America. 2012;**109**:E225-E233

[107] Benga I, Baltescu V, Tilinca R, Pavel O, Ghiran V, Muschevici D, et al. Plasma and cerebrospinal fluid concentrations of magnesium in epileptic children. Journal of the Neurological Sciences. 1985;**67**(1):29-34

[108] Gupta SK et al. Serum magnesium levels in idiopathic epilepsy. The Journal of the Association of Physicians of India. 1994;42(6):456-457

[109] Hall RCW, Joffe JR. Hypomagnesemia: Physical and psychiatric symptoms. JAMA. 1973;224(13):1749-1751

[110] Hardeland R, Pandi-Perumal SR, Cardinali DP. Melatonin. International Journal of Biochemistry & Cell Biology. 2006;38:313-316

[111] Di Bella L, Gualano L. Key aspects of melatonin physiology: Thirty years of research. Neuro Endocrinology Letters. 2006;27:425-432

[112] Gupta M, Gupta YK, Agarwal S. A randomized, double-blind, placebo controlled trial of melatonin add-on therapy in epileptic children on valproate monotherapy: Effect on glutathione peroxidase and glutathione reductase enzymes. British Journal of Clinical Pharmacology. 2004;58:542-547

[113] Gupta M, Kohli K, Gupta YK. Modulation of serum concentrations of melatonin by carbamazepine and valproate. Indian Journal of Physiology and Pharmacology. 2006;50:70-82

[114] Atroshi F, Erkki A, Westermarck T. The role of selenium in epilepsy and other neurological disorders. Epileptologia. 2007;15:211-224

[115] Ramaekers VT, Calomme M, Vanden BD, Makropoulos W. Selenium deficiency triggering interactable seizures. Neuropediatrics. 1994;25:217-223

[116] Ashrafi MR, Shabanian R, Abbaskhanian A. Selenium and intractable epilepsy: Is there any correlation? Pediatric Neurology. 2007;36:25-29

[117] Maertens P, Dyken P, Graf W. Free radicals, anticonvulsants, and the neuronal ceroid-lipofuscinoses. American Journal of Medical Genetics. 1995;57:225-228

[118] Hamed SA, Nabeshima T. The high atherosclerotic risk among epileptics: The athero-protective role of multivitamins. Journal of Pharmacological Sciences. 2005;98:340-353

[119] Tupeev IR, Kryzhanovskii GN, Nikushkin EV. The antioxidant system in the dynamic combined treatment of epilepsy patients with traditional anticonvulsant preparations and an antioxidant-alpha-tocopherol. Biulleten' Eksperimental'noĭ Biologii i Meditsiny. 1993;116:362-364

[120] Majkowski J. Epilepsy treatment and nutritional intervention. In: Atroshi F, editor. Pharmacology and Nutritional Intervention in the Treatment of Disease. Rijeka: IntechOpen; 2014. DOI: 10.5772/57484

[121] López J, González ME, Lorigados L. Oxidative stress markers in surgically treated patients with refractory epilepsy. Clinical Biochemistry. 2007;40:292-298

[122] Turkdogan D, Toplan S, Karakoc Y. Lipid peroxidation and antioxidative enzyme activities in childhood epilepsy. Journal of Child Neurology. 2002;17:673-676

[123] Groesbeck DK, Bluml RM, Kossoff EH. Long-term use of the ketogenic diet in the treatment of epilepsy. Developmental Medicine and Child Neurology. 2006;48(12):978-981

Chapter 7

Personalized Care: Prevention of Lifestyle Diseases

Tijjani Salihu Shinkafi and Shakir Ali

Additional information is available at the end of the chapter

http://dx.doi.org/10.5772/intechopen.92001

Abstract

Personalized care, which includes personalized medicine, personalized nutrition, and even personalized exercise, is a useful and a more effective method for the treatment and control of lifestyle diseases such as type 2 diabetes and cardiovascular diseases. The relationship between nutrients, diet and gene expression (commonly called as nutritional genomics or nutrigenomics) and precision or personalized medicine have received considerable attention of researchers, clinicians, drug developers, practitioners of traditional system of medicine, and regulatory agencies over the years. Many, if not all, of the common human debilitating conditions including cancer, obesity, cardiovascular diseases and diabetes are related directly or indirectly to an individual's nutritional status and its genetic make up. Understanding the interplay between diet and genes may help provide direction upon which personalized therapy can be used for the treatment and management of these catastrophic life-threatening conditions, including strategies for their prevention. In this era of human healthcare where the diagnosis of the disease and treatment of the patient are perceived to be patient-tailored, due to the differences in the genetic make-up of individuals and their lifestyle, personalized human healthcare could be the most effective method for the treatment and prevention of debilitating diseases with a high morbidity and mortality. This chapter provides an insight into the potential of individualized care in life-threatening complications.

Keywords: individualized care, precision medicine, lifestyle diseases, chronic inflammatory diseases

1. Introduction

Personalized or individualized care, which includes personalized medicine, as well as personalized nutrition and even personalized exercise, is an individual (patient)-centric, integrative, and holistic approach for the treatment and management of lifestyle diseases. Personalized

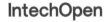

care, a term often used interchangeably with precision medicine (an essential piece of personalized care which specifically refers to the medical treatment of the patient) is a more comprehensive term (than personalized or precision medicine) that represents an overarching philosophy for patient care, taking the advantage of personalized medicine and pharmacogenomics, as well as personalized nutrition and exercise. Personalized medicine, as defined by Schleidgen et al. [1] as an emerging area of medical care seeking to improve stratification and timing of healthcare by utilizing biological information and biomarkers on the level of molecular disease pathways, genetics, proteomics, as well as metabolomics, is an essential piece of personalized care. The key issue of personalized or individualized medicine remains how a targeted therapy can be used to tackle rapidly increasing chronic health burden by maximizing therapeutic efficacy and minimizing drug toxicity risks for an individual. Since the completion of the human genome project in the year 2000, the field has continued to evolve over the years especially from pharmacogenetics to pharmacogenomics so as to effectively monitor the multigenic effect on drug response [2]. Realization of the limitation of pharmacogenetics leads to the emergence of pharmacogenomics, which determines how genes affect a person's response to drugs. This has opened up avenues for individualized identification of genetic variants using wide genome approaches through the use of latest and most recent methods, thus providing ways for determining molecular targets with the help of available DNA-based diagnostic screening tools [3].

A growing body of evidence has shown that chronic human diseases and conditions such as type 2 diabetes (T2D), cardiovascular diseases (CVD), atherosclerosis, obesity, and metabolic syndrome are associated with unhealthy lifestyle, which includes bad eating habits, physical inactivity, smoking, and exposure to stress [4]. A lifestyle modification with personalized nutrition and personalized physical activity is believed to play a central role in the prevention, management, and treatment of these life-threatening conditions [5]. Currently over 2500 genetic tests are available for the detection of diseases [6]. Ongoing efforts are being made to determine genetic risk of individuals to some of these diet-related conditions, like T2D and obesity, through available testing and screening methods so as to minimize the public health burden [7, 8]. Newer methods involving nanodiagnostic tools such as the DNA-based bionanosensors have recently emerged and are presumed to be safe and cost-effective with high specificity for early detection of the disease [9]. There is a vital need to educate the patients by the physicians and healthcare workers including the dietitians on the benefits of a well-balanced diet since failure to meet the nutritional requirements results in an array of conditions that occur due to the deficiency of certain nutrients. For example, the deficiencies of vitamins and minerals such as zinc, selenium, magnesium, chromium, and iron deficiencies have been reported in conditions like diabetes [10] and cystic fibrosis [11], especially among children. More recently, boron is getting recognition as an important trace element that may contribute significantly by mitigating the harmful effects in at least some of these diseases by augmenting the innate immune response and other mechanisms, such as stabilizing the complex membrane and macromolecular structures. Nutrient, especially the micronutrient deficiencies in early childhood or at a later stage may result in great economic burden that can lower a country's GDP [12]. Individualized nutrition and personalized care have the potential of a positive impact on the healthcare sector with certain changes in the system [13]. Some of the required changes may involve largely policy issues and healthcare infrastructural changes [14], as well as economic changes [15, 16] to lower the cost of medication.

2. Lifestyle diseases

Lifestyle factors such as bad eating habits, sedentary lifestyle, high-calorie diet and excessive alcohol intake increase the rate at which some or most chronic human diseases develop. Most of these diseases, which include cancer, diabetes and atherosclerosis, are a leading cause of death and pose great health and economic burden to the country [17]. Prevalence of diabetes, in particular, continues to increase in the world. Diabetes is projected to be the seventh leading cause of death by the year 2030 [18]. Lifestyle changes such as personalized exercise (physical activity), personalized diet (nutrigenomics), and relaxation techniques (meditation and yoga) can help prevent or at least minimize the occurrence, as well as the prevalence, of these diseases [4].

Lifestyle changes and somewhat drug intervention have profound effect on the development and progression of chronic human diseases, including the disease progress, for example, from the prediabetes stage to diabetes, or even diabetes-associated complications. However, it is not clear who may or may not respond appropriately to a particular therapy. This is because individuals are different. Lifestyle changes like healthy eating and physical activity can do a lot of wonder in preventing chronic diseases when coupled with individual awareness to disease through genetic risk testing and other methods. Personalized or individualized nutrition holds great promise in the future and can be used to identify associations between genes, nutrients, and a disease so as to improve public health [19].

3. Diet-related chronic conditions

3.1. Diet and physical activity

Diet and (lack of) physical activity constitute some of the major contributory factors for the development of chronic illnesses, both noncommunicable and communicable, directly impacting the immune system of the body and metabolism. Diseases like tuberculosis fail to develop if an individual's lifestyle is healthy with respect to diet and physical activity. In diet-related complications such as obesity and T2D, a complex interplay of several factors including both genetic predisposition and lifestyle of an individual has been reported [5, 19]. These factors can have serious devastating effects on health, as the appearance of one disease may increase the chance for another disease; for example, obesity alone may lead to an increase in T2D and CVD [20].

Diet-related diseases are generally chronic in nature and are often associated with age and type of diet (nutrition) [21]. Personalizing diet, i.e., increasing the nutritional quality of diet and genotyping (nutrigenomics), leads to achieving a better health [22]. Earlier, global guidelines on food, certain food groups, and other nutrient requirements of the population were recommended with the overall view of preventing or delaying the onset of diet-related diseases. Nowadays, with an increased understanding of genetic differences pertaining to nutritional requirements among individuals, scientists are making efforts to categorize these guidelines based on inter-individual variation in dietary response resulting in a personalized diet, thus preventing chronic diet-related conditions [21]. Over the years, a number of clinicians and researchers have tried to demonstrate the importance of dietary modifications to achieve healthy and sustainable weight loss among overweight and obese individuals. However, these attempts could not yield positive results because of different metabolic roles of macromolecules such as the lipid, protein and carbohydrate in energy homeostasis and differences in metabolism. These molecules have a great effect on metabolism, appetite, and thermogenesis, which support the idea of considering the fuel value provided by each macromolecule separately. At times, even when considered separately, nature and kind of food constituents matter. For example, a diet which can reduce the risk of T2D and CVD is important for people who already have the disease. In this case, a fiber-rich or nonstarch polysaccharide diet, like whole grain, legumes, fruits and vegetables, is the most appropriate diet.

A sedentary lifestyle equally contributes to lifestyle diseases. It has been identified as a link between obesity, diabetes, metabolic syndrome, CVD, and death [23]. Physical inactivity is widely believed to be the primary cause of most preventable chronic conditions including diabetes, obesity and CVD. Therefore, physical activity may delay or prevent these and other chronic conditions [24]. Weight loss is recognized as one of the baseline strategies employed to deal with chronic inflammatory diseases like diabetes and CVD [25]. Obese individuals are overweight and prone to develop chronic inflammatory diseases. A holistic approach focusing on changes in lifestyle including changes in diet to suit individual's needs, and physical activity, together with compatible precision medicine and ridding of the bad habits is bound to have beneficial effect on the management and prevention of life-threatening diseases and associated complications.

3.2. Type 2 diabetes

Individuals with type 2 diabetes are often faced with insulin resistance (IR) challenge arising from an accumulation of triglycerides in adipose tissues. Studies have shown that weight loss can bring significant improvement in IR both in T2D and in those with impaired glucose tolerance [26]. Nonetheless, there is an array of inter-individual variations with regard to improvement in insulin sensitivity and glycemia because of the individual response to changes in lifestyle factors such as the weight, diet and physical activity [5].

Increasing evidence has shown that single-nucleotide polymorphisms (SNPs) exist in diabetes [27, 28], which gives a lot of scope for the treatment based on genetic characteristics of an individual. These genetic differences are considered as markers of diabetes risk as they can be used to predict the disease and also to determine diabetes onset [29]. Nearly 80 genetic loci are thought to influence genetic susceptibility to both types of diabetes. An integral part of diabetes management and self-management education, medical nutrition therapy (MNT), was designed to provide patients with specific care as well as guidelines on lifestyle changes an individual can make and maintain in order to improve health [30]. Once individuals' basic nutritional requirements have been achieved, chances of developing disease are rare even for diabetics where nutrient supplementation may be an issue of concern [31].

3.3. Obesity

Management of obesity consists of the ability to lose weight either through exercise or personalized nutrition (non-pharmacological), or may involve the use of drugs. Due to individual genetic makeup and myriad of environmental factors, different individuals respond differently to exercise; some may even show resistance [32, 33]. Personalized exercise may help prevent unwanted individual response. In addition, identification of specific polymorphisms such as obesity-related SNPs may help find differences in dietary response to caloric restriction. Personalized nutrition is, therefore, expected to play a role in determining the kind and nature of diet suitable for different individuals owing to the environmental and genetic differences. Many of the diet-associated health burdens have been linked to SNPs, which is used to predict individual response to drugs in a population [34]. The most common examples of these polymorphisms are leptin/leptin receptor polymorphism (related to obesity gene), apolipoprotein (E and A1), which is related to CVD, and methylenetetrahydrofolate reductase (MTHR) related to folate metabolism [35].

3.4. Cardiovascular diseases

Cardiovascular diseases (CVDs) are a group of metabolic diseases arising from atherosclerosis [36]. CVDs account for the most common cause of morbidity and mortality in the world [36], with poorly controlled diabetes as one of the promoting factors. Newer technologies involving large-scale genotyping and sequencing have allowed for identification of heritable CVD risks which can be used in personalized treatment. Epigenetics and personalized attempts are increasingly proving beneficial and providing a new way to treat CVDs [37]. In the near future, it is hoped that the DNA sequence variants associated with CVD or which show association with the beneficial or adverse effects of medication and used to predict CVD risk may be identified and guide the decision of choosing the best medication and dose to individual patients.

3.5. Cancer

Much of the successful personalized treatments have been recorded in the area of oncology with many tumors and cancers being targeted with individualized regimens. Today, the world is witnessing a rapid progress in the upcoming field of personalized medicine with the emergence of genotyping industry for screening/testing, leading to an increased use of of precision medicines for cancer therapy. Many of these drugs are already available in the market and include kinase inhibitors [38]. Imatinib, lapatinib and erlotinib are some selective kinase inhibitors which are used to target anaplastic lymphoma [38].

3.6. Oral health and related diseases

Genomic information is increasing our understanding of oral health by providing an understanding of the disease etiology, thereby allowing easier diagnostic and a chance to take preventive measures to avoid the onset of oral diseases [39]. This is possible when genome analysis and disease risk assessment is started at childhood, as it gives room for proper planning for individualized prevention and monitoring strategies. By doing so, oral health and related problems like dental caries, periodontitis, and oral cancers may be detected at the onset and treated.

3.7. Osteoporosis

Osteoporosis is a complicated preventable syndrome that affects millions of peoples, especially women, in the world. Several personalized medicine intervention procedures are being investigated to identify the individuals with a high tendency to the disease. For instance, FRAX(R) is an algorithm that enables physicians to calculate the tendency for an individual patient risk for osteoporosis for 10 years, as well as helps in the selection of appropriate drug taking into consideration the choice of the patient [40]. Prognosis, treatment, and prevention of fractures would be easier when gene variants associated with osteoporosis are identified, leading to a more personalized approach/therapy [41].

4. Conclusion

Personalized care is at the verge of a revolution in healthcare sector, with potential to revolutionize the treatment, care and prevention of a number of debilitating life threatening diseases, some of which have been discussed in this chapter (**Figure 1**). When fully implemented, the treatment of patients can be individualized in strict accordance with their individual genetic make-up, rather than traditional "one-size-fits-all" pharmacology. A person's lifestyle, which decides the overall well-being of an individual, is crucial while implementing the approach

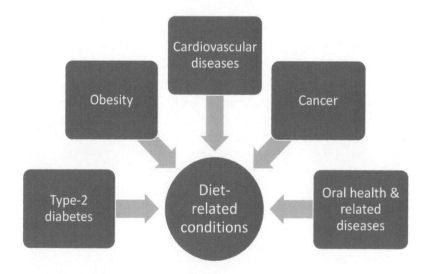

Figure 1. Diet-related conditions where personalized care can revolutionize the treatment, control and prevention of lifestyle diseases in human.

of personalized care of patients suffering from long-term lifestyle debilitating and morbid diseases through individualized nutrition, personal hygiene/oral health, and individualized needs that may be combined with relaxation techniques, such as meditation and yoga.

Acknowledgements

TSS has been a recipient of the India Council for Cultural Relations (ICCR) scholarship award and acknowledges ICCR for providing fellowship to pursue PhD under the supervision of SA.

Author details

Tijjani Salihu Shinkafi[1,2] and Shakir Ali[1]*

*Address all correspondence to: sali@jamiahamdard.ac.in

1 Department of Biochemistry, School of Chemical and Life Sciences, New Delhi, India

2 Department of Biochemistry, Faculty of Science, Usmanu Danfodiyo University Sokoto, Nigeria

References

[1] Schleidgen S, Klingler C, Bertram T, Rogowski WH, Marckmann G. What is personalized medicine: Sharpening a vague term based on a systematic literature review. BMC Medical Ethics. 2013;**14**:55

[2] Zaza G, Granata S, Mangino M, Grandaliano G, Schena FP. From, pharmacogenetics to pharmacogenomics: The start of a new era of personalized medicine in nephrology. Giornale Italiano di Nefrologia. 2010;**27**:353-366

[3] Vizirianakis IS. Challenges in current drug delivery from the potential application of pharmacogenomics and personalized medicine in clinical practice. Current Drug Delivery. 2004;**1**:73-80

[4] Minich DM, Bland JS. Personalized lifestyle medicine: Relevance for nutrition and lifestyle recommendations. Scientific World Journal. 2013;**2013**:129841

[5] Walker CG, Solis-Trapala I, Holzapfel C, Ambrosini GL, Fuller NR, et al. Modelling the interplay between lifestyle factors and genetic predisposition on markers of type 2 diabetes mellitus risk. PLoS One. 2015;**10**:e0131681

[6] Bray MS, Loos RJ, McCaffery JM, Ling C, Franks PW, et al. NIH working group report—Using genomic information to guide weight management: From universal to precision treatment. Obesity (Silver Spring). 2016;**24**:14-22

[7] Wang C, Gordon ES, Stack CB, Liu CT, Norkunas T, et al. A randomized trial of the clinical utility of genetic testing for obesity: Design and implementation considerations. Clinical Trials. 2014;**11**:102-113

[8] Cho AH, Killeya-Jones LA, O'Daniel JM, Kawamoto K, Gallagher P, et al. Effect of genetic testing for risk of type 2 diabetes mellitus on health behaviors and outcomes: Study rationale, development and design. BMC Health Services Research. 2012;**12**:16

[9] Abu-Salah KM, Zourob MM, Mouffouk F, Alrokayan SA, Alaamery MA, et al. DNA-based nanobiosensors as an emerging platform for detection of disease. Sensors (Basel). 2015;**15**:14539-14568

[10] Granados-Silvestre Mde L, Ortiz-Lopez MG, Montufar-Robles I, Menjivar-Iraheta M. Micronutrients and diabetes, the case of minerals. Cirugía y Cirujanos. 2014;**82**:119-125

[11] Sharma G, Lodha R, Shastri S, Saini S, Kapil A, et al. Zinc supplementation for one year among children with cystic fibrosis does not decrease pulmonary infection. Respiratory Care. 2016;**61**:78-84

[12] Win AZ. Micronutrient deficiencies in early childhood can lower a country's GDP: The Myanmar example. Nutrition. 2016;**32**:138-140

[13] Kornman KS, Duff GW. Personalized medicine: Will dentistry ride the wave or watch from the beach? Journal of Dental Research. 2012;**91**:8S-11S

[14] Abrahams E, Ginsburg GS, Silver M. The personalized medicine coalition: Goals and strategies. American Journal of Pharmacogenomics. 2005;**5**:345-355

[15] Antonanzas F, Juarez-Castello CA, Rodriguez-Ibeas R. Some economics on personalized and predictive medicine. The European Journal of Health Economics. 2014

[16] Abadi-Korek I, Glazer J, Granados A, Luxenburg O, Trusheim MR, et al. Personalized medicine and health economics: Is small the new big? A white paper. Israel Medical Association Journal. 2013;**15**:602-607

[17] Meetoo D. Chronic diseases: The silent global epidemic. The British Journal of Nursing. 2008;**17**:1320-1325

[18] Mathers CD, Loncar D. Projections of global mortality and burden of disease from 2002 to 2030. PLoS Medicine. 2006;**3**:e442

[19] Simopoulos AP. Nutrigenetics/nutrigenomics. Annual Review of Public Health. 2010;**31**: 53-68

[20] Migliaccio PA, Comuzzi M, Riefoli ML. Diet therapy of severe obesity. Annali Italiani di Chirurgia. 2005;**76**:417-423

[21] Konstantinidou V, Ruiz LA, Ordovas JM. Personalized nutrition and cardiovascular disease prevention: From Framingham to PREDIMED. Advances in Nutrition. 2014;**5**: 368S-371S

[22] German JB, Zivkovic AM, Dallas DC, Smilowitz JT. Nutrigenomics and personalized diets: What will they mean for food? Annual Review of Food Science and Technology. 2011;**2**:97-123

[23] Same RV, Feldman DI, Shah N, Martin SS, Al Rifai M, et al. Relationship between sedentary behavior and cardiovascular risk. Current Cardiology Reports. 2016;**18**:6

[24] Booth FW, Roberts CK, Laye MJ. Lack of exercise is a major cause of chronic diseases. Comprehensive Physiology. 2012;**2**:1143-1211

[25] Welty FK, Alfaddagh A, Elajami TK. Targeting inflammation in metabolic syndrome. Translational Research. 2016;**167**:257-280

[26] Lau DC, Teoh H. Current and emerging pharmacotherapies for weight management in prediabetes and diabetes. Canadian Journal of Diabetes. 2015;**39**(Suppl 5):S134-S141

[27] Yasuda K. Perspectives on postgenome medicine: Gene therapy for diabetes mellitus. Nihon Rinsho. 2001;**59**:157-161

[28] Scheen AJ. Towards a genotype-based approach for a patient-centered pharmacologic therapy of type 2 diabetes. Annals of Translational Medicine. 2015;**3**:S36

[29] Raciti GA, Nigro C, Longo M, Parrillo L, Miele C, et al. Personalized medicine and type 2 diabetes: Lesson from epigenetics. Epigenomics. 2014;**6**:229-238

[30] Burrowes JD. Incorporating ethnic and cultural food preferences in the renal diet. Advances in Renal Replacement Therapy. 2004;**11**:97-104

[31] Bonelli L, Puntoni M, Gatteschi B, Massa P, Missale G, et al. Antioxidant supplement and long-term reduction of recurrent adenomas of the large bowel. A double-blind randomized trial. Journal of Gastroenterology. 2013;**48**:698-705

[32] Bohm A, Weigert C, Staiger H, Haring HU. Exercise and diabetes: Relevance and causes for response variability. Endocrine. 2015;**51**(3):390-401

[33] Bouchard C, Antunes-Correa LM, Ashley EA, Franklin N, Hwang PM, et al. Personalized preventive medicine: Genetics and the response to regular exercise in preventive interventions. Progress in Cardiovascular Diseases. 2015;**57**:337-346

[34] Seedorf U, Schulte H, Assmann G. Genes, diet and public health. Genes & Nutrition. 2007;**2**:75-80

[35] Subbiah MT. Nutrigenetics and nutraceuticals: The next wave riding on personalized medicine. Translational Research. 2007;**149**:55-61

[36] Dokken BB. The pathophysiology of cardiovascular disease and diabetes: Beyond blood pressure and lipids. Diabetes Spectrum. 2008;**21**:160-165

[37] Musunuru K. Personalized genomes and cardiovascular disease. Cold Spring Harbor Perspectives in Medicine. 2015;**5**:a014068

[38] Settleman J. Cell culture modeling of genotype-directed sensitivity to selective kinase inhibitors: Targeting the anaplastic lymphoma kinase (ALK). Seminars in Oncology. 2009;**36**:S36-S41

[39] Eng G, Chen A, Vess T, Ginsburg GS. Genome technologies and personalized dental medicine. Oral Diseases. 2012;**18**:223-235

[40] Reginster JY, Neuprez A, Lecart MP, Beaudart C, Buckinx F, et al. Osteoporosis and personalized medicine. Revue Médicale de Liège. 2015;**70**:321-324

[41] Greene R, Mousa SS, Ardawi M, Qari M, Mousa SA. Pharmacogenomics in osteoporosis: Steps toward personalized medicine. Pharmacogenomics and Personalized Medicine. 2009;**2**:69-78

Chapter 8

Personalized Management of Selected Neurological Disorders

Shirley Ekvall, Tuomas Westermarck, Mari Havia and
Faik Atroshi

Additional information is available at the end of the chapter

http://dx.doi.org/10.5772/intechopen.92002

Abstract

Neurological disorders are medically complex diseases that affect the central and peripheral nervous systems. They can affect an entire neurological pathway or a single neuron. Some neurological problems can present years after a causative event. The World Health Organization reports that various types of neurological disorders affect millions of people around the world. So far, there are no therapies available to cure these disorders. Pharmacological and non-pharmacological interventions can at best relieve symptoms and perhaps delay the progression of the disease. However, there are a wide variety of helpful treatments for different disorders that may help an individual to learn better social skills and communication cues, in order to help them be able to interact socially, in a more natural fashion. For some neurological issues, the outlook can be quite good with treatment and adequate rehabilitation. Diet also plays an important role in the prevention of late-life cognitive decline. Deficits in cognition, low dietary quality and physical functioning, and cardio-metabolic risk factors are frequently reported in patients with neurological disorders. In this chapter we will briefly discuss research, as well as current opportunities and future prospects towards personalized medicine in relation to selected neurological disorders and diseases such as Down syndrome, neuronal ceroid lipofuscinoses (NCLs), and multiple sclerosis (MS).

Keywords: neurological disorders, free radicals, antioxidants, personalized medicine

1. Introduction

Genes are responsible for forming all of the neurons. However, they are certainly not the only factor determining how our brain develops and forms its inner connections. A combination of hereditary factors and environmental factors plays an important role in

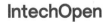

determining a neuron's final location [1]. Studies confirm that an active lifestyle maintains brain function [2]; thus, new research aims to develop lifestyle behaviors and medications that could improve normal brain development as well as repair damaged brains. Many neurological disorders emerge during the early years of development and may be diagnosed at birth or later, and their causes include congenital, chromosomal, and gene abnormalities, infections, immune disorders, and environmental factors such as nutritional deficiencies and toxins. The effectiveness of self-management interventions for people with long-term neurological conditions, in particular, Down syndrome (DS), neuronal ceroid lipofuscinosis (NCL), Duchenne muscular dystrophy (DMD), and multiple sclerosis (MS), has been reported. The effectiveness of various antioxidants on several neurodegenerative diseases in clinical trials has increasingly demonstrated that reactive oxygen species (ROS) and oxidative damage are important factors in the processes involved. Imbalanced defense mechanism of antioxidants and overproduction of free radicals from environment to living system lead to serious penalty resulting in neurodegeneration [3]. The current need for better interventions is highlighted, particularly the importance of providing condition-specific information. As the overall life expectancy across the globe has increased, the global community is now facing new challenges of improving quality of life and healthcare; however, advancements in medical technology have benefits and improved healthcare [4, 5]. This chapter provides an overview of the evidence of current findings; research limitations and future directions of research efforts are discussed in some neurological conditions such as DS, DMD, NCL, and MS.

2. Free radicals in the brain

Unlike many other tissues, the brain is a highly aerobic and totally oxygen-dependent tissue. Oxygen reduction produces reactive radical intermediates, such as superoxide and hydroxyl radicals which are thought to be the major agents of oxygen toxicity [6, 7]. Hydrogen peroxide is formed through dismutation of superoxide anion catalyzed by Cu-Zn and Mn forms of superoxide dismutase (SOD), both found in the central nervous system. In addition to Cu-Zn SOD (SOD-1), the activity of which is increased in DS, and hydrogen peroxide (H_2O_2) is generated in association with D- and L-amino acid oxidase, monoamine oxidase, α-hydroxyacid oxidase, xanthine oxidase, and cytochrome P-450 system.

Unlike charged oxygen radicals, H_2O_2, being rather unreactive and stable, rapidly crosses cell membranes. Cellular damage is accomplished when H_2O_2 decomposes to the highly reactive hydroxyl radical in reactions catalyzed by iron (II) or copper (I). If the scavenging of H_2O_2 and the contemporaneous prevention of hydroxyl radical formation do not take place, the hydroxyl radical may attack, e.g., fatty acid side chains, and start a chain reaction of lipid peroxidation. Lipid peroxidation causes gradual loss of membrane fluidity and membrane potential and increases membrane permeability to ions [6, 7]. Abnormalities in the fatty acid composition found in fetal DS brain phospholipids suggest that from the early stage of ontogenesis, lipoperoxidation may have a pathological significance [8, 9]. Oxidative degradation and polymerization of lipids lead to the accumulation of lipofuscin, the age pigment. Current evidence permits the interpretation that a high proportion of DS subjects later develop the neuropathological changes resembling Alzheimer's disease [10–12].

Considerable evidence has emerged in recent years implicating a role for oxygen free radicals in the initiation of cellular injury that leads to the development of several neurological disorders. The neonatal brain, with its high concentrations of unsaturated fatty acids (lipid content), high rate of oxygen consumption, and low concentrations of antioxidants, is particularly vulnerable to oxidative damage. Thus, increased oxidative stress has been implicated in various neurological disorders such as seizures, ischemia-reperfusion injury, and neurodegenerative diseases [13] such as Alzheimer's, Parkinson's, and amyotrophic lateral sclerosis (ALS, Lou Gehrig's disease). Free radical damage has been implicated in the initiation and propagation of seizure activity as well as the accompanying seizure-induced neuronal damage [14]. Therefore, antioxidants could play an important role in modulating susceptibility to seizure activity and seizure-induced neuronal injury.

Radical attack may also destroy membrane-bound enzymes and receptors, e.g., the binding of serotonin is decreased. However, the brain tends to need radical reactions for the generation of physiological responses. Cellular redox adjustments generally regulate functional sulfhydryl groups of proteins. There is evidence supporting the suggestion that free radical intermediates are involved, e.g., in the coupling between depolarization of the plasma membrane Ca^{2+} fluxes and neurotransmitter release [15, 16]. It has also been hypothesized that the elimination of neurofilaments at nerve terminals is regulated by oxygen radicals and that a contact of a growing neurite with a neighboring neuron induces the production of oxygen radicals. Rapid elimination of oxygen radicals during synaptogenesis would result in a reduced number of synaptic connections [17]. Accordingly, transgenic mice bearing the human SOD gene develop abnormalities in neuromuscular junctions of the tongue which closely resemble those of DS patients [18]. However, these abnormalities may be explained by a decreased level of superoxide anion as well as by increased formation of highly active and toxic hydroxyl radicals and singlet oxygen.

The regulation of glutathione (GSH) level (GSH/GSSG) through pentose phosphate pathway producing nicotinamide adenine dinucleotide phosphate (NADPH), GSH reductase, and glutathione peroxidase (GSHPx) contributes to the overall redox state of cells in brain [19]. The brain tends to need radical reactions as well as to possess specific or high endogenous levels of free radical scavengers such as dopamine, norepinephrine, catechol estrogens, taurine, and carnosine [20] in neurons. Carnosine is involved with GABA activity in the brain, and brain tissue contains high levels of carnosine, which is capable of reducing the oxidative, nitrosative, and glycemic stress to which the brain is especially vulnerable [21–23]. Oxidation and glycation produce inflammation and also contribute to cross-linking of proteins, including the Alzheimer's disease protein called amyloid-beta [24]. A study by Takahashi [25] demonstrated that homocarnosine levels were high in patients who responded to antileptic drugs. The functional balance between various free radical scavenger systems in the brain seems reasonable. Significant positive correlations between catalase and SOD levels have been reported in tissues of normal subjects excluding erythrocytes. Factors concomitantly influencing the variation of the activities of SOD, catalase, and GSHPx have been reported. Enzymes frequently called protective should rather be envisaged as being regulatory, controlling the levels of different states of oxygen reduction, phorbol esters, and strong superoxide producers through NADPH oxidase activation [26–29], inducing biosynthesis of polyamines [30, 31]. The role of polyamines is also associated with the architectural modeling of brain regions and generation of synaptic connections [32–34]. Thus effective scavenging of superoxide by excess SOD-1 may contribute even to the polyamine biosynthesis.

In addition to the complex enzyme systems, biochemical defenses include low molecular weight free radical scavengers and antioxidants. Lipid soluble vitamin E lowers the steady-state concentrations of many free radical species [35–39]. Ubiquinone may exert, similarly to vitamin E, a protective effect against lipid peroxidation [40]. The concentration of vitamin E in a fetal DS brain does not significantly differ from that of controls [41]. We have found the serum vitamin E concentrations of Down syndrome patients to be normal (1.01 + 0.35 vs. 1.13 + 0.39 mg/100 ml) [42]. In addition to conventional antioxidant systems, the brain has been found to contain specific or high endogenous levels of free radical scavengers such as dopamine, norepinephrine [43–45], catechol estrogens [20], carnosine [46], and taurine [47, 48]. The transport of taurine to platelets is impaired in DS [49]. Taurine and hypotaurine, found in high concentrations in the brain [50], could act as intracellular superoxide scavengers which would inhibit not only lipid peroxidation but also inactivation of SOD by both superoxide and H_2O_2 [51, 52]. The presence of 1–10 mM taurine protects cultured lymphoblastoid cells from the injurious effect of iron-ascorbate [48].

The role of dietary beta-carotene in the central nervous system is not elucidated. Beta-carotene acts as an antioxidant at low oxygen pressures [53–55]. Being converted to retinol or retinoic acid, it causes a marked decrease in superoxide generation. Through a still unknown mechanism, retinoic acid induces human neuroblastoma cell differentiation in vitro [56–58], and it also contributes to neural differentiation of embryonal carcinoma cells in vitro [59].

Serum β-carotene and vitamin A levels are generally normal in DS, although vitamin A levels lower than in normal subjects have also been reported. Relatively high carotene/vitamin A ratio suggests decreased efficiency in converting carotene to vitamin A. In addition the utilization of vitamin A in DS may be impaired at its site of action [60–62].

Thyroid hormones improve the cleaving of beta-carotene to vitamin A. This conversion to retinol is decreased in hypothyroidism. Thus, in hypothyroidism the vitamin A concentration decreases even when the dietary β-carotene remains the same or rises [63, 64].

3. Down syndrome

Down syndrome (DS), also known as trisomy 21, is a genetic disorder caused by the presence of all or part of a third copy of chromosome 21 [65]. It is one of the most common chromosome abnormalities in humans [66]. Globally, as of 2010, DS occurs in about 1 per 1000 births [67] and results in about 17,000 deaths [68].

In spite of the intensified antenatal diagnostics and termination of affected pregnancies, the prevalence of DS, first described in 1866, is still so high that it constitutes an important healthcare problem. DS phenotype is readily recognized at birth. Karyotype analysis confirms the diagnosis of DS associated with trisomy of chromosome 21. Since the further development of the child is predestined to be hampered by a multitude of clinical symptoms including mental retardation, premature aging, and immunological disorders such as hypothyroid states, attempts have been made to increase the understanding of the etiopathogenesis of the syndrome and to influence its progress.

The genetic imbalance due to an extra set of normal genes located in chromosome 21 means that the expression of these or actually of only some genes in the q arm leads to the disturbed development. Cumulative effects of increased amounts of primary gene products may be deleterious if no compensatory mechanisms exist. Genes of the q arm in chromosome 21, which may contribute to the DS pathology, include α/β interferon receptor, phosphoribosyl-glycinamide synthetase [69–72], cystathionine beta synthase [73], and cytoplasmic Cu-Zn superoxide dismutase (SOD-1) [74, 75].

DS, described in a karyotypically normal 18-month-old boy, has been explained by a micro-duplication of a chromosome 21 fragment (not exceeding 2000–3000 kilobase pairs) containing the SOD-1 gene [76, 77]. Further evidence of the involvement of additional SOD-1 gene in the neuropathological symptoms of DS has been derived from studies performed with transgenic cell lines and from mice carrying the human SOD gene [18, 78].

Consistent with the gene dosage effect, SOD-1 activity is increased in the cerebral cortex of DS fetuses as well as in erythrocytes, blood platelets, leukocytes, and fibroblasts of DS patients [79] (Thilakavathy et al. 2008). According to Sinet [75], elevated SOD-1 activity may constitute an oxygen free radical "stress." Usually SOD-1 protects cells from the harmful effects of oxygen radicals by catalyzing formation of H_2O_2 from O_2^- enzymes that remove excessive peroxides like catalase and glutathione peroxidase (GSHPx) [74]. NADPH is needed for the regeneration by glutathione reductase of glutathione (GSH), the utilization of which is increased via GSHPx as a defense against peroxide formation. Thus several enzymes with structural loci other than those of chromosome 21, including glutathione reductase, glutathione peroxidase, and glucose-6-phosphate dehydrogenase, show elevated activity in erythrocytes of DS patients [80, 81].

Some reports suggest that Both SOD GSHPx activities are increased in Down syndrome children [82]. It remains to be seen whether oxidative damage will still be related to the accumulation of aluminum silicates in the brain as well as to that of the senile plaques and tangles. Experiments have indicated that aluminum salts may not only accelerate Fe (II)-induced peroxidation of membrane lipids but do this especially in the brain [83]. Interestingly a high proportion of Down syndrome patients develop the neuropathological and clinical changes of AD suggesting a close pathogenetic relationship between these disorders. Thus the correction of antioxidant balance in AD by Se supplementation should be demonstrated by other means so as to direct it preventatively to those with a high risk of developing AD.

Balazs and Brooksbank [8] noticed that the adaptive response to elevated SOD-1 activity, i.e., increased GSHPx activity found in other tissues, is not detected in the fetal DS brain. The level of GSHPx activity in neural tissues seems to be as such too low to provide protection from peroxide-induced lesions [84]. Furthermore, if H_2O_2 production is high, catalase might be a superior scavenger, because restoration of glutathione becomes a limiting factor for the activity of GSHPx [85]. However, catalase level is normal in DS erythrocytes [72, 86], and its activity is practically absent in the brain tissue [87]. Consequently brain cells may be extremely susceptible to oxygen free radicals.

3.1. The pathophysiology of Down syndrome and the role of the thyroid gland

Thyroid hormone has a regulatory function on mitosis and differentiation of neural cells; hence, it is intimately involved in normal brain maturation [88–91]. Experimentally trijodo-thyronine enhances neural outgrowth in vitro [92, 94]. Even subclinical hypothyreosis during the postnatal period may contribute to the delayed and incomplete maturation of the cerebral and cerebellar cortices.

Increased prevalence of thyroid dysfunction is associated with DS in infants as well as in older children and adults [95–98]. Hypothyroidism is reported in 17–50% of the DS patients studied depending on the age and sex distribution of the population [98]. The relatively high incidence of autoimmune thyroiditis suggests that impaired immune surveillance is the primary mechanism in hypothyroidism [99]. Pueschel and Pezullo [98] conducted a study which showed that approximately 28% of their 151 DS patients had elevated antimicrosomal antibodies, and a highly significant correlation of antimicrosomal antibodies to T4 and to TSH was found. Recent studies indicate that antimicrosomal antibodies are mainly, if not exclusively, against thyroid peroxidase [100].

Thyroid peroxidase is a membrane-bound enzyme associated with the endoplasmic reticulum and the apical membrane of the thyroid cell. Immunoelectron microscopical observations of the thyroid microsomal antigen in the apical plasma membrane are compatible with the notion that microsomal antigen is identical with thyroid peroxidase [101–104].

SOD-1 system, which generates H_2O_2, is essential in the iodination and coupling reactions catalyzed by thyroid peroxidase [105–107]. However, an excess of H_2O_2 may inactivate the peroxidase complex [105–108]. The irreversible loss of catalytic activity, caused by H_2O_2 or by the reactive oxygen species generated, may result from oxidation of functionally important amino acid residues to carbonyl derivatives. This may also render the protein susceptible to proteolytic attack and to detachment of its cellular compartment. If so, the maintenance of the thyroid peroxidase function and its integrity would require correct steady-state production of H_2O_2 and strict control of its level. This requirement is mainly met with by GSHPx and catalase.

Antigenicity of the modified and disintegrated thyroid peroxidase should be recognized by helper lymphocytes only in the context of MHC Class 11 products coded by genes in the HLA-D region. This region normally expressed only by a restricted variety of cell types is found in autoimmune disorders in target cells. Thus an aberrant expression of HLA-DR antigen found on thyrocytes in Graves' and Hashimoto's disease indicates its potential importance in antigen presentation of thyroid autoimmune disorders [109, 110].

The presence and intensity of DR expression in Graves' thyroids correlate positively with the titer of microsomal antibodies. Curiously, in cultured thyroid cells, plant lectins are able to induce the expression of HLA-DR by a mechanism unrelated to the known mito-genic effects. On the other hand, the inducing effect of gamma-interferon (IFN-γ) could have a physiological significance (IFN-α and IFN-β did not induce Class II expression in thyrocytes) [111–113]:

• Release of IFNs and lymphokines, best candidates for inducers, must be triggered by other factors [111–113].

On the basis of the gene dosage effect, we suggest possible mechanisms for the sensitization of DS thyroids to autoimmunization:

• Viral challenge including enhanced production of oxygen radicals due to macrophage and neutrophil activity may exert additional requirement for GSHPx and selenium. If these needs are not met with overproduction of oxygen radicals and constitutive excess of both LFA-1 and its beta-chain, it may hinder normal immune response [111–114].

• Excess H_2O_2 causes fragmentation of thyroid peroxidase which detaches from the cell membrane and turns into an autoantigen.

• Increased expression of IFN-α/IFN-P receptors, the gene of which is found in chromosome 21, may sensitize thyrocytes to the induction of HLA-DR antigen by γ-IFN [111–113].

3.2. The impact of early hearing loss on language

Down syndrome occurs in approximately 1 in 600–800 live births [115] and remains the most common genetic abnormality seen in most otolaryngology practices. Down syndrome has a number of clinical problems associated with it [116–118]. The symptoms of DS vary from person to person, and people with the syndrome may have different problems at different times of their lives [119]. Hearing loss will affect many people with Down syndrome at some point in their lives. It has been reported that children with Down syndrome are at particular risk of some degree of hearing impairment due to a number of physiological differences. The authors concluded that there are a range of middle ear problems that can be treated successfully if the children are taken for routine cleaning and examination from birth [120]. Hearing losses affect 40–80% of individuals with DS [121–124]. In young children, the most common cause is conductive loss due to episodes of ear infection and otitis media with effusion (OME).

To determine the prevalence of hearing loss in newborn with Down syndrome, Tedeschi et al. [125] reported that newborn with Down syndrome have a higher prevalence of congenital hearing loss than the total neonatal population (15 vs. 0.25%). Individuals with Down syndrome are prone to otolaryngologic anomalies that complicate the diagnosis and classification of hearing impairment [126]. In children, hearing loss can affect educational, language-related, and emotional development. Even mild hearing loss can affect a child's articulation. It is reported that as many as 80% of people with Down syndrome will have some problem with hearing [127]. A retrospective and cross-sectional analysis was performed to evaluate the prevalence of OME in children with DS for consecutive age categories between 6 months and 12 years [128]. The authors concluded that a high prevalence of OME was found at the age of 1 year (66.7%), with a second peak prevalence of 60% at 6–7 years. A declining trend was seen in older children [128].

As with children, adults with DS may experience hearing loss due to glue ear. Picciotti et al. [129] assessed auditory function in adults with DS to evaluate the prevalence of hearing loss. The authors concluded that hearing loss is common in adults with DS and shows a pattern compatible with precocious aging of the hearing system.

3.3. Hearing and spoken language

Disorders impairing a patient's communication abilities may involve voice, speech, language, hearing, and/or cognition [130]. The effect of hearing difficulties on spoken language development has been demonstrated in many studies of the speech and language skills of children and teenagers with Down syndrome [131, 132].

Most individuals with DS also experience speech and language impairments although the severity of these is variable [133, 134]. Researchers studying language development in DS have measured hearing either directly tested or using pure tone audiometry to establish hearing thresholds [135] or, indirectly, using speech discrimination tasks [136–138]. Therefore, it suggested that speech and language therapy should be provided when children are found to have ongoing hearing difficulties and that joint audiology and speech and language therapy clinics could be considered for preschool children [138].

4. Duchenne muscular dystrophy

Duchenne muscular dystrophy (DMD) is one of the most severe myopathies, usually obvious by the age of 5, and evolves progressively until it causes disablement and death, around the age of 20 [139]. In young boys, DMD is caused by deletions or point mutations in the pre-mRNA for dystrophin that result in out-of-frame transcripts and hence a nonfunctional truncated dystrophin protein [140]. It is recessively inherited, linked to sex, and the gene determining DMD has been mapped in the Xp-21 locus [141]. It has an incidence of 1/3000–1/3500 male births and 1/3 of the cases coming from new mutation. Some affected individuals may develop intellectual disturbance due to unknown mechanism, so far. The sister of an affected individual has a 50% chance of carrying the defective gene [141]. The result of the dystrophic locus on the gene is the absence of dystrophin, a rod-shaped protein that is part of the muscle cytoskeleton. Death commonly results from involvement of the respiratory muscles. Dystrophin is present in the muscle of normal individuals and has been rarely, or not at all, detected in patients with DMD [142, 143]. The genetic alteration produces abnormality in the membrane of the muscular fibers that consists of a disturbance in the calcium transport (Ca^{2+}), inside the muscular fibers, which is the base mechanism of cellular degeneration and necrosis. There is fiber necrosis and replacement of fibers by fat. A nucleotide degradation and decreased muscle ATP and ADP content have been reported. The ATP is necessary to drive the Na^+/K^+ pump which maintains ionic gradients across the sarcolemma; resequester the Ca^{++} into the cisternae; and power contraction [144–146]. The production of ATP can be the result of anaerobic respiration, which breaks glucose down into ATP and lactic acid, or aerobic respiration when ATP, carbon dioxide, and water are formed. A second immediate reserve of energy exists in the form of creatine phosphate, which can donate phosphate to ADP to form ATP, becoming itself a creatine. In the resting muscle, glucose is stored as glycogen, and in such a muscle aerobic respiration synthesizes ATP from glucose or fatty acids.

Muscle dystrophy and mitochondrial dysfunction give rise to an amplification of stress-induced cytosolic calcium signals and an amplification of stress-induced reactive oxygen species (ROS) production, and increased oxidative stress within the cell damages the sarcolemma and eventually results in the death of the cell. Muscle fibers undergo necrosis and are ultimately replaced with adipose and connective tissue. In recent years, synthetic splice-switching oligonucleotides (SSO) have been developed as new treatments for DMD whereby an SSO is targeted to the pre-mRNA and mediates splicing redirection to restore the reading frame of the dystrophin gene via exon skipping and thus to generate a shorter but functional dystrophin protein isoform [140, 147–155]. Several SSO chemistries have been developed for exon skipping in DMD and other neuromuscular diseases [156, 157], but of these only two SSO chemical types have been used in clinical trials, namely, 2′-O-methyl phosphorothioates (2′-OMe/PS) [158] and phosphorodiamidate morpholino oligonucleotides (PMO) [159, 160].

Therapy of DMD has been an elusive goal. Studies with isolated myocytes have shown that lipid peroxidation with an enhanced free radical production can be activated by increasing Ca concentration [161–163]. Thus, several kinds of antioxidants have been proposed as a treatment since increased levels of thiobarbituric acid (TBA) reactive material has been found in the muscles and blood of DMD males [164]. We have previously reported that the biological half-life of ^{75}Se in DMD patients was significantly shorter than in healthy controls [165]. Low oxygen saturation in the muscle tissue may stimulate the Il-6 production, a cytokine, which is produced by contracting muscles and released into the blood. The blood circulation of the older Duchenne patients is particularly disturbed. Pedersen et al. [166] have demonstrated that Il-6 affects the metabolic genes, induction of lipolysis, inhibition of insulin resistance, and stimulation of cortisol production. In addition, carbohydrate supplementation during exercise was shown to inhibit the release of Il-6 from contracting muscles. Thus carnitine supplementation is indicated to the Duchenne patients, to make sure that the energy supply will be good [167].

Shimomura et al. [168] observed that a group of trained animals, part of which were coenzyme Q_{10} (CoQ$_{10}$)-treated, had to exercise for 30 min on treadmill, in downhill position. CoQ$_{10}$-treated animals had a higher level of CoQ$_{10}$ in their muscles, and the early rise in creatine kinase and lactic dehydrogenase plasma levels, due to the exercise, was evident at a remarkably significant lower extent, in the treated ones. Similar observations were also made in humans [169, 170]. Therefore we have been treating the Duchenne patients with CoQ$_{10}$. In our earlier work, we gave DMD patients sodium selenite, 0.05–0.1 mg Se kg^{-1} BW day^{-1}; α-tocopherol, 10–20 mg kg^{-1} BW day^{-1}; vitamin B$_2$, 0.2 mg kg^{-1} BW day^{-1}; vitamin B$_6$, 5 mg kg^{-1} BW day^{-1}; carnitine, 10–20 mg kg^{-1} BW day^{-1}; and ubiquinone-$_{10}$ (CoQ$_{10}$), 3 mg kg^{-1} BW day^{-1} [171]. We reported two siblings of whom the elder one got practically no antioxidants and the younger one has antioxidant treatment starting at the age of 6 years. The first one was wheelchair bound at the age of 8 years and deceased at the age of 17 years. However, at the age of 15 years, the younger brother was still able to walk without any assistance. At the age 19 years, he was to be a graduate student with the best scores of all seven subjects that he participated. At the age of 21 years, he was still able to swim a distance of 50 m without any assistance. At age of 30 years, he is still able to make computer art and to have art exhibitions of his own. There are also mothers who have made observations that the odor of lard characteristic of their DMD sons was cured during the antioxidant supplementation. Potential future developments therapy may be to produce functional amounts of dystrophin by skipping the mutated exon like what has been done in mdx dystrophic mouse [172–174].

5. Neuronal ceroid lipofuscinosis

Neuronal ceroid lipofuscinoses (NCLs) are clinically heterogeneous neurodegenerative lysosomal diseases [175–179]. NCLs are recessively inherited neurodegenerative lysosomal storage diseases. The neuronal ceroid lipofuscinoses are with a prevalence of 1 in 12,500 in some populations such as the USA and Northern Europe. Currently the classification is based on genetic defects, with 14 clinical subtypes and genetically separate neurodegenerative disorders that result from excessive accumulation of lipopigments (lipofuscin) in the body's tissues, and the most prevalent NCLs are CLN3 disease, classic juvenile and CLN2 disease, and classic late infantile [39, 176, 180–182]. Characteristics of the diseases are deposits of ceroid and lipofuscin pigments in the tissues, particularly in the neural tissue, visual failure, and progressive mental retardation; depending on the age of onset and clinical, electrophysiological, and neuropathological features, the NCLs can be subdivided into the infantile the late infantile, the juvenile and the adult type of NCL; however, the pathogenesis of NCL is still unknown.

5.1. Management of neuronal ceroid lipofuscinosis

Neuronal ceroid lipofuscinoses are a group of hereditary diseases caused by mutations in at least eight genes (CLN1-CLN8) [183, 184]. They are characterized by massive accumulation of autofluorescent lysosomal storage bodies in most cells and associated severe degeneration of the CNS [183]. There is no single, standard treatment for neuronal ceroid lipofuscinoses (NCLs), as there is currently no cure; however, a number of different treatments can be used to ease symptoms and encourage independence and better standards of general health [185]. Also there are certain medical problems that can affect someone with neuronal ceroid lipofuscinosis. However, a number of different treatments can be used to ease the symptoms and encourage independence and better standards of general health. These treatments are based on each individual's physical and intellectual needs as well as their personal strengths and limitations: enzyme replacement therapy, gene therapy, stem cells including tissue engineering, and medicine or metabolic therapy such as dietary restriction and immune biotherapy [186–190]. These modes of treatments have been used in many genetic diseases. Acetyl-L-carnitine (ALC) has been shown to be therapeutic in treatment of NCLs [191]. It was reported that ALC might rebalance the disorders underlying neuronal ceroid lipofuscinosis disease which are related to a disturbance in pH homeostasis [191].

The polyenic acid level with low levels of linoleic acid and an inverse relationship between GSHPx activity and the level of eicosatrienoic acid have been observed in juvenile neuronal ceroid lipofuscinosis (JNCL) [192]. The occurrence of the fluorescent pigments suggested the peroxidation of lipids in the etiology of NCL. It is likely that the diseased tissues peroxidized cause secondary damage more rapidly than normal tissues and cytotoxic end products of lipoperoxidation. On a weight basis, ceroid seen in JNCL patients binds five times more iron than the lipofuscin seen in normal elderly individuals. The increased levels of aluminum salts greatly enhance iron-dependent damage to membranes. Heiskala et al. [193] has confirmed the presence of complexable iron and copper in the CSF of patients with NCL and other neurological disorders, and when the pH value of the assay for iron was lowered, the NCL group had substantially more complexable iron in their CSFs. Interestingly aluminum has been observed in CSF and in ceroid lipofuscin pigments of the brain of NCL patients [194]. It is well established that damaged tissue release metals from protein-bound sites and these metals stimulate peroxidative damage to lipids and other biomolecules.

One of the most essential enzymes counteracting lipoperoxidation is the selenium-containing GSHPx. Two independent reports have demonstrated that erythrocyte GSHPx activity is decreased in JNCL patients [195]. This low GSHPx activity was reversed to normal level by selenium supplementation. The evaluation of sodium selenite absorption and losses before supplementation of JNCL patients has been studied by using total body counting for ^{75}Se detection. These studies showed that in three JNCL patients, about 55% of the administered ^{75}Se was eliminated during the first 11 days in the feces and about 10% in the urine [39]. Compared to healthy controls (42 and 7%, respectively), findings indicate a reduced absorption of selenium in JNCL patients contrary to a previous report. The low GSHPx activity in NCL patients may indeed reflect a low selenium intake most probably due to a disturbed absorption of selenium and secondary phenomena due to an inborn error of metabolism. Apart from the low selenium status, also very low vitamin E levels are found in the serum of advanced and hospitalized NCL patients. This can be explained by the recent finding of a pronounced reduction of apolipoprotein B as well as the whole fraction of very low-density lipoprotein (VLDL) in JNCL patients.

JNCL patients (genetically subgroups) have been given daily supplementation of sodium selenite (0.05–0.1 mg/Se/kg of BW), vitamin E (α-tocopherol acetate 0.014–0.05 g/kg BW), and vitamins B_2 (0.025–0.05 mg/kg BW) and B_6 (0.63–0.8 mg/kg BW). The benefits of the therapy are corroborated by the significant negative correlation of GSHPx activity with neurological dysfunction of motor performance, balance, coordination, and speech [196]. The mean age at death has been extended by 4 years as compared to that at the beginning of the century. As the best responders to antioxidant therapy show no neurological dysfunction at the age of over 20 years, there is no doubt that the life expectancy of JNCL patients receiving antioxidants, including selenium, will be significantly prolonged in the future [197]. Complications of the antioxidant therapy have been few and not severe. Six patients have experienced vomiting and nausea when the serum concentration of selenium reached the level of 0.45 to 0.5 mM. Serum levels up to 4.0 mM were usually well tolerated, as well as when the sodium selenite was changed to ebselen (2-phenyl-1,2,-benzisoselenazol-3(2H)-one).

6. Multiple sclerosis

Multiple sclerosis (MS) is a chronic autoimmune disease of the central nervous system, where suspected autoimmune attack causes nerve demyelination and progressive neuro-degeneration and should benefit from both anti-inflammatory and neuroprotective strate-gies [198]. MS affects an estimated 4.3 cases per 100,000 in Europe with a higher rate in Northern Europe [199]. Often it appears in individuals between 20 and 40 years of age and has a strong genetic component [200]. The disease course is benign in 10–15% of patients, and they do not need an assistive device for walking even after 20 years of MS [201, 202]. Low levels of polyenic acids are involved in the pathogenesis of both MS and JNCL. Earlier a decrease level of serum linoleate as well as unsaturated fatty acids of brain phospholipids in MS patients was shown [203, 204]. It has also been argued that supplementation with essential fatty acids may improve the clinical status of MS patients [205]. And as in NCL, the selenium may, by activating GSHPx (scavenger of organic peroxides), regulate the metabolic transformation of essential fatty acids and biotransformation of these to pros-taglandins, thromboxanes, and leukotrienes [206]. Curiously decreased GSHPx activities in erythrocytes have been found in female but not in male MS patients [207]. A significant association between the two haplotypes of the dopamine D2 receptor gene (DRD2) and the age of onset and/or diagnosis of MS was reported [208].

Current treatments for MS mainly target inflammatory processes, and there has been scant progress in treatments that enhance neuronal or glial regeneration. Can we predict the risk of serious side effects? This asks for the development of biomarkers, clinical, genetic, imag-ing, or immunological, that allow for a better stratification of patients [209]. The need for tailored therapeutics is especially imperative, as the consequences of an ineffective medica-tion might be irreversible dysfunction. However, it is obvious that treatment decisions in clinical practice must be made on an individual basis. This requires a personalized medicine approach in predicting disease activity in multiple sclerosis. Biomarkers that could predict disease course, treatment response, and risk of side effects would be highly appreciated. Despite extensive research over the last years, few biomarkers have made their way into clinical practice.

7. Advances in the development of novel antioxidant therapies

Earlier, through intervention efforts, patients with DS have received medical treatment and stimulation of sensory, motor, and cognitive areas [210]. In 1981, Harrell et al. [211] reported that the administration of a megavitamin mineral supplement to a heterogenous group of 16 men-tally retarded children, 4 of which had DS, had led to encouraging results. However, controlled double-blind studies on somewhat larger groups using similar megadoses of vitamins and minerals but no thyroid supplementation did not result in any beneficial effects [212–216]. However, these studies were devoid of a detailed theory of the mechanism of action, and the age distribution of the patients was disadvantageous in relation to possible targets in the developing brains.

Our primary survey and theory of antioxidant therapy in DS [42, 217] rest on the present concepts of the etiopathogenesis of DS [8, 79]. Earlier, selected antioxidants have been used, e.g., in the therapy of neuronal ceroid lipofuscinosis [218]. Prevention of free radical damage should be executed by agents focused on the tissue and cellular compartments and processes where the generation of free radicals is critical. In DS, elevated cytoplasmic SOD-1 activity causes free radical stress through H_2O_2. An excess of H_2O_2 may be activated in iron- or copper-catalyzed reactions to generate highly reactive hydroxyl radical (–OH) or singlet oxygen. The extent and nature of the damage depend on the precise site of the •OH production, which in turn depends on the intra- or extracellular location of the critical metal ions [7, 219].

However, GSHPx, which gives protection against elevated H_2O_2, is low in brains with intensive oxygen metabolism. Histochemical studies by Slivka and co-workers [220] are indicative of the relative absence of GSH in neuronal somata and locate GSH to non-neuronal elements and fibrous and terminal regions of neurons. Furthermore, in normal newborn infants, the activity of GSHPx is physiologically low [221, 222]. Just a reflection of this condition could be the low blood selenium level found in neonates [223]. Controversial results have been published on the level of selenium in plasma and erythrocytes of DS patients [79]. Peripherally decreased GSHPx activity may be corrected by selenium supplementation [224, 225]. Unlike catalase, benefit of optimal GSHPx activity is gained through its capability to reduce both H_2O_2 and organic hydroperoxides including lipid peroxides. The mean plasma selenium concentration in DS patients has been shown not to differ significantly from that of the control subjects although the GSHPx activity is 130% of the normal [226]. Neve and co-workers [227] reported normal erythrocyte but significantly decreased plasma selenium levels in 29 DS patients. These discrepancies may be explained by the differences in the population groups studied and by the distribution of the blood selenium pool. Only 10–15% of the erythrocyte selenium in man is reported to be incorporated into the GSHPx, whereas the corresponding value in rat is 75–85% [228].

We noticed in DS patients of different ages that the mean compensatory increase of erythrocyte GSHPx was lower than expected, 33.4 vs. 50%. The finding that the erythrocyte SOD/GSHPx ratio was higher than in healthy controls confirmed our belief of insufficient compensation [42, 217]. In DS the whole body retention of 5–8 kBq, ^{75}Se-sodium selenite, with 0.4 ug Se as carrier/kg BW, is estimated to be 53.3 ± 21.1%. Stable selenium supplementation increased ^{75}Se elimination indicating a saturated selenium pool in the body [229]. Selenium supplementation 0.025 mg Se/kg/d in the form of sodium selenite increased E-GSHPx activity by 28 (59.9% above normal). This was also demonstrated by the 23.9% decrease of SOD/GSHPx ratio ($P < 0.01$) [42, 217].

The consequences of selenium supplementation on the brain antioxidant balance, and thus its therapeutic value, are difficult to monitor. However, certain clinical, experimental, and in vitro observations may be indicative [230]. A highly positive correlation has been reported between erythrocyte GSHPx values and IQ in DS [231]. The plasma selenium concentration and erythrocyte GSHPx activity were found to be higher in DS girls than in DS boys, which is consistent with the finding of significantly higher IQ scores for female than for male DS patients. The positive correlation of E-GSHPx activity between DS subjects and their siblings suggests the influence of environmental and/or additional genetic factors [26, 230].

Estimates of the amount of selenium in the rat brain indicate that the GSHPx may account for only ⅕ of the total selenium in the brain [232]. The finding that selenoproteins other than GSHPx are distributed mainly in the brain and endocrine organs raises a question of their physiological role. After the administration of very small amounts of selenium, severely depleted rats retained in the brain and in the reproductive and several endocrine organs (including thyroid) a dose which was 20–50 times the dose found in adequately fed control animals. This indicates the existence of regulatory mechanisms which ensure a sufficient level of selenium in critical organs, above all in the brain and the thyroid even during depletion [91, 233].

In concentrations of 6×10^{-7} M, selenite induces a 30-fold increase of GSHPx activity in neuroblast cells in vitro [234]. Earlier studies on the rat liver suggested that selenium regulates the level of GSHPx mRNA as well as GSHPx protein concentration and GSHPx activity [235]. Concentrations of 10^{-5} M exert obvious toxic effects on nerve fibers in vitro [236]. Trace elements, as "doping impurities" in organic material, could be key variables that regulate conductivity in biological semiconduction structures [237]. We suggest that the abnormally high levels of copper and iron and the low level of zinc ion in erythrocytes and blood mononuclear cells are reflections of disturbed oxygen radical metabolism in DS. However, increased concentration of copper can be explained as gene dosage evident by the increased activity of SOD-1 [238]. Except for the decreased iron content in erythrocytes, the results were in accordance with an earlier study [239]. Ferrous-ion (Fe II) and copper-ion (Cu I) react with H_2O_2 producing •OH radicals [240, 241]. Titanium in erythrocytes may indicate insufficient protection by GSHPx. If titanium is present as Ti (IV), stable compounds may be formed with hydrogen peroxides and probably with superoxide anions to give 1:1 adducts [238]. The low plasma zinc concentration in DS children has been recognized in earlier studies as well [242, 243]. The homeostasis of zinc is regulated by the intestine. The absorption of zinc seems to be decreased in DS, mean retention of zinc being 30% compared with 58% in healthy adults. Stable zinc supplementation in one DS patient did not increase the 65Zn elimination, indicating an unsaturated zinc pool [229].

Interestingly, the primarily high blood mononuclear cell levels of copper decreased, whereas the concentration of iron and zinc was not affected during selenium supplementation [244]. No significant alterations were observed in the erythrocyte concentrations of magnesium, calcium, iron, copper, zinc, sulfur, titanium, and manganese. Aluminum was not found in erythrocytes nor in neutrophils of DS patients [238].

8. Brain antioxidant homeostasis in relation to selenium and GSHPx

In nature the availability of selenium, as a trace element, may be limited. GSHPx activity has been shown to reflect selenium status in deficient and adequate states [245]. On the other hand, protection against toxicity is likely to involve the alterations in GSH metabolism that occur in nutritional Se deficiency. A high concentration of erythrocyte glutathione in patients with neurological disorders has been reported [246–248]. However, regulatory mechanisms apparently exist which ensure that during periods of insufficient selenium intake, the content of the element is kept up above all in the brain and the reproductive and the endocrine organs.

Selenium seems to be somehow involved in the regulation of oxygen metabolism through its influence on a variety of enzymes. In concentrations of 6×10^{-7} to $\times 10^{-6}$ M, selenite induces a 30-fold increase of GSHPx activity in neuroblast cells in vitro. Other studies with the rat liver have suggested that Se status regulates the level of GSHPx mRNA as well as GSHPx protein concentration and GSHPx activity [235]. In concentrations of $0.7 - 2 \times 10^{-5}$ M, Se in the rat liver increases the activities of γ-glutamylcysteine synthetase, the first rate-limiting enzyme in GSH biosynthesis, and GSSG reductase, which catalyzes the reduction of GSSG to GSH [249]. In some species the induction of GSH S-transferase has been shown to occur as a result of Se deficiency. Hydrogen peroxide as the most stable and diffusible of the oxygen reduction intermediates may exert an influence on the expression of SOD, catalase, and GSHPx activities. The homeostasis in the oxidative metabolism and oxygen reduction may be distorted by different means either inherent or acquired. Depending on the spatial and temporal occurrence of the distortion, various neurological states are expressed. The developing brain is particularly susceptible to oxidative stress more so than the mature brain [250]. H_2O_2 accumulation has also been associated with increased injury in the superoxide dismutase-overexpressing neonatal murine brain, and greater cell death is seen when immature neurons are exposed to H_2O_2 than with mature neurons. Increased H_2O_2 accumulation may be the result of relative insufficiency of the endogenous enzyme GSHPx.

Under physiologic circumstances, the brain has efficient antioxidant defense mechanisms, including GSHPx, which converts potentially harmful H_2O_2 to oxygen and water at the expense of reduced GSH. Under oxidative stress, in the immature brain, endogenous levels of GSHPx may be inadequate for converting excess H_2O_2. Transgenic mice that overexpress GSHPx (hGPx-tg), when subjected to hypoxia-ischemia (HI), have less histologic brain injury than their WT littermates [19]. In addition, the cortex exhibits increased GSHPx enzyme activity at 24 h, whereas GSHPx activity remains unaltered in the WT brain. In addition, neurons cultured from the hGPx-tg brain are resistant to injury from exogenously applied H_2O_2 [251]. Neurons cultured from the hippocampus and cortex that are transfected (transfection describes the introduction of foreign material into eukaryotic cells) with genes for catalase and GSHPx also show protection from neurotoxic insults and a corresponding decrease in H_2O_2 accumulation [252]. These findings indicate that adequate GSHPx activity can ameliorate injury to the immature brain from oxidative stress due to H_2O_2.

It is well established that a previous stress to the brain can induce tolerance to subsequent injury, a phenomenon called personality change (PC). In neonatal rodents, protection against HI brain injury has been induced by PC with a period of hypoxia before the induction of HI [253]. The mechanisms of this protection have yet to be fully determined, but it has been established that a large number of genes are induced in response to hypoxia [254]. Many of these genes are regulated by the transcription factor hypoxia-inducible factor-1α (HIF-1α), perhaps most importantly vascular endothelial growth factor (VEGF) and erythropoietin (EPO). VEGF is upregulated after focal ischemic injury in the neonatal rat, in parallel with the induction of HIF-1α [255].

9. Current opportunities and future prospects towards personalized medicine

Neurological disorders are diseases that affect the central and peripheral nervous systems. They can affect an entire neurological pathway or a single neuron; the neurodegeneration describes the loss of neuronal structure and function [256]. They are caused by genetic mutations present during embryo or fetal development, although they may be observed later in life [257–259]. The mutations may be inherited from a parent's genome, or they may be acquired in utero. The risk factors for the diseases are diverse, including age, genetics, lifestyle, etc. Inflammatory conditions represent a major causative factor in numerous medically significant disorders. It can result from a range of stimuli from outside or within the body. However, these stimuli trigger cells and physiological processes within a host environment. It is believed that environmental exposures increase the risk of developing the disease. Even in inherited cases, exposure to toxins or other environmental factors may influence when symptoms of the disease appear or how the disease progresses [258, 260, 261].

With an increase in life span and decrease in death rate, the prevalence of these chronic recurring condition are rising all over the world. Moreover, no direct therapy/treatment is available now, which can reverse or retard the pathophysiological processes permanently. The medication (drug) regimen needs to be well integrated with healthy diet and lifestyle to attain high-quality and longer lives [262]. Therefore, the complex physiopathological mechanisms must now be clarified, and the immunological and genetical causes to neurological diseases must be investigated. New research on gene changes linked and gene therapy to neurological disorders is helping scientists better understand the disease, in which DNA or RNA is used as the pharmacological agent, defined as gene therapy [263]. Both genetic and environmental factors are known to influence susceptibility to diseases. Therefore, environmental factors may also have a protective effect.

The role of free radicals is well established in etiopathogenesis of neurological disorders. Some of the known antioxidants, which can prevent oxidation chronic recurring condition, have been studied [38, 39]. Recent developments in basic research have confirmed the relationship between etiopathogenesis and supplementation therapy with vitamins and trace elements. Supplementation therapy studies should be conducted. We need more clinical experience and a longer follow-up period with our neurological disorder patients receiving antioxidant therapy to reach more final conclusions concerning efficacy in the control of optimal development. Studies are now looking at the possible effects of these compounds more closely to develop related compounds that are even more potent and might be used as dietary supplements. However, so far, most research suggests that a balanced diet is of greater benefit than taking these substances as dietary supplements.

10. Personalized medicine approaches

Neurological diseases cannot be managed by using one single approach. These disorders, like all chronic diseases, are a complex metabolic system that is related to the way a patient's genes interact with their individual environment. Therefore, precise and reliable testing methods are needed including patient biomarkers, age, and genetic history. Oxidative stress has been linked to dozens of chronic conditions [264, 265]. Identifying the cause of oxidative stress such as emotional stressors, poor diet, smoking, metal toxicity [266], chemical exposure, and pesticides can be of help [266, 267]. To balance free radicals may require lifestyle and diet modifications such as antioxidant supplementation [268, 269].

There is no doubt that the nervous system is involved in the etiopathogenesis of various pathological states and diseases. Interactions between the nervous, endocrine, and immune systems might represent the anatomical and functional basis for understanding the pathways and mechanisms that enable the brain to modulate the progression of disease. For example, an increasing number of pharmacogenetic association studies in DS are being reported [270, 273]. Personalized medicine is an evidence-based, individualized medicine that delivers the right care to the right patient at the right time and results in measurable improvements in outcomes and a reduction on healthcare costs. However, in order to make personalized medicine effective, genomic techniques must be standardized and integrated into health systems and clinical workflow. Though personalizing drug treatment on the basis of individual genotype rather than ethnicity may be more appropriate, differences in allele frequencies across continents should be considered when designing clinical trials of new drugs [270]. For example, new therapies for treating DS require quality of life measurement, such as the use of stem cells in order to develop treatments which may improve the intelligence of those affected with the syndrome [274]. Other methods being studied include the use of antioxidants, gamma secretase inhibition, adrenergic agonists, and memantine [275–279].

Author details

Shirley Ekvall[1], Tuomas Westermarck[2*], Mari Havia[3] and Faik Atroshi[4†]

*Address all correspondence to: t.westermarck@gmail.com

1 University Affiliated Cincinnati Center for Developmental Disabilities, Children's Hospital Medical Center, University of Cincinnati, Cincinnati, OH, USA

2 Rinnekoti Foundation, Espoo, Finland

3 Helsinki University Central Hospital, Helsinki, Finland

4 Department of Pharmacology and Toxicology, University of Helsinki, Finland

† Deceased.

References

[1] Eliot L. What's Going on in There? How the Brain and Mind Develop in the First Five Years of Life. New York: Bantam Books; 1999

[2] Ornstein R, Thompson RF. The Amazing Brain. Boston: Houghton Mifflin; 1984. pp. 23-27

[3] Floyd RA. Antioxidants, oxidative stress, and degenerative neurological disorders. Proceedings of the Society for Experimental Biology and Medicine. 1999;**222**(3):236-245

[4] Dillon K, Prokesch S. Global challenges in health care: Is rationing in our future? Harvard Business Review. 2010

[5] Yager P, Domingo GJ, Gerdes J. Point-of-care diagnostics for global health. Annual Review of Biomedical Engineering. 2008;**10**:107-144

[6] Gutteridge JM, Westermarck T, Halliwell B. Oxygen radical damage in biological systems. In: Johnson JE Jr, Walford R, Harman O, Miquel J, editors. Free Radicals. Aging and Degenerative Diseases. New York: Alan R. Liss; 1985. pp. 99-139

[7] Halliwell B, Gutteridge JM. The importance of free radicals and catalytic metal ions in human diseases. Molecular Aspects of Medicine. 1985;**8**(2):89-193

[8] Balazs R, BWL B. Neurochemical approaches to the pathogenesis of Down's syndrome. Journal of Mental Deficiency Research. 1985;**29**:1-14

[9] Brooksbank BW, Balazs R. Superoxide dismutase and lipoperoxidation in down's syndrome fetal brain. Developmental Brain Research. 1984;**16**:37-44

[10] Mann DMA. Alzheimer's disease and Down's syndrome. Histopathology. 1988;**13**(2): 125-137

[11] Ness S, Rafii M, Aisen P, Krams M, Silverman W, Manji H. Down's syndrome and Alzheimer's disease: Towards secondary prevention. Nature Reviews. Drug Discovery. 2012;**11**(9):655-656

[12] Rafii MS, Aisen PS. Advances in Alzheimer's disease drug development. BMC Medicine. 2015;**13**:62

[13] Bains JS, Shaw CA. Neurodegenerative disorders in humans: The role of glutathione in oxidative stress-mediated neuronal death. Brain Research. Brain Research Reviews. 1997;**25**(3):335-358

[14] Halliwell B. Role of free radicals in the neurodegenerative diseases: Therapeutic implications for antioxidant treatment. Drugs & Aging. 2001;**18**(9):685-716

[15] Chaudhari N, Roper SD. The cell biology of taste. The Journal of Cell Biology. 2010;**190**(3): 285-296

[16] Zoccarato F, Pandolfo M, Deana R, Alexandre A. Inhibition by some phenolic antioxidants of Ca2+ uptake and neurotransmitter release from brain synaptosomes. Biochemical and Biophysical Research Communications. 1987;**146**(2):603-610

[17] Elomaa E, Virtanen I. Is the mental deterioration In Down's syndrome linked to impaired terminal degradation of neurofilaments? Med. Hypotheses. 1985;**16**: 171-172

[18] Avraham KB, Schickler M, Sapoznikov D, Yarom R, Groner Y. Down's syndrome: Abnormal neuromuscular junction in tongue of transgenic mice with elevated levels of human Cu/Zn-superoxide dismutase. Cell. 1988;**54**(6):823-829

[19] Sheldon R, Jiang X, Francisco C, Christen S, Vexler ZS, Tauber MG, et al. Manipulation of antioxidant pathways in neonatal murine brain. Pediatric Research. 2004;**56**(4):656-662

[20] Nakano M, Sugioka K, Naito I, Takekoshi S, Niki E. Novel and potent antioxidants on membrane phospholipid peroxidation: 2-hydroxyestrone and 2-hydroxyestradiol. Biochemical and Biophysical Research Communications. 1987;**142**:919-924

[21] Calabrese V, Colombrita C, Guagliano E, Sapienza M, Ravagna A, Cardile V, et al. Protective effect of carnosine during nitrosative stress in astroglial cell cultures. Neurochemical Research. 2005;**30**(6-7):797-807

[22] Guiotto A, Calderan A, Ruzza P, Borin G. Carnosine and carnosine-related antioxidants: A review. Current Medicinal Chemistry. 2005;**12**(20):2293-2315

[23] Reddy VP, Garrett MR, Perry G, Smith MA. Carnosine: A versatile antioxidant and antiglycating agent. Science of Aging Knowledge Environment. 2005;**2005**(18):pe12

[24] Dukic-Stefanovic S, Schinzel R, Riederer P, Münch G. AGES in brain ageing: AGE-inhibitors as neuroprotective and anti-dementia drugs? Biogerontology. 2001;**2**(1):19-34

[25] Takahashi H. Studies on homocarnosine in cerebrospinal fluid in infancy and childhood. Part I. Homocarnosine level in cerebrospinal fluid of normal infants and children. Brain & Development. 1981;**3**(3):255-261

[26] Björnsdottir H, Granfeldt D, Welin A, Bylund J, Karlsson A. Inhibition of phospholipase A(2) abrogates intracellular processing of NADPH-oxidase derived reactive oxygen species in human neutrophils. Experimental Cell Research. 2013;**319**(5):761-774

[27] Dechatelet LR, Shirley PS, Johnston RB. Effect of phorbol myristate acetate on the oxidative metabolism of human polymorphonuclear leukocytes. Blood. 1976;**47**: 545-5543

[28] Suzuki Y, Lehrer RI. NAD(P)H oxidase activity in human neutroph1ls stimulated by phorbol myristate acetate. Journal of Clinical Investigation. 1980;**66**:1409-1418

[29] Tepperman BL, Soper BD, Chang Q. Effect of protein kinase C activation on intracellular Ca^{2+} signaling and integrity of intestinal epithelial cells. European Journal of Pharmacology. 2005;**518**(1):1-9

[30] Han NR, Kim HM, Jeong HJ. Thymic stromal lymphopoietin is regulated by the intracellular calcium. Cytokine. 2012;**59**(2):215-217

[31] O'Brien TG, Simsiman RC, Boutwell RK. Induction of the polyamine-biosynthetic enzymes in mouse epidermis by tumorpromoting agents. Cancer Research. 1975;**35**:1662

[32] Greenwood MP, Greenwood M, Paton JF, Murphy D. Control of polyamine biosynthesis by Antizyme inhibitor 1 is important for transcriptional regulation of arginine vasopressin in the male rat hypothalamus. Endocrinology. 2015;**156**(8):2905-2917

[33] Jasper TW, Luttge WG, Benton TB, Garnica AD. Polyamines in the developing mouse brain. Developmental Neuroscience. 1982;**5**:233-242

[34] Slotkin TA, Bartolome J. Role of ornithine decarboxylase and the polyamines in nervous system development: A review. Brain Research Bulletin. 1986;**17**:307-320

[35] Niki E, Traber MG. A history of vitamin E. Annals of Nutrition & Metabolism. 2012;**61**:207-212

[36] Niki E. Lipid peroxidation: Physiological levels and dual biological effects. Free Radical Biology & Medicine. 2009;**47**:469-484

[37] Nishikimi M, Yamada H, Yagi K. Oxidation by superoxide of tocopherol dispersed in aqueous media with deoxycholate. Biochimica et Biophysica Acta. 1980;**627**(1):101-108

[38] Płonka-Półtorak E, Zagrodzki P, Nicol F, Kryczyk J, Bartoń H, Westermarck T, et al. Antioxidant agents and physiological responses in adult epileptic patients treated with lamotrigine. Pharmacological Reports. 2013;**65**(1)

[39] Westermarck T, Johansson E, Atroshi F. Antioxidants may slow down the progress of neuronal ceroid lipofuscinosis (NCL, BATTEN'S disease) including epilepsy. Epileptologia. 2006;**14**(Suppl 1):119

[40] Ernster L. Ubiquinone: Redox coenzyme, hydrogen carrier, antioxidant. In: Folkers K, Yamamura Y, editors. Biomedical and Clinical Aspects of Coenzyme A. Vol. 4. Amsterdam: Biomedical Press; 1984. pp. 3-13

[41] Metcalfe T, Bowen DM, Muller DPR. Vitamin E concentrations in human brain of patients with Alzheimer's disease, fetuses with Down's syndrome, centenarians, and controls. Neurochemical Research. 1989;**14**:1209

[42] Antila E, Nordberg UR, Westermarck T. Antioxidant therapy in Down syndrome (OS). A theory and primary survey. In: Selenium in Biology and Medicine. Fourth International Symposium, July 18-21, 1988. W-Germany: University of TUbingen; 1988

[43] Feeney DM, Sutton RL. Pharmacotherapy for recovery of function after brain injury. Critical Reviews in Neurobiology. 1987;**3**:135-197

[44] Goldstein LB. Effects of amphetamines and small related molecules on recovery after stroke in animals and man. Neuropharmacology. 2000;**39**:852-859

[45] Misra HP, Fridovich I. The role of superox1de anion in the autoxidation of epinephrine and a simple assay for superoxide dismutase. Journal of Biological Chemistry. 1972;**247**:3170-3175

[46] Kohen R, Yamamoto Y, Cundy KC, Ames BN. Antioxidant activity of carnosine, homocarnosine, and anserine present in muscle and brain. Proceedings of the National Academy of Sciences of the United States of America. 1988;**85**(9):3175-3179

[47] Oja SS, Kontro P. Taurine. In: Lajtha A, editor. Handbook of Neurochemistry. Vol. 3. New York: Plenum Press; 1983. pp. 501-553

[48] Pasantes-Morales H, Wright CE, Gaull GE. Taurine protection of lymphoblastoid cells from iron-ascorbate induced damage. Biochemical Pharmacology. 1985;**34**(12):2205-2207

[49] Boullin DJ, Airaksinen EM, Paasonen M. Platelet taurine in Down's syndrome. Medical Biology. 1975;**53**:184-186

[50] Perry TL, Hansen S, Berry K, Mok C, Lesk D. Free amino acids and related compounds in b1ops1es of human brain. Journal of Neurochemistry. 1971;**18**:521-528

[51] Alvarez JG, Storey BT. Taurine, hypotaurine, epinephrine and albumin inhibit lipid peroxidation in rabbit spermatozoa and protect against loss of motility. Biology of Reproduction. 1983;**29**:548-555

[52] Sinet PM, Garber P. Inactivation of the human CuZn superoxide dismutase during exposure to O-2, and H_2O_2. Archives of Biochemistry and Biophysics. 1981;**212**:411-416

[53] Britton G. Structure and properties of carotenoids in relation to function. The FASEB Journal. 1995;**9**:1551-1558

[54] Burton GW, Ingolod KU. Beta-carotene: An unusual type of lipid antioxidant. Science. 1984;**224**:569-573

[55] Chen CH, Han RM, Liang R, Fu LM, Wang P, Ai XC, et al. Direct observation of the β-carotene reaction with hydroxyl radical. The Journal of Physical Chemistry. B. 2011;**115**(9):2082-2089

[56] Maden M. Retinoic acid in the development, regeneration and maintenance of the nervous system. Nature Reviews. Neuroscience. 2007;**8**:755-765

[57] Mey J. New therapeutic target for CNS injury? The role of retinoic acid signaling after nerve lesions. Journal of Neurobiology. 2006;**66**:757-779

[58] Sidell N, Sarafian T, Kelly M, Tsuchida T, Hausler M. Retinoic acid-induced differentiation of human neuroblastoma: a cell variant system showing two distinct responses. Experimental Cell Biology. 1986;**54**:287-300

[59] Jetten AM. Induction of differentiation of embryonal carcinoma cells by retinoids. In: Sherman MI, editor. Retinoids and Cell Differentiation. Boca Raton, Florida: CRC Press Inc.; 1986. pp. 105-136

[60] Pueschel SM, Hillemeier C, Caldwell M, Senft K, Mevs C, Pezzullo JC. Vitamin a gastrointestinal absorption in persons with Down's syndrome. Journal of Mental Deficiency Research. 1990;**34**(Pt 3):269-275

[61] Roizen NJ. Complementary and alternative therapies for Down syndrome. Mental Retardation and Developmental Disabilities Research Reviews. 2005;**11**:149-155

[62] Underwood BA. Vitamin A deficiency disorders: International efforts to control a preventable "pox". The Journal of Nutrition. 2004;**134**:S231-S236

[63] Mandal SK, Dastidar AG. Carotene and retinol levels in the diagnosis of hypothyroidism. The Journal of the Association of Physicians of India. 1985;**33**(10):654-655

[64] Mondul AM, Weinstein SJ, Bosworth T, Remaley AT, Virtamo J, Albanes D. Circulating thyroxine, thyroid-stimulating hormone, and hypothyroid status and the risk of prostate cancer. PLoS One. 2012;**7**(10):e47730. DOI: 10.1371/journal.pone.0047730. Epub October 30, 2012

[65] Patterson D. Molecular genetic analysis of Down syndrome. Human Genetics. 2009; **126**(1):195-214

[66] Malt EA, Dahl RC, Haugsand TM, Ulvestad IH, Emilsen NM, Hansen B, et al. Health and disease in adults with Down syndrome. Tidsskrift for den Norske laegeforening: Tidsskrift for Praktisk Medicin, NY Raekke. 2013;**133**(3):290-294

[67] Weijerman ME, de Winter JP. Clinical practice. The care of children with Down syndrome. European Journal of Paediatrics. 2010;**169**(12):1445-1452

[68] Lozano R, Naghavi M, Foreman K, Lim S, Shibuya K, Aboyans V, et al. Global and regional mortality from 235 causes of death for 20 age groups in 1990 and 2010: A systematic analysis for the Global Burden of Disease Study 2010. Lancet. 2012;**380**(9859):2095-2128

[69] Antonarakis SE, Lyle R, Dermitzakis ET, Reymond A, Deutsch S. Chromosome 21 and Down syndrome: From genomics to pathophysiology. Nature Reviews. Genetics. 2004;**5**:725-738

[70] Epstein CJ, Cox DR, Epstein LB. Mouse trisomy 16: An animal model of human trisomy 21 (Down syndrome). Annals of the New York Academy of Sciences. 1985;**450**:157-168

[71] Lott IT, Dierssen M. Cognitive deficits and associated neurological complications in individuals with Down's syndrome. Lancet Neurology. 2010;**9**:623-633

[72] Mccoy EE, Sneddon JM. Cell biological aspects of Down's syndrome. In: Fedoroff S, Hertz L, editors. Advances in Cellular Neurobiology. Vol. 4. New York: Academic Press; 1983. pp. 249-266

[73] Chadefaux B, Rethore MO, Raoul O, Ceballos I, Poisson-Nier M, Gilgenkranz S, et al. Cystathionine beta synthase. gene dosage effect in trisomy 21. Biochemical and Biophysical Research Communications. 1985;**128**:40-44

[74] Marucci G, Morandi L, Bartolomei I, Salvi F, Pession A, Righi A, et al. Amyotrophic lateral sclerosis with mutation of the Cu/Zn superoxide dismutase gene (SOD1) in a patient with Down syndrome. Neuromuscular Disorders. 2007;**17**:673-676

[75] Sinet PM. Metabolism of oxygen derivatives in Down's syndrome. Annals of the New York Academy of Sciences. 1982;**396**:83-94

[76] Eckmann-Scholz C, Bens S, Kolarova J, et al. DNA-methylation profiling of fetal tissues reveals marked epigenetic differences between chorionic and amniotic samples. PLoS One. 2012;**7**(6):e39014

[77] Huret JL, Delabar JM, Marlhens F, Aurias A, Nicole A, Berthier M, et al. Down syndrome with duplication of a region of chromosome 21 containing the CuZn superoxide dismutase gene without detectable karyotypic abnormality. Human Genetics. 1987;**75**(3):251-257

[78] Elroy-Stein O, Groner Y. Impaired neurotransmitter uptake in PC12 cells overexpressing human Cu/Zn-superoxide dismutase—Implication for gene dosage effects in Down syndrome. Cell. 1988;**52**:259-267

[79] Kedziora J, Bartosz G. Down's syndrome. A pathology involving the lack of balance of reactive oxygen species. Free Radical Biology and Medicine. 1988;**4**:317-330

[80] Francke U. Gene dosage studies in Down syndrome. A review. In Trisomy 21 (Down syndrome) F.F. de la Cruz, P.S. Gerald, editors. University Park Press, Baltimore, 1981, 237-251

[81] Ordonez FJ, Rosety M, Rosety-Rodriguez M. Regular exercise did not modify significantly superoxide dismutase activity in adolescents with Down's syndrome. British Journal of Sports Medicine. 2006;**40**(8):717-718

[82] Sulthana MS, Kumar NS, Sridhar MG, Bhat VB, Rao RK. Antioxidant enzyme activity in children with Down syndrome. Current Pediatric Research. 2012;**16**(1):43-47

[83] Kuroda Y, Kobayashi K, Ichikawa M, Kawahara M, Muramoto K. Application of long-term cultured neurons in aging and neurological research: Aluminum neurotoxicity, synaptic degeneration and Alzheimer's disease. Gerontology. 1995;**41**(Suppl 1):2-6

[84] De Marchena O, Guarnieri M, McKhann G. Glutathione peroxidase levels in brain. Journal of Neurochemistry. 1974;**22**(5):773-776

[85] Brawn K, Fridovich I. Superoxide radical and superoxide dismutases: Threat and defence. Acta Physiologica Scandinavica. 1980;**492**(Suppl):9-18

[86] Mattiei JF, Baeteman MA, Baret A, Ardissone JP, Rebuffel P, Giraud F. Erythrocyte superoxide dismutase and redox enzymes in trisomy 21. Acta Paediatrica Scandinavica. 1982;**71**:589-591

[87] Sailer N. Enzymes. In: Lajtha A, editor. Handbook of Neuro-chemistry. Vol. 1. New York: Plenum Press; 1969. pp. 325-468

[88] Ahmed RG. Hypothyroidism and brain developmental players. Thyroid Research. 2015;**8**:2

[89] Andersen SL, Olsen J, Wu CS, Laurberg P. Psychiatric disease in late adolescence and young adulthood. Foetal programming by maternal hypothyroidism? Clinical Endocrinology. 2014;**81**:126-133

[90] Bass NH, Pelton EW, Young E. Defective maturation of cerebral cortex: An inevitable consequence of dysthyroid states during early postnatal life. In: Grave GD, editor. Thyroid Hormones and Brain Development. New York: Raven Press; 1977. pp. 199-214

[91]   Moog NK, Entringer S, Heim C, Wadhwa PD, Kathmann N, Buss C. Influence of maternal thyroid hormones during gestation on fetal brain development. Neuroscience. 2017;**342**:68-100

[92]   Anderson RB, Newgreen DF, Young HM. Neural crest and the development of the enteric nervous system. Advances in Experimental Medicine and Biology. 2006;**589**:181-196

[93]   Barakat-Walter I. Role of thyroid hormones and their receptors in peripheral nerve regeneration. Journal of Neurobiology. 1999;**40**:541-559

[94]   Romijn HJ, Habets AM, Mud MT, Wolters PS. Nerve outgrow the synaptogenes is and bioelectric activity in fetal rat cerebral cortex tissue cultured in serum-free chemically defined medium. Developmental Brain Research. 1982;**2**:583-589

[95]   Fort P, Lifshitz F, Bellisario R, Davis J, Lanes R, Pugliese M, et al. Abnormalities of thyroid function in infants with Down syndrome. The Journal of Pediatrics. 1984;**104**(4):545-549

[96]   Karlsson B, Gustafsson J, Hedov G, Ivarsson S, Anneren G. Thyroid dysfunction in Down syndrome: Related to age and thyroid autoimmunity. Archives of Disease in Childhood. 1998;**73**:242-245

[97]   Kennedy RL, Jonest TH, Cukle HS. Down's syndrome and the thyroid. Clinical Endocrinology. 1992;**37**:471-476

[98]   Pueschel SM, Pezzullo JC. Thyroid dysfunction in Down syndrome. American Journal of Diseases of Children. 1985;**139**:636-639

[99]   Tuysuz B, Beker DB. Thyroid dysfunction in children with Down's syndrome. Acta Paediatrica. 2001;**90**:1389-1393

[100] Ruf J, Czarnocka B, De Micco C, Dutoit C, Ferrand M, Carayon P. Thyroid peroxidase is the organ-specific 'microsomal' autoantigen involved in the thyroid autoimmunity. Acta Endocrinologica. 1987;**281**:49-56

[101] Karakosta P, Alegakis D, Georgiou V, Roumeliotaki T, Fthenou E, Vassilaki M, et al. Thyroid dysfunction and autoantibodies in early pregnancy are associated with increased risk of gestational diabetes and adverse birth outcomes. The Journal of Clinical Endocrinology and Metabolism. 2012;**97**:4464-4472

[102] McLachlan SM, Rapoport B. The molecular biology of thyroid peroxidase: Cloning, expression and role as autoantigen in autoimmune thyroid disease. Endocrine Reviews. 1992;**13**:192-206

[103] Nilsson M, Molne J, Karlsson FA, Ericson LE. Immunoelectron microscopic studies on the cell surface location of the thyroid microsomal antigen. Molecular and Cellular Endocrinology. 1987;**53**:177-186

[104] Weetman AP, McGregor AM. Autoimmune thyroid disease: Further developments in our understanding. Endocrine Reviews. 1994;**15**:788-830

[105] Boelaert K, Horacek J, Holder RL, Watkinson JC, Sheppard MC, Franklyn JA. Serum thyrotropin concentration as a novel predictor of malignancy in thyroid nodules investigated by fine-needle aspiration. The Journal of Clinical Endocrinology & Metabolism. 2006;**91**(11):4295-4301

[106] Corvilain B, Van Sande J, Laurent E. The H_2O_2-generating system modulates protein iodination and the activity of the pentose phosphate pathway in dog thyroid. Endocrinology. 1991;**128**:779-785

[107] Nunez J, Pommier J. Formation of thyroid hormones. In: Munson PL, Diczfalusy E, Glover J, Olson RE, editors. Vitamins and Hormones. Advances in Research and Applications. New York: Academic Press; 1982. pp. 175-229

[108] Stanley JA, Neelamohan R, Suthagar E, Vengatesh G, Jayakumar J, Chandrasekaran M, et al. Lipid peroxidation and antioxidants status in human malignant and non-malignant thyroid tumours. Human and Experimental Toxicology. 2016;**35**(6):585-597

[109] Prabhakar BS, Bahn RS, Smith TJ. Current perspective on the pathogenesis of graves' disease and ophthalmopathy. Endocrine Reviews. 2003;**24**:802-835

[110] Weetman AP. Autoimmune thyroid disease: Propagation and progression. European Journal of Endocrinology. 2003;**148**:1-9

[111] Bonmort M, Ullrich E, Mignot G, Jacobs B, Chaput N, Zitvogel L. Interferon-gamma is produced by another player of innate immune responses: The interferon-producing killer dendritic cell (IKDC). Biochimie. 2007;**89**(6-7):872-877

[112] Pujol-Borrell R, Todd I. Inappropriate HLA class II in autoimmunity: is it the primary event? In: Doniach D, Botazzo GF, editors. Bai/liere Clinical Immunology and Allergy. London: Batlliere Tindal; 1987. pp. 1-27

[113] Tatsuta T, Sugawara S, Takahashi K, Ogawa Y, Hosono M, Nitta K. Leczyme: A new candidate drug for cancer therapy. BioMed Research International. 2014;**2014**:421415. DOI: 10.1155/2014/421415. Epub April 23, 2014

[114] Taylor GM. Altered expression of lymphocyte functional antigen in Down syndrome. Immunology Today. 1987;**8**:366-369

[115] Blaser S, Propst EJ, Martin D, Feigenbaum A, James AL, Shannon P, et al. Inner ear dysplasia is common in children with Down syndrome (trisomy 21). The Laryngoscope. 2006;**116**(12):2113-2119

[116] Foresta C, Ferlin A, Gianaroli L, Dallapiccola B. Guidelines for the appropriate use of genetic tests in infertile couples. European Journal of Human Genetics. 2002;**10**:303-312

[117] Gravholt CH, Juul S, Naeraa RW, Hansen J. Prenatal and postnatal prevalence of turner syndrome: A registry study. British Medical Journal. 1996;**312**:16-21

[118] Moore SW. Down syndrome and the enteric nervous system. Pediatric Surgery International. 2008;**24**:873-883

[119] Bull MJ, the Committee on Genetics. Health supervision for children with Down syndrome. Pediatrics. 2011;**128**:393-406

[120] Sacks B, Wood A. Hearing disorders in children with Down syndrome. Down Syndrome News and Update. 2003;**3**(2):38-41

[121] Dahle AJ, McCollister FP. Hearing and otologic disorders in children with Down syndrome. American Journal of Mental Deficiency. 1986;**90**(6):636-642

[122] Davies B. Auditory disorders. In: Stratford B, Gunn P, editors. New Approaches to Down Syndrome. London: Cassell; 1996. pp. 100-121

[123] Marcell MM, Cohen S. Hearing abilities of Down syndrome and other mentally handicapped adolescents. Research in Developmental Disabilities. 1992;**13**(6):533-551

[124] Roizen N. Hearing loss in children with Down syndrome: A review. Down Syndrome Quarterly. 1997;**1997**(2):1-4

[125] Tedeschi AS, Roizen NJ, Taylor HG, Murray G, Curtis CA, Parikh AS. The prevalence of congenital hearing loss in neonates with Down syndrome. The Journal of Pediatrics. 2015;**166**(1):168-171

[126] McPherson B, Lai SP, Leung KK, Ng IH. Hearing loss in Chinese school children with Down syndrome. International Journal of Pediatric Otorhinolaryngology. 2007;**71**:1905-1915

[127] Shott SR. Down syndrome: Common paediatric ear, nose and throat problems. Down Syndrome Quarterly. 2000;**5**(2):1-6

[128] Maris M, Wojciechowski M, Van de Heyning P, Boudewyns A. A cross-sectional analysis of otitis media with effusion in children with Down syndrome. European Journal of Pediatrics. 2014;**173**(10):1319-1325

[129] Picciotti PM, Carfi A, Anzivino R, Paludetti G, Conti G, Brandi V, et al. Audiologic assessment in adults with Down syndrome. American Journal on Intellectual and Developmental Disabilities. 2017;**122**:333-341

[130] Miller RM, Groher ME, Yorkston KM, et al. Speech, language, swallowing, and auditory rehabilitation. In: JA DL, Gans BM, editors. Rehabilitation Medicine: Principles and Practice. 3rd ed. Philadelphia, PA: Lippincott-Raven; 1998

[131] Buckley SJ. The significance of hearing loss for children with Down syndrome. Down Syndrome News and Update. 2003;**3**(2):37-37

[132] Miller JF, Leddy M, Leavitt LA, editors. Improving the Communication of People with Down Syndrome. Baltimore: Paul Brookes Publishing; 1999

[133] Abbeduto L, Brady N, Kover ST. Language development and fragile X syndrome: Profiles, syndrome-specificity, and within-syndrome differences. Mental Retardation and Developmental Disabilities Research Reviews. 2007;**13**(1):36-46

[134] Abbeduto L, Murphy MM, Cawthon SW, Richmond EK, Weissman MD, Karadottir S, et al. Receptive language skills of adolescents and young adults with down or fragile X syndrome. American Journal of Mental Retardation. 2003;**108**(3):149-160

[135] Chapman RS, Schwartz SE, Bird EK. Language skills of children and adolescents with Down syndrome: I. Comprehension. Journal of Speech and Hearing Research. 1991;**34**(5):1106-1120

[136] Jarrold C, Baddeley AD. Short-term memory for verbal and Visuospatial information in Down's syndrome. Cognitive Neuropsychiatry. 1997;**2**(2):101-122

[137] Keller-Bell Y, FOX RA. A preliminary study of speech discrimination in youth with Down syndrome. Clinical Linguistics & Phonetics. 2007;**21**:305-317

[138] Laws G, Hall A. Early hearing loss and language abilities in children with Down syndrome. International Journal of Language & Communication Disorders. 2014;**49**(3): 333-342

[139] Rowland LP. Clinical perspective: Phenotypic expression. In: Strohman RC, Wolf S, editors. Muscular Dystrophy, Gene Expression in Muscle. New York, NY: Plenum Press; 1985. pp. 3-5

[140] O'Donovan L, Okamoto I, Arzumanov AA, Williams DL, Deuss P, Gait MJ. Parallel synthesis of cell-penetrating peptide conjugates of PMO toward exon skipping enhancement in Duchenne muscular dystrophy. Nucleic Acid Therapeutics. 2015;**25**(1):1-10

[141] Swash M, Heathfield KW. Quadriceps myopathy: A variant of the limb-girdle dystrophy syndrome. Journal of Neurology, Neurosurgery, and Psychiatry. 1983;**46**:355-357

[142] Beam KG. Duchenne muscular dystrophy. Localizing the gene product. Nature. 1988;**333**(6176):798-799

[143] Hoffman EP, Fischbeck KH, Brown RH, Johnson M, Medori R, Loike JD, et al. Characterization of dystrophin in muscle-biopsy specimens from patients with Duchenne's or Becker's muscular dystrophy. The New England Journal of Medicine. 1988;**318**(21):1363-1368

[144] Bers DM. Cardiac excitation-contraction coupling. Nature. 2002;**415**:198-205

[145] Fabiato A. Time and calcium dependence of activation and inactivation of calcium-induced release of calcium from the sarcoplasmic reticulum of a skinned canine cardiac Purkinje cell. The Journal of General Physiology. 1985;**85**:247-289

[146] Terentyev D, Viatchenko-Karpinski S, Gyorke I, Terentyeva R, Gyorke S. Protein phosphatases decrease sarcoplasmic reticulum calcium content by stimulating calcium release in cardiac myocytes. The Journal of Physiology. 2003;**552**:109-118

[147] Dominski Z, Kole R. Restoration of correct splicing in thalassemic pre-mRNA by antisense oligonucleotides. Proceedings of the National Academy of Sciences of the United States of America. 1993;**90**:8673-8677

[148] Douglas AGL, Wood MJA. Splicing therapy for neuromuscular disease. Molecular and Cellular Neurosciences. 2013;**56**:169-185

[149] Kole R. Modification of pre-mRNA splicing by antisense oligonucleotides. Acta Biochimica Polonica. 1997;**44**:231-237

[150] Kole R, Vacek M, Williams T. Modification of alternative splicing by antisense therapeutics. Oligonucleotides. 2004;**14**:65-74

[151] Lacerra G, Sierakowska H, Carestia C, Fucharoen S, Summerton J, Weller D, et al. Restoration of hemoglobin a synthesis in erythroid cells from peripheral blood of thalassemic patients. Proceedings of the National Academy of Sciences of the United States of America. 2000;**97**(17):9591-9596

[152] Muntoni F, Wood MJA. Targeting RNA to treat neuromuscular disease. Nature Reviews. 2011;**10**:621-637

[153] Suwanmanee T, Sierakowska H, Lacerra G, Svasti S, Kirby S, Walsh CE, et al. Restoration of human beta-globin gene expression in murine and human IVS2-654 thalassemic erythroid cells by free uptake of antisense oligonucleotides. Molecular Pharmacology. 2002;**62**(3):545-553

[154] Wilton SD, Fall AM, Harding PL, McClorey G, Coleman C, Fletcher S. Antisense oligonucleotide-induced exon skipping across the human dystrophin gene transcript. Molecular Therapy. 2007;**15**(7):1288-1296

[155] Wilton SD, Lloyd F, Carville K, Fletcher S, Honeyman K, Agrawal S, et al. Specific removal of the nonsense mutation from the mdx dystrophin mRNA using antisense oligonucleotides. Neuromuscular Disorders. 1999;**9**(5):330-338

[156] Järver P, O'Donovan L, Gait MJ. A chemical view of oligonucleotides for exon skipping and related drug applications. Nucleic Acid Therapeutics. 2014;**24**:37-47

[157] Koo T, Wood MJA. Clinical trials using antisense oligonucleotides in Duchenne muscular dystrophy. Human Gene Therapy. 2013;**24**:479-488

[158] Goemans NM, Tulinius M, van den Akker JT, Burm BE, Ekhart PF, Heuvelmans N, et al. Systemic administration of PRO051 in Duchenne's muscular dystrophy. New England Journal of Medicine. 2011;**364**:1513-1522

[159] Cirak S, Arechavala-Gomeza V, Guglieri M, Feng L, Torelli S, Anthony K, et al. Exon skipping and dystrophin restoration in patients with Duchenne muscular dystrophy after systemic phosphorodiamidate morpholino oligomer treatment: An open-label, phase 2, dose-escalation study. Lancet. 2011;**378**(9791):595-605

[160] Mendell J, Rodino-Klapac LR, Sahenk Z, Roush K, Bird L, Lowes LP, et al. Eteplirsen for the treatment of Duchenne muscular dystrophy. Annals of Neurology. 2013;**74**:637-647

[161] Hunter MI, Brzeski MS, De Vane PJ. Superoxide dismutase, glutathione peroxidase and thiobarbituric acid-reactive compounds in erythrocytes in Duchenne muscular dystrophy. Clinica Chimica Acta. 1981;**115**:93-98

[162] Hunter MI, Mohamed JB. Plasma antioxidants and lipid peroxidation products in Duchenne muscular dystrophy. Clinica Chimica Acta. 1986;**155**(2):123-131

[163] Jackson MJ, Coakley J, Stokes M, Edwards RH, Oster O. Selenium metabolism and supplementation in patients with muscular dystrophy. Neurology. 1989;**39**(5):655-659

[164] Jackson M, Edwards RH. Free radicals and trials of antioxidant therapy in muscle disorders. Advances in Experimental Medicine and Biology. 1990;**264**:485-491

[165] Westermarck T, Rahola T, Kallio AK, Suomela M. Long term turnover of selenite-Se in children with motor disorders. Klinische Pädiatrie. 1982;**194**:301-302

[166] Pedersen BK, Steensberg A, Fischer C, Keller C, Keller P, Plomgaard P, et al. Searching for the exercise factor: Is IL-6 a candidate? Journal of Muscle Research and Cell Motility. 2003;**24**(2-3):113-119

[167] Le Borgne F, Guyot S, Logerot M, Beney L, Gervais P, Demarquoy J. Exploration of lipid metabolism in relation with plasma membrane properties of duchenne muscular dystrophy cells: Influence of L-carnitine. PLoS One. 2012;**7**(11)

[168] Shimomura Y, Suzuki M, Sugiyama S, Hanaki Y, Ozawa T. Protective effect of coenzyme Q10 on exercise-induced muscular injury. Biochemical and Biophysical Research Communications. 1991;**176**:349-355

[169] Belardinelli R, Muçaj A, Lacalaprice F, Solenghi M, Seddaiu G, Principi F, et al. Coenzyme Q10 and exercise training in chronic heart failure. European Heart Journal. 2006;**27**(22):2675-2681

[170] Littarru GP, Tiano L. Clinical aspects of coenzyme Q10: An update. Nutrition. 2010;**26**(3): 250-254

[171] Westermarck T, Atroshi F. Dietary approaches to patients with Duchenne muscular dystrophy (DMD), patients with spielmeyer-sergen disease, and patients with epilepsy. Trace Elements in Medicine. 2005;**6**(2):27-32

[172] Lu A, Poddar M, Tang Y, Proto JD, Sohn J, Mu X, et al. Rapid depletion of muscle progenitor cells in dystrophic mdx/utrophin−/− mice. Human Molecular Genetics. 2014;**23**(18):4786-4800

[173] Lu QL, Mann CJ, Lou F, Bou-Gharios G, Morris GE, Xue SA, et al. Functional amounts of dystrophin produced by skipping the mutated exon in the mdx dystrophic mouse. Nature Medicine. 2003;**9**(8):1009-1014

[174] van Deutekom JC, van Ommen GJ. Advances in Duchenne muscular dystrophy gene therapy. Nature Reviews. Genetics. 2003;**4**(10):774-783

[175] Bennett MJ, Rakheja D. The neuronal ceroid-lipofuscinoses. Developmental Disabilities Research Reviews. 2013;**17**(3):254-259

[176] Mole SE. Batten's disease: Eight genes and still counting? Lancet. 1999;**354**:443-445

[177] Pardo CA, Rabin BA, Palmer DN, Price DL. Accumulation of the adenosine triphosphate synthase subunit C in the mnd mutant mouse. A model for neuronal ceroid lipofuscinosis. The American Journal of Pathology. 1994;**144**(4):829-835

[178] Persaud-Sawin DA, Mousallem T, Wang C, Zucker A, Kominami E, Boustany RM. Neuronal ceroid lipofuscinosis: A common pathway? Pediatric Research. 2007;**61**(2): 146-152

[179] Santavuori P, Haltia M, Rapola J, Raitta C. Infantile type of so-called neuronal ceroid lipofuscinosis part 1. A clinical study of 15 patients. Journal of the Neurological Sciences. 1973;**18**:257-267

[180] Bäckman ML, Santavuori PR, Aberg LE, Aronen ET. Psychiatric symptoms of children and adolescents with juvenile neuronal ceroid lipofuscinosis. Journal of Intellectual Disability Research. 2005;**49**(Pt 1):25-32

[181] Crystal RG, Sondhi D, Hackett NR, Kaminsky SM, Worgall S, Stieg P, et al. Clinical protocol. Administration of a replication-deficient adeno-associated virus gene transfer vector expressing the human CLN2 cDNA to the brain of children with late infantile neuronal ceroid lipofuscinosis. Human Gene Therapy. 2004;**15**:1131-1154

[182] Narayan SB, Pastor JV, Mitchison HM, Bennett MJ. CLN3L, a novel protein related to the batten disease protein, is overexpressed in Cln3−/− mice and in batten disease. Brain. 2004;**127**(Pt 8):1748-1754

[183] Mole SE, Williams RE, Goebel HH. Correlations between genotype, ultrastructural morphology and clinical phenotype in the neuronal ceroid lipofuscinoses. Neurogenetics. 2005;**6**:107-126

[184] Winchester B, Vellodi A, Young E. The molecular basis of lysosomal storage diseases and their treatment. Biochemical Society Transactions. 2000;**28**(2):150-154

[185] Hawkins-Salsbury JA, Cooper JD, Sands MS. Pathogenesis and therapies for infantile neuronal ceroid lipofuscinosis (infantile CLN1 disease). Biochimica et Biophysica Acta. 2013;**1832**(11):1906-1909

[186] Dhar S, Bitting RL, Rylova SN, Jansen PJ, Lockhart E, Koeberl DD, et al. Flupirtine blocks apoptosis in batten patient lymphoblasts and in human postmitotic CLN3- and CLN2-deficient neurons. Annals of Neurology. 2002;**51**(4):448-466

[187] Kohan R, Cismondi IA, Oller-Ramirez AM, et al. Therapeutic approaches to the challenge of neuronal ceroid lipofuscinoses. Current Pharmaceutical Biotechnology. 2011;**12**(6):867-883

[188] Lönnqvist T, Vanhanen SL, Vettenranta K, Autti T, Rapola J, Santavuori P, et al. Hematopoietic stem cell transplantation in infantile neuronal ceroid lipofuscinosis. Neurology. 2001;**57**(8):1411-1416

[189] Neverman NJ, Best HL, Hofmann SL, Hughes SM. Experimental therapies in the neuronal ceroid lipofuscinoses. Biochimica et Biophysica Acta. 2015;**1852**(10 Pt B):2292-2300

[190] Sands MS. Considerations for the treatment of infantile neuronal ceroid lipofuscinosis (infantile batten disease). Journal of Child Neurology. 2013;**28**(9):1151-1158

[191] Traina G, Bernardi R, Cataldo E, Macchi M, Durante M, Brunelli M. In the rat brain acetyl-L-carnitine treatment modulates the expression of genes involved in neuronal ceroid lipofuscinosis. Molecular Neurobiology. 2008;**38**(2):146-152

[192] Banerjee P, Dasgupta A, Siakotos AN, Dawson G. Evidence for lipase abnormality: High levels of free and triacylglycerol forms of unsaturated fatty acids in neuronal ceroid-lipofuscinosis tissue. American Journal of Medical Genetics. 1992;**42**:549-554

[193] Heiskala H, Gutteridge J, Westermarck T, Alanen T, Santavuori P. Bleomycin-detectable iron and phenanthroline-detectable copper in the cerebrospinal fluid of patients with neuronal ceroid-lipofuscinoses. American Journal of Medical Genetics. Supplement. 1988;**5**:193-202

[194] Johansson E, Lindh U, Westermarck T, Heiskala H, Santavuori P. Altered elemental profiles in neuronal ceroid lipofuscinosis. Journal of Trace Elements and Electrolytes in Health and Disease. 1990;**4**(3):139-142

[195] Hall NA, Lake BD, Dewji NN, Patrick AD. Lysosomal storage of subunit c of mitochondrial ATP synthase in Batten's disease (ceroid-lipofuscinosis). The Biochemical Journal. 1991;**275**:269-272

[196] Piattella L, Cardinali C, Zamponi N, Papa O. Spielmeyer-Vogt disease: Clinical and neurophysiological aspects. Child's Nervous System. 1991;**7**(4):226-230

[197] Santavuori P, Heiskala H, et al. Experience over 17 years with antioxidant treatment in Spielmeyer-Sjogren's disease. American Journal of Medical Genetics—Part A. 1988;**5**(Suppl):265-274

[198] Compston A, Coles A. Multiple sclerosis. Lancet. 2002;**359**:1221-1231

[199] Pugliatti M, Rosati G, Carton H, Riise T, Drulovic J, Vécsei L, et al. The epidemiology of multiple sclerosis in Europe. European Journal of Neurology. 2006;**13**(7):700-722

[200] Haegert DG, Marrosu MG. Genetic susceptibility to multiple sclerosis. Annals of Neurology. 1994;**36**(Suppl 2):S204-S210

[201] Skoog B, Runmarker B, Winblad S, Ekholm S, Andersen O. A representative cohort of patients with non-progressive multiple sclerosis at the age of normal life expectancy. Brain. 2012;**135**:900-911

[202] Skoog B, Tedeholm H, Runmarker B, Odén A, Andersen O. Continuous prediction of secondary progression in the individual course of multiple sclerosis. Multiple Sclerosis and Related Disorders. 2014;**3**(5):584-592

[203] Belin J, Pettet N, Smith AD, Thompson RH, Zilkha KJ. Linoleate metabolism in multiple sclerosis. Journal of Neurology, Neurosurgery, and Psychiatry. 1971;**34**(1):25-29

[204] Thompson RH. Fatty acid metabolism in multiple sclerosis. Biochemical Society Symposium. 1972;**35**:103-111

[205] Schwarz S, Leweling H. Multiple sclerosis and nutrition. Multiple Sclerosis. 2005; **11**(1):24-32

[206] Simopoulos AP. Omega-3 fatty acids in inflammation and autoimmune diseases. Journal of the American College of Nutrition. 2002;**21**(6):495-505

[207] Clausen J, Jensen GE, Nielsen SA. Selenium in chronic neurologic diseases. Multiple sclerosis and Batten's disease. Biological Trace Element Research. 1988;**15**:179-203

[208] Gade-Andavolu R, MacMurray JP, Blake H, Muhleman D, Tourtellotte W, Comings DE. Association between the gamma-aminobutyric acid A3 receptor gene and multiple sclerosis. Archives of Neurology. 1998;**55**(4):513-516

[209] Derfuss T. Personalized medicine in multiple sclerosis: Hope or reality? BMC Medicine. 2012;**10**:116

[210] Pueschel SM. Therapeutic approaches in Down syndrome. In: Delacruz FF, Gerald PS, editors. Trisomy 21 (Down syndrome). Baltimore: University Park Press; 1981. pp. 217-224

[211] Harrell RF, Capp RH, Davis DR, Peerless J, Ravitz LR. Can nutritional supplements help mentally retarded children? An exploratory study. Proceedings of the National Academy of Sciences of the United States of America. 1981;**78**(1):574-578

[212] Anjos T, Altmäe S, Emmett P, Tiemeier H, Closa-Monasterolo R, Luque V, et al. Nutrition and neurodevelopment in children: Focus on NUTRIMENTHE project. European Journal of Nutrition. 2013;**52**(8):1825-1842

[213] Bennet FC, McClelland S, Kriegsmann EA, Andrus LB, Sells CJ. Vitamin and mineral supplementation in Down's syndrome. Pediatrics. 1983;**72**:707-713

[214] Kozlowski BW. Megavitamin treatment of mental retardation in children: A review of effects on behavior and cognition. Journal of Child and Adolescent Psychopharmacology. 1992;**2**(4):307-320

[215] Schaevitz L, Berger-Sweeney J, Ricceri L. One-carbon metabolism in neurodevelopmental disorders: using broad-based nutraceutics to treat cognitive deficits in complex spectrum disorders. Neuroscience and Biobehavioral Reviews. 2014;**46**(Pt 2):270-284. DOI: 10.1016/j.neubiorev.2014.04.007. Epub April 23, 2014

[216] Smith GF, Spiker D, Peterson CP, Cicchetii D, Justine P. Use of megadoses of vitamins and minerals in Down syndrome. The Journal of Pediatrics. 1984;**105**:228-234

[217] Antila, E., Nordberg, U-R., Syvaosa, E-L. and Westermarck, T. Selenium therapy in Down syndrome (OS). A theory and a clinical trial. In Antioxidants in Therapy and Preventive Medicine (I. Emerit, L. Packer and C. Auclair). Plenum Pub. Co., New York. 1989.

[218] Antila E, Westermarck T. On the etiopathogenesis and therapy of Down syndrome. The International Journal of Developmental Biology. 1989;**33**:183-188

[219] Halliwell B, Gutteridge JM. Oxygen toxicity, oxygen radicals, transition metals and disease. Biochemical Journal. 1984;**9**:1-14

[220] Slivka A, Mytilineou C, Cohen G. Histochemical evaluation of glutathione in brain. Brain Research. 1987;**409**:275-284

[221] Miller DS. Hereditary hemolytic anemias. Pediatric Clinics of North America. 1972;**19**:865-887

[222] Rocha JC, Martins MJ. Oxidative stress in phenylketonuria: Future directions. Journal of Inherited Metabolic Disease. 2012;**35**(3):381-398

[223] Westermarck T, Raunu P, Kirjarinta M, Lappalainen L. Selenium content of who le blood and serum in adults and children of different ages from different parts of Finland. Acta Pharmacologica et Toxicologica. 1977;**40**:465-475

[224] Thompson CD, Robinson MF, Campbell DR, Rea HM. Effect of prolonged supplementation with daily supplements of selenomethionine and sodium selenite on glutathione peroxidase activity in blood of New Zealand residents. The American Journal of Clinical Nutrition. 1982;**36**:24-31

[225] Westermarck T, Sandholm M. Decreased erythrocyte glutathione peroxidase activity in neuronal ceroid lipofuscinosis (NCL)-corrected with selenium supplementation. Acta Pharmacologica et Toxicologica. 1977;**40**:70-74

[226] Anneren G. Down's syndrome. A metabolic and endocrinological study. Acta Universitatis Upsaliensis. 1984;**483**(VI):1-15, Uppsala

[227] Neve J, Sinet PM, Molle L, Nicole A. Selenium, zinc and copper in Down's syndrome (trisomy 21): Blood levels and relations with glutathione peroxidase and superoxide dismutase. Clinica Chimica Acta. 1983;**133**:209-214

[228] Beilstein MA, Butler IA, Whang ER. Metabolism of 70 Se-selenite by rhesus monkeys. In: Friberg L, Nordberg G, Falke GF, Vouk V, editors. Handbook on the Toxicology of Metals. Amsterdam: Biomedical Press; 1984. pp. 482-520

[229] Westermarck T, Rahola T, Suomela M, Alanen T, Puhakainen M. Biological half-life of Se-selenite and Zn-chloride in Down syndrome patients. In: Mills CF, Bremner I, Chesters JK, editors. Proceedings of the Fifth International Symposium on Trace Elements in Man and Animals. Farnham Royal, Slough SL2 3BN, UK: Commonwealth Agricultural Bureaux; 1985. pp. 792-795

[230] Ani C, Grantham-McGregor S, Muller D. Nutritional supplementation in Down syndrome: Theoretical considerations and current status. Developmental Medicine and Child Neurology. 2000;**42**(3):207-213

[231] Sinet PM, Lejeune J, Jerome H. Trisomy 21 (Down's syndrome). Glutathione peroxidase. Hexose monophosphate shunt and IQ. Life Sciences. 1979;**24**:29-34

[232] Prohaska JR, Ganther HE. Selenium and glutathione peroxidase in developing rat brain. Journal of Neurochemistry. 1976;**27**:1379-1387

[233] Behne O, Hilmert H, Scheid S, Gessner H, Elger W. Evidence for specific selenium target tissues and new biologically important selenoproteins. Biochimica et Biophysica Acta. 1988;**966**:12-21

[234] Germain GS, Arneson RM. Selenium induced glutathione peroxidase activity in mouse neuroblastoma cells. Biochemical and Biophysical Research Communications. 1977;**79**:119-123

[235] Saedi MS, Smith CG, Frampton J, Chambers I, Harrison PR, Sunde RA. Effect of selenium status on MRNA levels for glutathione peroxidase in rat liver. Biochemical and Biophysical Research Communications. 1988;**153**:855-861

[236] Lindner G, Grosse G. Effect of a selenium compound (Na_2SeO_3) on nerve tissue in vitro. Zeitschrift für Mikroskopisch-Anatomische Forschung. 1985;**99**(4):627-638

[237] Parantainen J, Atroshi F. Trace elements as possible keys to biological semiconduction. In: n1 Conf. on Medical. Biochemical and Chemical Aspects of Free Radicals. 1988. 1 (Abstr)

[238] Antila E, Nordberg UR, Syvaoja EL, Westermarck T. Selenium therapy in Down syndrome (DS): A theory and a clinical trial. Advances in Experimental Medicine and Biology. 1990;**264**:183-186

[239] Anneren G, Johansson E, Lindh U. Trace elemental profiles in individual blood cells from patients with Down's syndrome. Acta Paediatrica Scandinavica. 1985;**74**:259-263

[240] Adewuyi YG. Sonochemistry in environmental remediation. 1. Combinative and hybrid sonophotochemical oxidation processes for the treatment of pollutants in water. Environmental Science & Technology. 2005;**39**(10):3409-3420

[241] Dunford HB. Free radicals in iron-containing systems. Free Radical Biology & Medicine. 1987;**3**(6):405-421

[242] Halsted JA, Smith JC Jr. Plasma-zinc in health and disease. Lancet. 1970;**1**:322-324

[243] Milunsky A, Hackley M, Halsted JA. Plasma erythrocyte and leucocyte zinc levels in Down's syndrome. Journal of Mental Deficiency Research. 1970;**14**:99-105

[244] Malakooti N, Pritchard MA, Adlard PA, Finkelstein DI. Role of metal ions in the cognitive decline of Down syndrome. Frontiers in Aging Neuroscience. 2014;**6**:136

[245] Thomson CD. Assessment of requirements for selenium and adequacy of selenium status: A review. European Journal of Clinical Nutrition. 2004;**58**:391-402

[246] Atroshi F, Westermarck T. High concentrations of erythrocyte glutathione in patients with neurological disorders: Possible clinical implications. In: Rice-Evans C, editor. Free Radical Oxidant Stress & Drug Action. London: Richelieu Press; 1987. pp. 419-424

[247] Atroshi F, Parantainen J, Sankari S, Österman T. Prostaglandin and glutathione peroxidase in bovine mastitis. Research in Veterinary Science. 1986;**40**:361-366

[248] Atroshi F, Sankari S, Työppönen J, Parantainen J. Inflammation related changes in trace elements, GSH-metabolism, prostaglandins and sialic acid. In: Hurly LS, Keen CL, Lonnerdal B, Rucker RB, editors. Trace Elements in Man and Animals 6. New York, London: Plenum Press; 1988. pp. 97-99

[249] Chung A-S, Maines MD. Effect of selenium on glutathione metabolism. Induction of gamma-glutamylcysteine synthetase and glutathione reductase in the rat liver. Biochemical Pharmacology. 1981;30:3217-3223

[250] LaFemina MJ, Sheldon RA, Ferriero DM. Acute hypoxia-ischemia results in hydrogen peroxide accumulation in neonatal but not adult mouse brain. Pediatric Research. 2006;59:680-683

[251] McLean CW, Mirochnitchenko O, Claus CP, Noble-Haeusslein LJ, Ferriero DM. Overexpression of glutathione peroxidase protects immature murine neurons from oxidative stress. Developmental Neuroscience. 2005;27:169-175

[252] Wang H, Cheng E, Brooke S, Chang P, Sapolsky R. Over-expression of antioxidant enzymes protects cultured hippocampal and cortical neurons from necrotic insults. Journal of Neurochemistry. 2003;87:1527-1534

[253] Miller BA, Perez RS, Shah AR, Gonzales ER, Park TS, Gidday JM. Cerebral protection by hypoxic preconditioning in a murine model of focal ischemia reperfusion. Neuroreport. 2001;12:1663-1669

[254] Bernaudin M, Tang Y, Reilly M, Petit E, Sharp FR. Brain genomic response following hypoxia and re-oxygenation in the neonatal rat. Identification of genes that might contribute to hypoxia-induced ischemic tolerance. The Journal of Biological Chemistry. 2002;277:39728-39738

[255] Mu D, Jiang X, Sheldon RA, Fox CK, Hamrick SE, Vexler ZS, et al. Regulation of hypoxia-inducible factor 1 alpha and induction of vascular endothelial growth factor in a rat neonatal stroke model. Neurobiology of Disease. 2003;14:524-534

[256] Zellweger H. Genetic aspects of neurological disease. Archives of Internal Medicine. 1965;115:387-397

[257] Boyer SH, Fainer DC. Genetics and diseases of muscle. The American Journal of Medicine. 1963;35:622-631

[258] Cannon JR, Greenamyre JT. The role of environmental exposures in neurodegeneration and neurodegenerative diseases. Toxicological Sciences. 2011;124(2):225-250

[259] Mckusick VA. Medical genetics 1962. Journal of Chronic Diseases. 1963;16:457-634

[260] Hunter DJ. Gene-environment interactions in human diseases. Nature Reviews. Genetics. 2005;6:287-298

[261] van der Mei IA, Otahal P, Simpson S Jr, Taylor B, Winzenberg T. Meta-analyses to investigate gene-environment interactions in neuroepidemiology. Neuroepidemiology. 2014;42(1):39-49

[262]　Kaipainen P, Westermarck T, Kaski M, Iivanainen M, Atroshi F. Determination of levetiracetam in patients with epilepsy and intellectual disability. European Journal of Pharmaceutical Sciences. 2006;**28**(Suppl 1):S38

[263]　Simonato M, Bennett J, Boulis NM, Castro MG, Fink DJ, Goins WF, et al. Progress in gene therapy for neurological disorders. Nature Reviews. Neurology. 2013;**9**(5):277-291

[264]　Poulsen HE. Oxidative DNA modifications. Experimental and Toxicologic Pathology. 2005;**57**(Suppl 1):161-169

[265]　Villamena FA. Chemistry of reactive species. In: Villamna FA, editor. Molecular Basis of Oxidative Stress–Chemistry, Mechanism, and Disease Pathogenesis. Hoboken: John Wiley & Sons, Inc.; 2013. pp. 1-48

[266]　Atroshi F, Tallberg T, Abdulla VM, Westermarck T. The impact of heavy metals on health with special emphasis on cadmium carcinogenesis. In: Behera B, Panda SP, editors. Natural Resource Conservation and Environment Management. New Delhi: APH Publishing Corporation; 2010. pp. 1-12

[267]　Antila E, Mussalo-Rauhamaa H, Kantola M, Atroshi F, Westermarck T. Association of cadmium with human breast cancer. Science of the Total Environment. 1996;**186**:251-256

[268]　Crohns M, Westermarck T, Atroshi F. Prostate cancer, inflammation and antioxidants. In: Hamilton G, editor. Advances in Prostate Cancer. Croatia: InTech; 2013. pp. 401-421

[269]　Tallberg T, Atroshi F. Prostate cancer, the long search for etiologic and therapeutic factors: Dietary supplementation avoiding invasive treatment. In: Spiess PE, editor. Prostate Cancer: From Bench to Bedside. Croatia: InTech Publisher; 2011. pp. 33-52

[270]　Daly AK. Pharmacogenetics of drug metabolizing enzymes in the United Kingdom population: Review of current knowledge and comparison with selected European populations. Drug Metabolism and Personalized Therapy. 2015;**30**(3):165-174

[271]　Mann MW, Pons G. Various pharmacogenetic aspects of antiepileptic drug therapy: A review. CNS Drugs. 2007;**21**(2):143-164

[272]　Rabin KR, Whitlock JA. Malignancy in children with trisomy 21. The Oncologist. 2009;**14**(2):164-173

[273]　Rieder MJ, Carleton B. Pharmacogenomics and adverse drug reactions in children. Frontiers in Genetics. 2014;**5**:78

[274]　Goodman MJ, Brixner DI. New therapies for treating Down syndrome require quality of life measurement. American Journal of Medical Genetics—Part A. 2013;**161A**(4):639-641

[275]　Costa AC, Scott-McKean JJ. Prospects for improving brain function in individuals with Down syndrome. CNS Drugs. 2013;**27**(9):679-702

[276]　Vosslamber S, van Baarsen LG, Verweij CL. Pharmacogenomics of IFN-beta in multiple sclerosis: Towards a personalized medicine approach. Pharmacogenomics. 2009;**10**(1):97-108

[277] Weinshenker BG. Natural history of multiple sclerosis. Annals of Neurology. 1994;**36**(S1,Suppl):S6-S11

[278] WHO. Genes and Human Disease, Genes and Chromosomal Diseases. 1211 Geneva 27, Switzerland: WHO PRESS; 2015

[279] WHO. Neurological Disorders: Public Health Challenges. 1211 Geneva 27, Switzerland: WHO PRESS; 2006

Reactive Oxygen Species and Selenium in Epilepsy and in Other Neurological Disorders

Erkki Antila, Tuomas Westermarck, Arno Latvus and
Faik Atroshi

Additional information is available at the end of the chapter

http://dx.doi.org/10.5772/intechopen.92003

Abstract

Oxidative stress has been implicated in epilepsy and various neurodegenerative disorders. In this review, we elaborate oxidative stress-mediated neuronal loss and assess the role of selenium in some neurological disorders including epilepsy. Selenium as an essential trace element has attracted the attention of many researchers because of its potentialities in human health. It has an important role in the brain, immune response, defense against tissue damage, and thyroid function. Selenium forms part of the active site of the peroxide-destroying enzyme glutathione peroxidase (GSHPx), and it also has other functions, for example in biotransformation and detoxification. Functional and clinical consequences of selenium deficiency states in neurological diseases have been described, and the selenium requirement, which is influenced by various processes, has been discussed. Wide variations have been found in selenium status in different parts of the world, and populations or groups of patients exposed to marginal deficiency are more numerous than was previously thought. Chronic diseases, such as neurological disorders, heart disease, diabetes, cancer, aging, and others, are reported to associate with markers of oxidative damage. It is, therefore, not unreasonable to suggest that antioxidants would alleviate the oxidative damage, resulting in health improvements. In recent years, accumulated evidence in nutrigenomics, laboratory experiments, clinical trials, and epidemiological data have established the role of selenium in a number of conditions. Most of these effects are related to the function of selenium in the antioxidant enzyme systems. Current research activities in the field of human medicine and nutrition are devoted to the possibilities of using selenium as an adjuvant for the treatment of degenerative or free radical diseases such as neurological disorders, inflammatory diseases, and cancer.

Keywords: selenium, antioxidants, oxidative stress, pathogenesis of neurological disorders

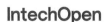

1. Introduction

Selenium is a trace mineral essential to human health, which has an important role in the immune response, defense against tissue damage, and thyroid function. Improving selenium status could help protect against overwhelming tissue damage and infection in critically ill adults [1–4]. Selenium is incorporated into proteins to make selenoproteins, which are important antioxidant enzymes. The antioxidant properties of selenoproteins help prevent cellular damage from free radicals. Free radicals are natural by-products of oxygen metabolism that may contribute to the development of chronic diseases such as cancer and heart disease [5, 6]. There is evidence that selenium deficiency may contribute to development of a form of hypothyroidism and a weakened immune system. Specific diseases have been associated with selenium deficiency such as Keshan and Kashin-Beck disease, which results in osteoarthropathy and myxedematous endemic cretinism, which results in mental retardation [7, 8].

In recent years, considerable evidence has emerged implicating a role for oxygen free radicals in the initiation of cellular injury which can lead to the development of several neurological disorders. The neonatal brain, with its high concentrations of unsaturated fatty acids (lipid content), high rate of oxygen consumption, and low concentrations of antioxidants, is particularly vulnerable to oxidative damage. Thus, increased oxidative stress has been implicated in various neurological disorders such as seizures, ischemia-reperfusion injury, and neurodegenerative diseases [9, 10] such as Alzheimer's, Parkinson's, and Lou Gehrig's disease. Free radical damage has been implicated in the initiation and propagation of seizure activity as well as the accompanying seizure-induced neuronal damage [11]. Therefore, antioxidants could play an important role in modulating susceptibility to seizure activity and seizure-induced neuronal injury.

The use of selenium as a supplement in neurological disorders has been reported. The rationale for selenium supplementation comes from the nutrient's role as an antioxidant [12], working primarily as a component of glutathione peroxidase, an important cellular protector against free radical damage. Furthermore, selenium deficiency is known to result in neuromuscular disease. Attempts have been taken to relate selenium to different neurological disorders as epilepsy, phenylketonuria and maple syrup urine disease, Parkinson's disease, amyotrophic lateral sclerosis, neuronal ceroid lipofuscinoses, myotonic dystrophy, multiple sclerosis, Down syndrome (DS), and Alzheimer's disease [13, 14]. The relevant connection between selenium and the majority of these disorders rests on clinical observations during selenium supplementation alone or in combination with other antioxidants.

2. Selenium distribution in humans

Due to the uneven geographic distribution of selenium in soil, the amount of whole-body selenium in adult humans was reported to differ in different countries [15–18]. At normal dietary levels, the highest selenium concentration was detected in reindeer liver and kidney, followed by the spleen, pancreas, heart, brain, lung, bone, and skeletal muscle. Selenium concentration in the human body was also found to vary with age. For instance, selenium concentration in fetal brain decreased with age but increased with age postnatally. Blood selenium levels were negatively correlated with age in healthy adults, and the same was documented for 40 patients with dementia of the Alzheimer type (DAT). Furthermore, Ejima et al. [19] reported that selenium concentrations varied in different adult human brain regions.

3. Selenium in the brain

Neurochemical aspects of selenium have been widely reported. In this approach to the etio-pathogenetic role of selenium in CNS diseases, teleological ideas are explicitly correlated to the paradigm of oxygen toxicity. The brain differs from many other tissues, being a highly aerobic and totally oxygen-dependent tissue. Oxygen reduction produces reactive radical intermediates, i.e., singlet oxygen, a superoxide radical which is thought to be a major agent of oxygen toxicity. Hydrogen peroxide, H_2O_2, is formed through dismutation of a singlet oxygen catalyzed by Cu-Zn and Mn forms of superoxide dismutase, both found in CNS tissues. Other hydrogen peroxide-generating enzymes are associated with D- and L-amino acid oxidase, monoamine oxidase, a-hydroxyacid oxidase, xanthine oxidase, and cytochrome P-450 system.

Unlike charged oxygen radicals being a rather unreactive and stable, H_2O_2 rapidly crosses cell membranes. Cellular damage is accomplished when H_2O_2 decomposes to the highly reactive hydroxyl radical in iron(II) or copper(I) catalyzed reactions. Scavenging of H_2O_2 and contemporaneous prevention of hydroxyl radical formation occurs predominantly at two cellular sites, in the peroxisomes and in the cytoplasm by catalase and GSHPx (GSHPx, glutathione/hydrogen peroxide oxidoreductase, EC 1.11.1.9), respectively. If this is not done, the hydroxyl radical may attack the fatty acid side chains and start a chain reaction of lipid peroxidation. Lipid peroxidation causes gradual loss of membrane fluidity and membrane potential and increases membrane permeability to ions. Radical attack may also destroy membrane-bound enzymes and receptors, e.g., the binding of serotonin is decreased. Oxidative degradation and polymerization of lipids leads to the accumulation of lipofuscin, the age pigment. The presence of catalytic iron and copper complexes in human CSF, and the high iron content of brain, suggests that they are very sensitive to oxygen radical generation.

The crucial role of selenium as a trace element in the nervous tissue has been associated with a selenoenzyme glutathione peroxidase. Selenium is thought to be present at the active site of GSHPx in its selenolate form as selenocysteine [20]. The fairly homogenous distribution of selenium in the human brain corresponds well with the regions of the highest and lowest GSHPx activity found in the rat brain. However, estimates of the amounts of selenium in rat brain have indicated that GSHPx may account for only 1/5 of the total Se found in the brain [21]. Most of the selenium is bound to proteins and not to amino acids or nucleic acids [22]. Selenoproteins, other than GSHPx, found in the brain and the reproductive and the endocrine organs seem to serve as a priority pathway of the element during inadequate selenium intake. The function of selenium in proteins has been explained in terms of semiconduction [23]. It is possible although not yet proven that selenium may have this or some other special functions outside of GSHPx too.

Observations suggest that free radical intermediates may be involved in the coupling between depolarization of the plasma membrane, Ca^{2+} fluxes, and neurotransmitter release [24]. In general, cellular redox adjustments regulate functional sulfhydryl groups of proteins. Therefore, cellular prooxidant states may be involved in the generation of physiological responses. This means that the adjustment of redox equilibrium in CNS is a far more delicate phenomenon than just a tendency to a normal balance.

The regulation of GSH level (GSH/GSSG) through pentose phosphate pathway producing NADPH, GSH-reductase, and GSHPx contributes to the overall redox state of cells in the brain [25]. The brain tends to need radical reactions as well as to possess specific or high endogenous levels of free radical scavengers such as dopamine, norepinephrine, and catechol estrogens, taurine and carnosine [26], in neurons. Carnosine is involved with GSBA activity in the brain, and a study by Takahashi [27] demonstrated that homocarnosine levels were high in patients who responded to antiepileptic drugs. The functional balance between various free radical scavenger systems in the brain seems reasonable. Significant positive correlations between catalase and SOD levels have been reported in tissues of normal subjects excluding erythrocytes. Factors concomitantly influencing the variation of the activities of SOD, catalase, and GHSPx have been reported. Enzymes frequently called a protective should rather be envisaged as being regulatory, controlling the levels of different states of oxygen reduction.

4. Brain antioxidant homeostasy in relation to selenium and GSHPx

As a trace element in nature, the availability of selenium may be limited. GSHPx activity has been shown to reflect selenium status in deficient and adequate states [6]. On the other hand, protection against toxicity is likely to involve the alterations in GSH metabolism that occur in nutritional Se deficiency. High concentrations of erythrocyte glutathione in patients with neurological disorders have been reported [28]. However, regulatory mechanisms apparently exist which ensure that during periods of insufficient selenium intake, the content of the element is kept up above all in the brain and the reproductive and endocrine organs.

Yoshida et al. [29] reported a comprehensive method for identifying the selenium-binding proteins using PenSSeSPen as a model of the selenium metabolite, selenotrisulfide (RSSeSR, STS), which was applied to a complex cell lysate generated from the rat brain. The authors stated that a thiol-containing protein at m/z 15155 in the brain cell lysate was identified as the cystatin-12 precursor (CST12) from a rat protein database search and a tryptic fragmentation experiment. CST12 belongs to the cysteine proteinase inhibitors of the cystatin superfamily that are of interest in mechanisms regulating the protein turnover and polypeptide production in the central nervous system and other tissues. Consequently, CST12 is suggested to be one of the cytosolic proteins responsible for the selenium metabolism in the brain [29].

Selenium seems to be somehow involved in the regulation of oxygen metabolism through its influence on a variety of enzymes. In concentrations of 6×10^{-7} to $\times 10-6$ M, selenite induces a 30-fold increase of GSHPx activity in neuroblast cells in vitro. Other studies with the rat liver have suggested that Se status regulates the level of GSHPx mRNA as well as regulates GSHPx protein concentration and GSHPx activity [30]. In concentrations of $0.7–2 \times 10^{-5}$ M, Se in rat liver increases the activities of g-glutamylcysteine synthetase, the first rate-limiting enzyme in GSH biosynthesis, and GSSG-reductase, which catalyzes the reduction of GSSG to GSH [31]. In some species the induction of GSH-S-transferase has been shown to occur as a result of Se deficiency. H_2O_2 as the most stable and diffusible of the oxygen reduction intermediates may exert an influence on the expression of SOD, catalase, and GSHPx activities. GSHPx, which exists in several forms that differ in their primary structure and localization, catalyzes the reduction of hydrogen peroxide and organic hydroperoxide by glutathione and functions in the protection of cells against oxidative damage [32]. The homeostasy in the oxidative metabolism and oxygen reduction may be distorted by different means, either inherent or acquired. Depending on the spatial and temporal occurrence of the distortion, various neurological states are expressed.

The developing brain is particularly susceptible to oxidative stress, more so than the mature brain [33]. H_2O_2 accumulation has also been associated with increased injury in superoxide dismutase-overexpressing neonatal murine brain, and greater cell death is seen when immature neurons are exposed to H_2O_2 than mature neurons. Increased H_2O_2 accumulation may be the result of relative insufficiency of the endogenous enzyme GSHPx.

Under physiologic circumstances, the brain has efficient antioxidant defense mechanisms, including GSHPx, which converts potentially harmful H_2O_2 to oxygen and water at the expense of reduced GSH. Under oxidative stress, in the immature brain, endogenous levels of GSHPx may be inadequate for converting excess H_2O_2. Transgenic mice that overexpress GSHPx (hGPx-tg), when subjected to hypoxic-ischemic (HI), have less histologic brain injury than their Wt littermates [25]. In addition, the cortex exhibits increased GSHPx enzyme activity at 24 h, whereas GSHPx activity remains unaltered in the Wt brain. In addition, neurons cultured from GSHPx-tg brain are resistant to injury from exogenously applied H_2O_2 [34]. Neurons cultured from the hippocampus and cortex that are transfected (transfection describes the introduction of foreign material into eukaryotic cells) with genes for catalase and GSHPx also show protection from neurotoxic insults and a corresponding decrease in H_2O_2 accumulation [35]. These findings indicate that adequate GSHPx activity can ameliorate injury to the immature brain from oxidative stress due to H_2O_2.

It is well established that previous stress to the brain can induce tolerance to subsequent injury, a phenomenon called personality change (PC). In neonatal rodents, protection against HI brain injury has been induced by PC with a period of hypoxia before the induction of HI [36]. The mechanisms of this protection have yet to be fully determined, but it has been established that a large number of genes are induced in response to hypoxia [37]. Several of these genes are regulated by the transcription factor hypoxia-inducible factor-1α (HIF-1α) and perhaps most importantly vascular endothelial growth factor (VEGF) and erythropoietin (EPO). VEGF is upregulated after focal ischemic injury in the neonatal rat, in parallel with induction of HIF-1α [38, 39].

5. Aging, dementia, and Alzheimer's disease

Major interest in CNS selenium is related to aspects of oxidative stress and aging. The decrease in cerebral blood flow, glucose utilization, and oxygen consumption common to many dementias results from abnormalities of brain structure with a high oxidative capacity. During mental activity, regional cerebral oxidative metabolism and regional cerebral blood flow increase in several areas of the brain. In dementia of the Alzheimer type, brain blood flow and oxidative metabolism are reduced. This situation may lead to loss of balance between prooxidants and antioxidants [40]. The role of H_2O_2 in the etiology of Alzheimer's disease has been reported [41, 42]. Furthermore, the activities of catalase and GSHPx decrease with aging in intact animals. Some reports suggest that the SOD activity is significantly greater in Alzheimer cell fibroblasts. Both GSHPx and SOD activities in the erythrocytes of AD have been reported to be normal, while other studies show significantly higher erythrocyte SOD level in AD [43]. It remains to be seen whether oxidative damage will still be related to the accumulation of aluminum silicates in the brain as well as to that of the senile plaques and tangles. Experiments have indicated that aluminum salts may not only accelerate Fe(II)-induced peroxidation of membrane lipids but do this especially in the brain [44, 45].

In order to evaluate the peroxidative stress in dementias, autopsy brain samples should be studied for GSHPx, SOD, catalase, and selenium. A direct causal relationship between brain antioxidant defenses and dementia in aging and Alzheimer's disease is hard to demonstrate because of the extremely slow process. Interestingly a high proportion of Down syndrome patients develop the neuropathological and clinical changes of AD, suggesting a close patho-genetic relationship between these disorders. Thus, the correction of antioxidant balance in AD by Se supplementation should be demonstrated by other means so as to direct it preventatively to those with a high risk of developing AD.

In Alzheimer's disease the H_2O_2 molecule should be considered a therapeutic target for treatment of the oxidative stress associated with the disease. The actions of H_2O_2 include modification of DNA, proteins, and lipids, all of which are effects seen in an Alzheimer's disease brain, possibly contributing to the loss of synaptic function characteristic of the disease. Future research and development of agents that specifically target the H_2O_2 molecule or enzymes involved in its metabolism may provide the future route to Alzheimer's disease therapy [42].

6. Down syndrome

Trisomy 21 (Down syndrome) is the most common genetic cause of learning disability in humans [46], occurring in about 1 per 1000 babies born each year [47]. Postmortem studies have reported neuronal depletion and structural abnormalities of the brain during late gestation and early postnatal life [48]. Down syndrome was found to have increased activity of superoxide dismutase without a compensatory increase in glutathione peroxidase activity [49]. However, there is no evidence to support the use of antioxidant or folinic acid supplements in children with Down syndrome [50].

Increased primary gene products which may contribute to the pathology of DS include cytoplasmic CuZn-superoxide dismutase (SOD). Consistent with the gene dosage effect, SOD activity is increased by 50%, leading to noxious concentrations of H_2O_2, while brain GSHPx remains normal. The overall redox state in other tissues is corrected by an adaptive increase of GSHPx activity. This means that the brain is especially susceptible to oxygen free radical stress. Our primary survey of specific antioxidant therapy with selenium [51] rests on this theory.

The whole-body retention of 5–8 kBq ^{75}Se-sodium selenite with 0.4 g Se as carrier/kg body weight in DS patients has been earlier estimated to be 53.3 + 21.1%. Stable Se supplementation increased ^{75}Se elimination, indicating a saturated Se pool in the body. Twenty-four patients aged 1–41 years were either given selenium supplements of 0.025 mg Se/kg/d in the form of sodium selenite or given placebo or no preparation. The serum levels of selenium indicated no real deficiency as compared to the normal healthy population. However, the mean compensatory increase of erythrocyte GSHPx activity before supplementation was lower than expected. Because of difficulties in obtaining brain biopsies, variables found in the plasma and erythrocyte samples were used as indicators of antioxidant balance. Sinet et al. [52] have reported a high positive correlation between erythrocyte GSHPx values and the intelligence quotient in DS patients. Because of this and the difficulties in testing changes of IQ which is one of the most decisive clinical goals of therapy, we found it reasonable to follow changes of E-GSHPX. Selenium supplementation increased E-GSHPx activity by 28% (59.9% above normal). The correction is sensitive to adequate Se supplementation as indicated by SOD/GSHPx index which decreased by 23.9% (P < 0.01) [51]. Interestingly the primarily high serum and blood mononuclear cell levels of cupric and ferrous ions decreased, and that of zinc ions increased during supplementation. In conclusion we believe that the patients have benefited from the selenium supplementation through optimization of their antioxidant protection by GSHPx.

7. Selenium and epilepsy

An epilepsy syndrome is a complex of signs and symptoms defining a unique condition [53]. Oxidative stress and generation of reactive oxygen species are strongly implicated in a number of neuronal and neuromuscular disorders, including epilepsy. The functions of selenium as an antioxidant trace element are believed to be carried out by selenoproteins that possess antioxidant activities and the ability to promote neuronal cell survival. Selenoproteins are important for normal brain function, and decreased function of selenoproteins may lead to impaired cognitive function and neurological disorders [54].

Free radicals and lipoperoxidation reactions seem to be involved in epileptic seizure developing after brain hemorrhage of different kinds. There is an association between hemosiderin deposition and post-traumatic epilepsy. An extravasation of blood and hemolysis of erythrocytes result in the decompartmentalization of free iron and accelerate the rates of lipoperoxidation and superoxide-dependent formation of OH radicals, which are propagated by reperfusion and reoxygenation in postischemic tissue injury. Simultaneously the activity of GSHPx in the ischemic tissue is decreasing. Selenium and other antioxidants have been observed to prevent synergistically the lipoperoxidation in animals and in man. Pretreatment of rats with vitamin E and selenium prior to iron injections has been shown to prevent the development of seizures to a high degree in a large percentage of experimental rats [55]. There are also reports of the normalization of the EEG of patients with the juvenile type of neuronal ceroid lipofuscinosis (JNCL) after vitamin E and sodium selenite supplementation. In addition, the onset of epilepsy is significantly earlier among JNCL patients not given this antioxidant therapy (11.1 year) than patients receiving antioxidant therapy (13.6 year) [56].

Numerous evidences suggest that selenium may ameliorate some of the adverse metabolic consequences of valproic acid. Valproic acid therapy has been shown to deplete plasma selenium levels, a cofactor required for glutathione peroxidase activity. Selenium supplement may help lower ammonia level in patients with valproate-induced hyperammonemia over long-term treatment. Selenium deficiency may lead to the loss of seizure control, even when the patient is remained on the same dose of valproic acid [57, 58]. Furthermore, Ashrafi et al. [59] concluded that the measurement of serum selenium in patients with intractable epilepsy should be considered.

8. Juvenile type of neuronal ceroid lipofuscinosis

The neuronal ceroid lipofuscinoses (NCL) are a group of recessively inherited neurodegenerative-lysosomal storage diseases of infancy, with an estimated occurrence of 1 in 12,500 live births [60–62]. Characteristics of the diseases are deposits of ceroid and lipofuscin pigments in the tissues, particularly in the neural tissue, visual failure, and progressive mental retardation. Depending on the age of onset and clinical, electrophysiological, and neuropathological features, the NCLs can be subdivided into the infantile, the late infantile, the juvenile, and the adult type of NCL. The pathogenesis of NCL is unknown. The polyenic acid level with low levels of linoleic acid and an inverse relationship between GSHPx activity and the level of eicosatrienoic acid has been observed in JNCL [63].

The occurrence of the fluorescent pigments suggested the peroxidation of lipids in the etiology of NCL. It is likely that the diseased tissues peroxidize more rapidly than normal tissues and cytotoxic end products of lipoperoxidation cause secondary damage. On a weight basis, ceroid seen in JNCL patients binds five times more iron than the lipofuscin seen in normal elderly individuals. The increased levels of aluminum salts greatly enhance iron-dependent damage to membranes. Heiskala et al. [64] have confirmed the presence of complexable iron and copper in the CSF of patients with NCL and other neurological disorders, and when the pH value of the assay for iron was lowered, the NCL group had substantially more complexable iron in their CSFs. Interestingly aluminum has been observed in CSF and in ceroid lipofuscin pigments of the brain of NCL patients [65]. It is well established that damaged tissue releases metals from protein-bound sites and these metals stimulate peroxidative damage to lipids and other biomolecules.

One of the most essential enzymes counteracting lipoperoxidation is the selenium-containing GSHPx. Two independent reports have demonstrated that erythrocyte GSHPx activity is decreased in JNCL patients [66, 67]. This low GSHPx activity was reversed to normal level by selenium supplementation.

The evaluation of sodium selenite absorption and losses before supplementation of JNCL patients has been studied by using total body counting for ^{75}Se detection. These studies showed that in three JNCL patients, about 55% of the administered ^{75}Se was eliminated during the first 11 days in the feces and about 10% in the urine [68]. Compared to healthy controls (n = 2, percentages 42% and 7%, respectively), findings indicate a reduced absorption of selenium in JNCL patients contrary to a previous report. The low GSHPx activity in NCL patients may indeed reflect a low selenium intake, most probably due to a disturbed absorption of selenium and secondary phenomena due to an inborn error of metabolism. Apart from the low selenium status, also very low vitamin E levels are found in the serum of advanced and hospitalized NCL patients. This can be explained by the recent finding of a pronounced reduction of apo-protein B as well as the whole fraction of very low density lipoprotein (VLDL) in JNCL patients.

JNCL patients (genetically subgroups) have been given daily supplementation of sodium selenite (0.05–0.1 mg/Se/kg of b.w.), vitamin E (α-tocopherol acetate 0.014–0.05 g/kg b.w.), vitamin B_2 (0.025–0.05 mg/kg b.w.), and vitamin B_6 (0.63–0.8 mg/kg b.w.). The benefits of the therapy are corroborated by the significant negative correlation of GSHPx activity with neurological dysfunction of motor performance, balance, coordination, and speech [69]. The mean age at death has been extended by 4 years as compared to that at the beginning of the century. As the best responders to antioxidant therapy show no neurological dysfunction at the age of over 20 years, there is no doubt that the life expectancy of JNCL patients receiving antioxidants, including selenium, will be significantly prolonged in the future [70]. Complications of the antioxidant therapy have been few and not severe. Six patients have experienced vomiting and nausea when the serum concentration of selenium reached the level of 4.5–5 M. Serum levels up to 4.0 M were usually well tolerated as well as when the sodium selenite was changed to EbselenR (2-Phenyl-1,2-benzoselenazol-3-one).

9. Multiple sclerosis (MS)

Multiple sclerosis is a severe neurodegenerative disease of polygenic etiology affecting the central nervous system. Low levels of polyenic acids are involved in the pathogenesis of both MS and JNCL [71, 72]. In 1972 Thompson et al. found decreased levels of serum linoleate as well as unsaturated fatty acids of brain phospholipids in MS patients. It has also been shown that supplementation with essential fatty acids may improve the clinical status of young MS patients diagnosed early. As in NCL, the selenium may by activating GSHPx (scavenger of organic peroxides) regulate the metabolic transformation of essential fatty acids and biotransformation of these to prostaglandins, thromboxanes, and leukotrienes. Curiously decreased GSHPx activities in erythrocytes have been found in female but not in male MS patients [73].

Blood selenium levels have been reported to be lower in MS patients than in healthy controls [74–76]. However, selenium concentration has been shown to be normal in plasma and erythrocytes but lowered in platelets of MS patients. Impaired Se status has been found in MS largely in the connection of severe protein-calorie malnutrition. Treatment of MS with Se supplementation does not seem warranted in the absence of demonstrated deficiency. Thus, in the reported selenium-containing antioxidant treatments, the clinical benefit to the course of MS has remained open to speculation.

10. Neurotoxicity

10.1 Mercury intoxication

Mercury is well known for its severe toxicity especially by inhalation [77]. People exposure to Hg is mainly due to environmental pollution and the consumption of fish or other aquatic product [78]. Chronic mercury poisoning is characterized by neurological and psychological symptoms, such as tremor, restlessness, personality changes, anxiety, sleep disturbance, and depression. Symptoms are reversible after cessation of exposure. Because of the blood-brain barrier, there is no central nervous involvement related to inorganic mercury exposure [79]. Selenium interacts in the body with a wide range of toxic metals such as arsenic, cadmium, mercury, copper, silver, and lead. It has been shown to be highly effective in animals in preventing brain damage of organic and inorganic mercury. In postmortem brain samples from persons exposed to mercury vapors, mercury and selenium were found at a molar ratio of approximately 1. This indicates that the brain is the target organ in human exposure to mercury vapors. Mercury and selenium react in various ways. The role of brain selenium in inorganic heavy metal toxicity is thought to be minimal [80, 81]. Mercuric ion bound to selenium is proposed to form a biologically inert complex, leading to increased body burden of both elements. This reaction seems to take place only when a threshold of mercury exposure is exceeded. Selenium influences the oxidation rate of elemental mercury in cases of low GSHPx activity; decreased mercury oxidation may lead to increased brain uptake. Selenium may also together with vitamin E counteract mercury-induced lipid peroxidation.

11. Other CNS diseases related to selenium

11.1 Parkinson's disease

Parkinson's disease (PD) is a chronic and progressive movement disorder, meaning that symptoms continue and worsen over time. Oxidative stress is also thought to have a pathogenic role in Parkinson's disease [82, 83]. Selenium protects cellular elements from oxidative damage and may participate in redox-type reactions. Low plasma selenium concentrations are associated with subtle neurological impairments reflected in soft neurological signs [84, 85]. Plasma Se was the only statistically significant difference of up to 16 elements identified for PD patients [86] relative to Alzheimer's disease patients. Redox-active role is evidenced by an increased lipid peroxidation and reduced glutathione levels [87] and high concentration of iron and free radical generation via autocatalytic mechanisms within neuromelanin-containing catecholaminergic neurons in the substantia nigra. In addition, the observation that exogenous administration of cysteine, N-acetyl cysteine, or glutathione decreased the neurotoxic effects of 6-hydroxydopamine in vitro and in vivo reinforces this hypothesis [88].

11.2 Tardive dyskinesia

Tardive dystonia (TD), a rarer side effect after longer exposure to antipsychotics, is characterized by local or general, sustained, involuntary contraction of a muscle or muscle group, with twisting movements, generally slow, which may affect the limbs, trunk, neck, or face [89, 90]. This condition is characterized by involuntary movements. These abnormal movements most often occur around the mouth. The disorder may range from mild to severe. For some people, it cannot be reversed, while others recover partially or completely. Tardive dyskinesia is seen most often after long-term treatment with antipsychotic medications. Other names for this specific disorder are linguofacial dyskinesia, oral-facial dyskinesia, tardive dystonia, tardive oral dyskinesia, and TD. Many preclinical and clinical studies have investigated the possible role of selenium and other antioxidants. These studies suggest that free radicals are probably involved in the pathogenesis of TD and that vitamin E and selenium could be efficacious in its treatment.

11.3 Duchenne muscular dystrophy

Muscular dystrophy (MD) is a group of genetic diseases involving progressive weakness and degeneration of the muscles that control movement. In some forms of MD, the heart muscles and other involuntary muscles, as well as other organs, are also affected. There are nine distinct types of MD, with myotonic the most common form among adults and Duchenne the most common form among children, primarily affecting males. MD is an incurable, often fatal disease. It is usually obvious by the age of 5 and evolves progressively until it causes disablement and death, around the age of 20. Death commonly results from involvement of the respiratory muscles. It is recessively inherited and linked to sex, and the gene determining DMD has been mapped in the Xp-21 locus. It has an incidence of 1/3000–1/3500 male births, and one third of the cases come from new mutation. Some affected individuals may develop intellectual disturbance due to unknown mechanism, so far. The sister of an affected individual has a 50% chance of carrying the defective gene. The result of the dystrophic locus on the gene is the absence of dystrophin, a rod-shaped protein that is part of the muscle cytoskeleton.

The genetic alteration produces abnormality in the membrane of the muscular fibers that consists of a disturbance in the calcium transport (Ca^{2+}), inside the muscular fibers, which is the base mechanism of cellular degeneration and necrosis. There is fiber necrosis and replacement of fibers by fat. A nucleotide degradation, and decreased muscle ATP and ADP content, has been reported. The ATP is necessary to drive the Na+/K+ pump, which maintains ionic gradients across the sarcolemma; re-sequester the Ca^{2+} into the cisternae; and have power contraction. The production of ATP can be the result of anaerobic respiration, which breaks glucose down into ATP and lactic acid, or aerobic respiration when ATP, carbon dioxide, and water are formed. A second immediate reserve of energy exists in the form of creatine phosphate, which can donate phosphate to ADP to form ATP, becoming itself creatine. In the resting muscle, glucose is stored as glycogen, and in such a muscle aerobic respiration synthesizes ATP from glucose or fatty acids.

Therapy of DMD has been an elusive goal. Studies with isolated myocytes have shown that lipid peroxidation with an enhanced free radical production can be activated by increasing Ca concentration. Low oxygen saturation in the muscle tissue may stimulate the Il-6 production, a cytokine, which is produced by contracting muscles and released into the blood. The blood circulation of the older Duchenne patients is particularly disturbed. Pedersen et al. [91] have demonstrated that Il-6 affects the metabolic genes, induction of lipolysis, inhibition of insulin resistance, and stimulation of cortisol production. In addition, carbohydrate supplementation during exercise was shown to inhibit the release of Il-6 from contracting muscle. Thus carnitine supplementation is indicated to the Duchenne patients, to make sure that the energy supply will be good.

Johansson et al. [92] hypothesized that increased production of interleukin-6 (IL-6) and tumor necrosis factor-alpha (TNF-alpha) may be important underlying mechanisms in myotonic dystrophy. Patients with high body fat mass had significantly increased insulin levels and decreased morning levels of cortisol, ACTH, and testosterone. IL-6 and TNF-alpha levels are increased, and adrenocortical hormone regulation is disturbed in MD. Adiposity may contribute to these disturbances, which may be of importance for decreased adrenal androgen hormone production and metabolic, muscular, and neuropsychiatric dysfunction in MD [92]. Henríquez-Olguín et al. [93] reported that IL-6 is a key metabolic modulator that is released by the skeletal muscle to coordinate a multisystemic response (liver, muscle, and adipocytes) during physical exercise; the alteration of this response in dystrophic muscles may contribute to an abnormal response to contraction and exercise.

Thus, several kinds of antioxidants have been proposed as a treatment since increased levels of thiobarbituric acid (TBA) reactive material have been found in the muscles and blood of DMD boys [94]. Increased amounts of pentane are expelled by the DMD patients [95]. We have previously reported that the biological half-life of ^{75}Se in DMD patients was significantly shorter than in healthy controls [96]. We also reported that patients with myotonic muscular dystrophy, the most common form of muscular dystrophy in adults, show improvement in muscular force and function when treated with selenium and vitamin E [97].

Shimomura et al. [98] observed a group of trained animals, part of which were coenzyme Q10 treated and had to exercise for 30 min on treadmill, in downhill position. CoQ10-treated animals had higher level of CoQ10 In their muscles, and the early rise in creatine kinase and lactic dehydrogenase plasma levels, due to the exercise, was evident at a remarkably significant lower extent, in the treated ones. Similar observations were also made in humans [99]. Therefore we have been treating the Duchenne patients with CoQ10. We have been given two siblings of whom the elder one got practically no antioxidants and the younger one whose antioxidant treatment started at the age of 6 years. Nutrient supplement protocol for DMD patients included sodium selenite 0.05-0.1 mg Se kg^{-1} b.w. day^{-1} ; alpha-tocopherol, 10-20 mg kg^{-1} b.w. day^{-1}; vitamin B2, 0.2 mg kg^{-1} b.w. day^{-1}; vitamin B6, 5 mg kg^{-1} b.w. day^{-1}; L-carnitine 10–20 mg kg^{-1} b.w. day^{-1}; ubiquinone-10 (coenzyme Q10) 3 mg kg^{-1} b.w. day^{-1} [100]. In the future the therapy may be by producing functional amounts of dystrophin by skipping the mutated exon like what has been done in the mdx dystrophic mouse [101].

12. Personalized gene therapy

The analytical power of modern methods for DNA analysis has outstripped our capability to interpret and understand the data generated. It is vital that we understand the mechanisms through which mutations affect biochemical pathways and physiological systems [102]: major bcr-abl mRNA nucleic acid amplification assay, genetic analysis of progressive muscular dystrophy, genetic analysis of rearranged immunoglobulin gene, and genetic analysis of malignant tumor. The promise of personalized medicines is enormous, particularly for rare disease [103, 104]. The genetic diversity of Emery-Dreifuss muscular dystrophy (EDMD) predicts that a cure will ultimately depend upon the individual's defect at the gene level, making this an ideal candidate for a precision medicine approach [105]. Ataluren known as PTC124 is a drug for the treatment of Duchenne muscular dystrophy caused by a nonsense mutation (nmDMD) and cystic fibrosis caused by a nonsense mutation (nmCF). PTC124 can lead to restoration of some dystrophin expression in human Duchenne muscular dystrophy muscles with mutations resulting in premature stops [106]. Eteplirsen, a phosphoramidite morpholino sequence complementary to a portion of exon 51, is designed to force the exclusion of exon 51 from the mature DMD mRNA. Similar drugs targeting other DMD exons are under development and could theoretically restore reading frame in majority of patients. The fact that such drugs rely on specific sequence information and target the proximate cause of the disease makes these one of the first examples of precision genetic medicine [104, 107].

A common denominator to the spectrum of neurological disorders and selenium seems to be oxygen toxicity. Difficulties exist in giving proper weight to the interaction of the components of a complex system like the brain's antioxidant defense. The presence of multiple and contemporaneous control mechanisms means that a dysregulated system is impaired not only in one but more regulatory or homeostatic mechanism. Supplementation by a single factor like selenium or together with other antioxidants may to a limited extent sustain these mechanisms. However, much more basic research should be done before these complexities can be better understood. The neurological diseases reviewed above have provided the theoretical framework for the continued investigation of the efficacy of the pharmacological manipulation of glutathione concentration and synthesis in treatment of these diseases [108–110].

Acknowledgements

In memoriam of Faik Atroshi (1949–2019)

Our dear friend, collaborator in research and present coauthor Dr Faik Atroshi, PhD, born on September 22, 1949 in Mosul passed unexpectedly away on February 25, 2019. He was until his retirement docent in University of Helsinki, Senior Researcher in Pharmacology and Toxicology, Adjunct Professor in Clinical Genetics and Clinical Nutrition, and Visiting Professor at different international universities. He will be remembered as an exceptionally dedicated and respectable scientist as well as an inspirational mentor and collaborator. We will miss his enthusiasm, creativity, and desire to continuously learn and to integrate knowledge from various fields of biomedicine.

Abbreviations

DAT	dementia of the Alzheimer type
LPO	lipid peroxides
SOD	superoxide dismutase
CAT	catalase
GSH	glutathione
GSHPx	glutathione peroxidase
Zn	zinc
Cu	copper
Cu-Zn SOD	copper zinc superoxide dismutase
ROS	reactive oxygen species
CNS	central nervous system
DHP	enzyme dehydropeptidase
TNF	tumor necrosis factor
GR	glutathione reductase
GSH	glutathione
ADC	arginine decarboxylase
ODC	ornithine decarboxylase
NADPH	nicotinamide adenine dinucleotide phosphate
GST	glutathione-S-transferases
GSSG	oxidized glutathione
AD	Alzheimer's disease
·OH	hydroxyl radical
E-GSHPx	erythrocyte glutathione peroxidase
EEG	electroencephalogram activation: EEG is an essential component in the evaluation of epilepsy
CSF	cerebrospinal fluid
JNCL	juvenile neuronal ceroid lipofuscinosis
MS	multiple sclerosis

Author details

Erkki Antila[1*], Tuomas Westermarck[2], Arno Latvus[3] and Faik Atroshi[4†]

*Address all correspondence to: erkki.antila@pp.fimnet.fi

1 Medical Center Kruunuhaka, Helsinki, Finland

2 Rinnekoti Research Center, Espoo, Finland

3 Helsinki, Finland

4 Department of Pharmacology and Toxicology, University of Helsinki, Finland

† Deceased.

References

[1] Rayman MP. The importance of selenium to human health. Lancet. 2000;356(9225): 233-241

[2] Weiss G, Carver PL. Role of divalent metals in infectious disease susceptibility and outcome. Clinical Microbiology and Infection. Jan 2018;24(1):16-23

[3] Winkel LH, Johnson CA, Lenz M, Grundl T, Leupin OX, Amini M, et al. Environmental selenium research: From microscopic processes to global understanding. Environmental Science & Technology. 2012;46(2):571-579

[4] Fairweather-Tait SJ, Bao Y, Broadley MR, Collings R, Ford D, Hesketh JE, et al. Selenium in human health and disease. Antioxidants & Redox Signaling. 2011;14:1337-1383

[5] Prabhu KS, Lei XG. Selenium. Advances in Nutrition. 2016;7(2):415-417

[6] Thomson CD. Assessment of requirements for selenium and adequacy of selenium status: A review. European Journal of Clinical Nutrition. 2004;58:391-402

[7] Ellis DR, Salt DE. Plants, selenium and human health. Current Opinion in Plant Biology. 2003;6:273-279

[8] Iwasa K, Kanzaki N, Fujishiro T, Hayashi S, Hashimoto S, Kuroda R, et al. Arthroscopic ankle arthrodesis for treating osteoarthritis in a patient with kashin-beck disease. Case Reports in Medicine. 2014;2014:931278

[9] Bains JS, Shaw CA. Neurodegenerative disorders in humans: The role of glutathione in oxidative stress-mediated neuronal death. Brain Research. Brain Research Reviews. 1997;25:335-358

[10] Paglia G, Miedico O, Cristofano A, Vitale M, Angiolillo A, Chiaravalle AE, et al. Distinctive pattern of serum elements during the progression of Alzheimer's disease. Scientific Reports. 2016;6:22769

[11] Halliwell B. Role of free radicals in the neurodegenerative diseases: Therapeutic implications for antioxidant treatment. Drugs & Aging. 2001;**18**(9):685-716

[12] Cameron A, Rosenfeld J. Nutritional issues and supplements in amyotrophic lateral sclerosis and other neurodegenerative disorders. Current Opinion in Clinical Nutrition and Metabolic Care. 2002;**5**(6):631-643

[13] Olson D, Westermarck T, Ekvall SW. Seizures and epilepsy. In: Ekvall SW, Ekvall VK, editors. Pediatric Nutrition in Chronic Diseases and Developmental Didsorders. 2nd ed. New York: Oxford University Press; 2005. pp. 93-96 (Chapter 10)

[14] Sinha I, Karagoz K, Fogle RL, Hollenbeak CS, Zea AH, Arga KY, et al. "Omics" of selenium biology: A prospective study of plasma proteome network before and after selenized-yeast supplementation in healthy men. OMICS. 2016;**20**(4):202-213

[15] Lemire M, Fillion M, Barbosa F Jr, Guimarães JR, Mergler D. Elevated levels of selenium in the typical diet of Amazonian riverside populations. Science of the Total Environment. 2010;**408**(19):4076-4084

[16] Schiavon M, Pilon-Smits EA. The fascinating facets of plant selenium accumulation—Biochemistry, physiology, evolution and ecology. The New Phytologist. 2017;**213**(4):1582-1596

[17] Xun P, Bujnowski D, Liu K, Morris JS, Guo Z, He K. Distribution of toenail selenium levels in young adult Caucasians and African Americans in the United States: The CARDIA Trace Element Study. Environmental Research. 2011;**111**(4):514-519

[18] Zachara BA, Pawluk H, Bloch-Boguslawska E, Sliwka KM, Korenkiewicz J, Skok Z, et al. Tissue level, distribution, and total body selenium content in healthy and diseased humans in Poland. Archives of Environmental Health. 2001;**56**:461-466

[19] Ejima A, Watanabe C, Koyama H, Matsuno K, Satoh H. Determination of selenium in the human brain by graphite furnace atomic absorption spectrometry. Biological Trace Element Research. 1996;**54**:9-21

[20] Wajner M, Latini A, Wyse ATS, Dutra-Filho CS. The role of oxidative damage in the neuropathology of organic acidurias: Insights from animal studies. Journal of Inherited Metabolic Disease. 2004;**27**(4):427-448

[21] Larsen PR, Berry MJ. Nutritional and hormonal regulation of thyroid hormone deiodinases. Annual Review of Nutrition. 1995;**15**:323-352

[22] Wrobel JK, Power R, Toborek M. Biological activity of selenium: Revisited. IUBMB Life. 2016;**68**(2):97-105

[23] Parantainen J, Sankari S, Atroshi F. Biological functions of silicon, selenium and glutathione peroxidase (GSH Px) explained in terms of semiconduction. In: Hurly LS, Keen CL, Bo L, Rucker RB, editors. Trace Elements in Man and Animals 6. New York & London: Plenum Press; 1988. pp. 359-360

[24] Hall ED, Yonkers PA. Attenuation of motor nerve terminal repetitive discharge by the 21-aminosteroid tirilazad: Evidence of a neural calcium antagonist action. Brain Research. 1998;**779**(1-2):346-349

[25] Sheldon R, Jiang X, Francisco C, Christen S, Vexler ZS, Tauber MG, et al. Manipulation of antioxidant pathways in neonatal murine brain. Pediatric Research. 2004;**56**(4):656-662

[26] Nakano M, Sugioka K, Naito I, Takekoshi S, Niki E. Novel and potent antioxidants on membrane phospholipid peroxidation: 2-hydroxy estrone and 2-hydroxy estradiol. Biochemical and Biophysical Research Communications. 1987;**142**:919-924

[27] Takahashi H. Studies on homocarnosine in cerebrospinal fluid in infancy and childhood. Part II. Homocarnosine levels in cerebrospinal fluid from children with epilepsy, febrile convulsion or meningitis. Brain and Development. 1981;**3**:263-270

[28] Atroshi F, Westermarck T. High concentrations of erythrocyte glutathione in patients with neurological disorders: Possible clinical implications. In: Rice-Evans C, editor. Free Radical Oxidant Stress & Drug Action. London: Richelieu Press; 1987. pp. 419-424

[29] Yoshida S, Hori E, Ura S, Haratake M, Fuchigami T, Nakayama M. A comprehensive analysis of selenium-binding proteins in the brain using its reactive metabolite. Chemical & Pharmaceutical Bulletin (Tokyo). 2016;**64**(1):52-58

[30] Saedi MS, Smith CG, Frampton J, Chambers I, Harrison PR, Sunde RA. Effect of selenium status on MRNA levels for glutathione peroxidase in rat liver. Biochemical and Biophysical Research Communications. 1988;**153**:855-861

[31] Chung A-S, Maines MD. Effect of selenium on glutathione metabolism. Induction of gamma-glutamylcysteine synthetase and glutathione reductase in the rat liver. Biochemical Pharmacology. 1981;**30**:3217-3223

[32] Takebe G, Yarimizu J, Saito Y, Hayashi T, Nakamura H, Yodoi J, et al. A comparative study on the hydroperoxide and thiol specificity of the glutathione peroxidase family and selenoprotein P. The Journal of Biological Chemistry. 2002;**277**:41254-41258

[33] LaFemina MJ, Sheldon RA, Ferriero DM. Acute hypoxia-ischemia results in hydrogen peroxide accumulation in neonatal but not adult mouse brain. Pediatric Research. 2006;**59**:680-683

[34] McLean CW, Mirochnitchenko O, Claus CP, Noble-Haeusslein LJ, Ferriero DM. Overexpression of glutathione peroxidase protects immature murine neurons from oxidative stress. Developmental Neuroscience. 2005;**27**:169-175

[35] Wang H, Cheng E, Brooke S, Chang P, Sapolsky R. Over-expression of antioxidant enzymes protects cultured hippocampal and cortical neurons from necrotic insults. Journal of Neurochemistry. 2003;**87**:1527-1534

[36] Miller BA, Perez RS, Shah AR, Gonzales ER, Park TS, Gidday JM. Cerebral protection by hypoxic preconditioning in a murine model of focal ischemiareperfusion. NeuroReport. 2001;**12**:1663-1669

[37] Bernaudin M, Tang Y, Reilly M, Petit E, Sharp FR. Brain genomic response following hypoxia and re-oxygenation in the neonatal rat. Identification of genes that might contribute to hypoxia-induced ischemic tolerance. Journal of Biological Chemistry. 2002;**277**:39728-39738

[38] Mu D, Jiang X, Sheldon RA, Fox CK, Hamrick SE, Vexler ZS, et al. Regulation of hypoxia-inducible factor 1 alpha and induction of vascular endothelial growth factor in a rat neonatal stroke model. Neurobiology of Disease. 2003;**14**:524-534

[39] Song H, Ren X, Liu P. Distribution and inhibition effect of seleno-L-methionine on 4T1 mouse mammary carcinoma. International Journal of Physiology, Pathophysiology an d Pharmacology. 2015;**7**(2):76-86

[40] Berman K, Brodaty H. Tocopherol (Vitamin E) in Alzheimer's disease and other neuro-degenerative disorders. CNS Drugs. 2004;**18**(12):807-825

[41] Huebbe P, Jofre-Monseny L, Boesch-Saadatmandi C, Minihane AM, Rimbach G. Effect of apoE genotype and vitamin E on biomarkers of oxidative stress in cultured neuronal cells and the brain of targeted replacement mice. Journal of Physiology and Pharmacology. 2007;**58**(4):683-698

[42] Milton NGN. Role of hydrogen peroxide in the aetiology of Alzheimer's disease: Implications for treatment. Drugs and Aging. 2004;**21**(2):81-100

[43] Chang YT, Chang WN, Tsai NW, Huang CC, Kung CT, Su YJ, et al. The roles of bio-markers of oxidative stress and antioxidant in Alzheimer's disease: A systematic review. BioMed Research International. 2014;**2014**: Article ID 182303, 14 p. DOI: 10.1155/2014/182303

[44] Kuroda Y, Kobayashi K, Ichikawa M, Kawahara M, Muramoto K. Application of long-term cultured neurons in aging and neurological research: Aluminum neuro-toxicity, synaptic degeneration and Alzheimer's disease. Gerontology. 1995;**41**(Suppl 1):2-6

[45] Sumathi T, Shobana C, Kumari BR, Nandhini DN. Protective role of Cynodon dactylon in ameliorating the aluminium-induced neurotoxicity in rat brain regions. Biological Trace Element Research. 2011;**144**(1-3):843-853

[46] Malt EA, Dahl RC, Haugsand TM, Ulvestad IH, Emilsen NM, Hansen B, et al. Health and disease in adults with Down syndrome. Tidsskrift for den Norske laegeforening: Tidsskrift for praktisk medicin, ny raekke. 2013;**133**(3):290-294

[47] Weijerman ME, de Winter JP. Clinical practice. The care of children with Down syn-drome. European Journal of Paediatrics. 2010;**169**(12):1445-1452

[48] Becker L, Mito T, Takashima S, Onodera K. Growth and development of the brain in Down syndrome. Progress in Clinical and Biological Research. 1991;**373**:133-152

[49] Brooksbank BW, Balazs R. Superoxide dismutase, glutathione peroxidase and lipoper-oxidation in Down's syndrome fetal brain. Brain Research. 1984;**318**:37-44

[50] Ellis JM, Tan HK, Gilbert RE, Muller DP, Henley W, Moy R, et al. Supplementation with antioxidants and folinic acid for children with Down's syndrome: Randomised controlled trial. BMJ. 2008;**336**(7644):594-597

[51] Antila E, Nordberg UR, Syvaoja EL, Westermarck T. Selenium therapy in Down syndrome (DS): A theory and a clinical trial. Advances in Experimental Medicine and Biology. 1990;**264**:183-186

[52] Sinet PM, Lejeune J, Jerome H. Trisomy 21 (Down's syndrome), glutathione peroxidase, hexose monophosphate shunt and IQ. Life Sciences. 1979;**24**:29-34

[53] Guerrini R. Valproate as a mainstay of therapy for pediatric epilepsy. Pediatric Drugs. 2006;**8**(2):113-129

[54] Pillai R, Uyehara-Lock JH, Bellinger FP. Selenium and selenoprotein function in brain disorders. IUBMB Life. 2014;**66**(4):229-239

[55] Willmore LJ. Post-traumatic epilepsy: Cellular mechanisms and implications for treatment. Epilepsia. 1990;**31**(Suppl 3):S67-S73

[56] Santavuori P, Westermarck T, Rapola J, Pohja P, Moren R, Lappi M, et al. Antioxidant treatment in Spielmeyer-Sjögren disease. Acta Neurologica Scandinavica. 1985;**71**:136-145

[57] Humphreys S, Murti G, Holmes MD. Selenium deficiency and valproate-induced hyperammonemia: 1.320. Epilepsia. 2004;**45**(Suppl 7):122-123

[58] Płonka-Półtorak E, Zagrodzki P, Nicol F, Kryczyk J, Bartoń H, Westermarck T, et al. Antioxidant agents and physiological responses in adult epileptic patients treated with lamotrigine. Pharmacological Reports. 2013;**65**(1):99-106

[59] Ashrafi MR, Shabanian R, Abbaskhanian A, Nasirian A, Ghofrani M, Mohammadi M, et al. Selenium and intractable epilepsy: Is there any correlation? Pediatric Neurology. 2007;**36**(1):25-29

[60] Herrmann P, Druckrey-Fiskaaen C, Kouznetsova E, Heinitz K, Bigl M, Cotman SL, et al. Developmental impairments of select neurotransmitter systems in brains of Cln3(Deltaex7/8) knock-in mice, an animal model of juvenile neuronal ceroid lipofuscinosis. Journal of Neuroscience Research. 2008;**86**(8):1857-1870

[61] Kyttala A, Lahtinen U, Braulke T, Hofmann SL. Functional biology of the neuronal ceroid lipofuscinoses (NCL) proteins. Biochimica et Biophysica Acta. 2006;**1762**:920-933

[62] Mole SE. Batten disease: Four genes and still counting. Neurobiology of Disease. 1998;**1998**(5):287-303

[63] Banerjee P, Dasgupta A, Siakotos AN, Dawson G. Evidence for lipase abnormality: High levels of free and triacylglycerol forms of unsaturated fatty acids in neuronal ceroid-lipofuscinosis tissue. American Journal of Medical Genetics. 1992;**42**(4):549-554

[64] Heiskala H, Gutteridge JMC, Westermark T, Alanen T, Santavuori P. Bleomycin-detectable iron and phenanthroline-detectable copper in the cerebrospinal fluid of

patients with neuronal ceroid-lipofuscinoses. American Journal of Medical Genetics. Supplement. 1988;5:193-202

[65] Johansson E, Lindh U, Westermarck T, Heiskala H, Santavuori P. Altered elemental profiles in neuronal ceroid lipofuscinosis. Journal of Trace Elements and Electrolytes in Health and Disease. 1990;4(3):139-142

[66] Benedict JW, Sommers CA, Pearce DA. Progressive oxidative damage in the central nervous system of a murine model for juvenile Batten disease. Journal of Neuroscience Research. 2007;85(13):2882-2891

[67] Hall NA, Lake BD, Patrick AD. Recent biochemical and genetic advances in our under-standing of Batten's disease (ceroid-lipofuscinosis). Developmental Neuroscience. 1991;13(4-5):339-344

[68] Westermarck T, Erkki A, Faik A. Vitamin E therapy in neurological diseases. In: Packer L, Fuchs J, editors. Vitamin E in Health and Disease. New York, Basel, Hong Kong: Marcel Dekker; 1993. pp. 799-806

[69] Piattella L, Cardinali C, Zamponi N. Papa O Spielmeyer-Vogt disease: Clinical and neu-rophysiological aspects. Child's Nervous System. 1991;7(4):226-230

[70] Santavuori P, Heiskala H, Westermark T, Sainio K, Moren R. Experience over 17 years with antioxidant treatment in Spielmeyer-Sjögren disease. American Journal of Medical Genetics. Supplement. 1988;5:265-274

[71] Gourraud PA, Harbo HF, Hauser SL, Baranzini SE. The genetics of multiple sclerosis: An up-to-date review. Immunological Reviews. 2012;248(1):87-103

[72] Lvovs D, Favorova OO, Favorov AV. A polygenic approach to the study of polygenic diseases. Acta Naturae. 2012;4(3):59-71

[73] Clausen J, Jensen GE, Nielsen SA. Selenium in chronic neurologic diseases. In: Schrauzer GN, editor. Biological Trace Element Research. Clifton, New Jersey: The Humana Press; 1988. pp. 179-203

[74] Komatsu F, Kagawa Y, Kawabata T, Kaneko Y, Kudoh H, Purvee B, et al. Influence of essential trace minerals and micronutrient insufficiencies on harmful metal overload in a Mongolian patient with multiple sclerosis. Current Aging Science. 2012;5(2):112-125

[75] Mai J, Sorensen PS, Hansen JC. High dose antioxidant supplementation to MS patients. Effects on glutathione peroxidase, clinical safety, and absorption of selenium. Biological Trace Element Research. 1990;24(2):109-117

[76] Socha K, Kochanowicz J, Karpińska E, Soroczyńska J, Jakoniuk M, Mariak Z, et al. Dietary habits and selenium, glutathione peroxidase and total antioxidant status in the serum of patients with relapsing-remitting multiple sclerosis. Nutrition Journal. 2014;13:62

[77] Kosnett M. Mercury. In: Olson K, editor. Poisoning & Drug Over-dose. NY, USA: The McGraw-Hill Companies, Inc; 2012. pp. 271-276

[78] McNutt M. Mercury and health. Science. 2013;**341**:1430-1430

[79] Jarup L. Heavy metals in the environment. Paediatric and Perinatal Epidemiology. 2003;**17**(2):221-222

[80] Nehru B, Dua R. The effect of dietary selenium on lead neurotoxicity. Journal of Environmental Pathology, Toxicology and Oncology. 1997;**16**(1):47-50

[81] Ruszkiewicz J, Albrecht J. Changes in the mitochondrial antioxidant systems in neurodegenerative diseases and acute brain disorders. Neurochemistry International. 2015;**88**:66-72

[82] Dézsi L, Vécsei L. Monoamine oxidase B inhibitors in Parkinson's disease. CNS & Neurological Disorders—Drug Targets. 2017. [Epub ahead of print]

[83] Lacher SE, Slattery M. Gene regulatory effects of disease-associated variation in the NRF2 network. Current Opinion in Toxicology. 2016;**1**:71-79

[84] Dominiak A, Wilkaniec A, Jęśko H, Czapski GA, Lenkiewicz AM, Kurek E, et al. Selol, an organic selenium donor, prevents lipopolysaccharide-induced oxidative stress and inflammatory reaction in the rat brain. Neurochemistry International. 2017;**108**:66-77

[85] Shahar A, Patel KV, Semba RD, Bandinelli S, Shahar DR, Ferrucci L, et al. Plasma selenium is positively related to performance in neurological tasks assessing coordination and motor speed. Movement Disorders. 2010;**25**(12):1909-1915

[86] McIntosh KG, Cusack MJ, Vershinin A, Chen ZW, Zimmerman EA, Molho ES, et al. Evaluation of a prototype point-of-care instrument based on monochromatic X-ray fluorescence spectrometry: Potential for monitoring trace element status of subjects with neurodegenerative disease. Journal of Toxicology and Environmental Health. Part A. 2012;**75**(21):1253-1268

[87] Delanty N, Dichter M. Antioxidant therapy in neurologic disease. Archives of Neurology. 2000;**57**(9):1265-1270

[88] Soto-Otero R, Mendez-Alvarez E, Hermida-Ameijeiras A, et al. Autoxidation and neurotoxicity of 6-hydroxydopamine in the presence of some antioxidants: Potential implication in relation to the pathogenesis of Parkinson's disease. Journal of Neurochemistry. 2000;**74**:1605-1612

[89] Burke RE, Fahn S, Jankovic J, Marsden CD, Lang AE, Gollomp S, et al. Tardive dystonia: Late-onset and persistent dystonia caused by antipsychotic drugs. Neurology. 1982;**32**(12):1335-1346

[90] Rakesh G, Muzyk A, Szabo ST, Gupta S, Pae CU, Masand P. Tardive dyskinesia: 21st century may bring new treatments to a forgotten disorder. Annals of Clinical Psychiatry. 2017;**29**(1):e9-e20

[91] Pedersen BK, Steensberg A, Fischer C, Keller C, Keller P, Plomgaard P, et al. Searching for the exercise factor: Is IL-6 a candidate? Journal of Muscle Research and Cell Motility. 2003;**24**(2-3):113-119

[92] Johansson A, Carlström K, Ahrén B, Cederquist K, Krylborg E, Forsberg H, et al. Abnormal cytokine and adrenocortical hormone regulation in myotonic dystrophy. The Journal of Clinical Endocrinology and Metabolism. 2000;**85**(9):3169-3176

[93] Henríquez-Olguín C, Altamirano F, Valladares D, López JR, Allen PD, Jaimovich E. Altered ROS production, NF-κB activation and interleukin-6 gene expression induced by electrical stimulation in dystrophic mdx skeletal muscle cells. Biochimica et Biophysica Acta. 2015;**1852**(7):1410-1419

[94] Jackson MJ, Edwards RHT. Free radicals and trials of antioxidant therapy in muscle diseases. Advances in Experimental Medicine and Biology. 1990;**1990**(264):485-491

[95] Grinio LP, Orlov ON, Prilipko LL, Kagan VE. Lipid peroxidation in children with Duchenne's hereditary myopathy. Bulletin of Experimental Biology and Medicine. 1984;**98**:423-425

[96] Westermarck T, Rahola T, Kallio A-K, Suomela M. Long term Turnover of selenite-Se in children with motor disorders. Klinische Pädiatrie. 1982;**194**:301-302

[97] Westermarck T, Aberg L, Santavuori P, Antila E, Edlund P, Atroshi F. Evaluation of the possible role of coenzyme Q10 and vitamin E in juvenile neuronal ceroid-lipofuscinosis (JNCL). Molecular Aspects of Medicine. 1997;**18**(Suppl):S259-S262

[98] Shimomura Y, Suzuki M, Sugiyama S, et al. Protective effect of coenzyme Q10 on exercise induced muscular injury. Biochemical and Biophysical Research Communications. 1991;**176**:349-355

[99] Littarru GP, Tiano L, et al. Clinical aspects of coenzyme Q 10: An update. Nutrition. 2010;**26**:250-254

[100] Westermarck T, Antila E, Kaksonen S, Laakso J, Härkönen M, Atroshi F. Long-term follow-up of two Duchenne muscle dystrophy patients treated with antioxidants. In: Hiramatsu M, Yoshikawa T, Inoue M, editors. Food and Free Radicals. New York, London: Plenum Press; 1997. pp. 161-163

[101] Lu QL, Mann CJ, Lou F, Bou-Gharios G, Morris GE, et al. Functional amounts of dystrophin produced by skipping the mutated exon in the mdx dystrophic mouse. Nature Medicine. 2003;**9**(8):1009-1014

[102] Bonthron DT, Foulkes WD. Genetics meets pathology—An increasingly important relationship. The Journal of Pathology. 2017;**241**(2):119-122

[103] Lim LE, Rando TA. Technology insight: Therapy for Duchenne muscular dystrophy-an opportunity for personalized medicine? Nature Clinical Practice. Neurology. 2008;**4**(3):149-158

[104] Miceli MC, Nelson SF. The case for eteplirsen: Paving the way for precision medicine. Molecular Genetics and Metabolism. 2016;**118**(2):70-71

[105] Pillers DA, Von Bergen NH. Emery-Dreifuss muscular dystrophy: A test case for precision medicine. The Application of Clinical Genetics. 2016;**9**:27-32

[106] Nelson SF, Crosbie RH, Miceli MC, Spencer MJ. Emerging genetic therapies to treat Duchenne muscular dystrophy. Current Opinion in Neurology. 2009;**22**(5):532-538

[107] Mendell JR, Goemans N, Lowes LP, Alfano LN, Berry K, Shao J, et al. Longitudinal effect of eteplirsen versus historical control on ambulation in Duchenne muscular dystrophy. Annals of Neurology. 2016;**79**(2):257-271

[108] Atroshi F, Antila E, Westermarck T. The role of selenium in epilepsy and other neurological disorders. Epileptologia. 2007;**15**:211-224

[109] Dworkin RH. Linoleic acid and multiple sclerosis. Lancet. 1981;**1**(8230):1153-1154

[110] Tiano L, Padella L, Santoro L, Carnevali P, Principi F, Brugè F, et al. Prolonged coenzyme Q10 treatment in Down syndrome patients: Effect on DNA oxidation. Neurobiology of Aging. 2012;**33**(3):626.e1-626.e8

Chapter 10

Zinc in Human Health

Ananda S. Prasad

Additional information is available at the end of the chapter

http://dx.doi.org/10.5772/intechopen.92005

Abstract

The essential role of zinc in human health was first suggested by our studies in growth-retarded Iranian villagers in 1961. Our later studies in 1963 established conclusively that zinc was essential for human and that zinc deficiency resulted in severe growth retardation, hypogonadism in males, immune dysfunctions, and cognitive function impairment. The suggestion that zinc was an essential element for humans remained very controversial, but in 1974, the USA National Academy of Sciences declared zinc as an essential element for humans and established the recommended dietary allowances. In 1978, the FDA and other regulatory agencies made it mandatory to include zinc in total parenteral nutrition fluids, which resulted in saving many lives. During the past five decades, tremendous progress has been made in the understanding of the biochemical role of zinc, and we now know that zinc therapy has impacted significantly on human health and diseases. In this review, I plan to present a brief historical review of the discovery of zinc as an essential element for humans, the clinical manifestations of zinc deficiency, its therapeutic impact on human health and diseases, biomarkers of human zinc deficiency, and its biochemical role.

Keywords: zinc, anti-inflammatory agent, antioxidant agent, oxidative stress, inflammatory cytokines

1. Historical review

In 1869, Raulin [1] reported for the first time that zinc was essential for the growth of *Aspergillus niger*. In 1926, it was reported that zinc was required for the growth of the plants, and in 1934, it was shown to be a growth factor for the rats [2].

I received my training in medicine as a clinical scientist under Professor Cecil James Watson at the University of Minnesota Medical School. The purpose of this training was to train

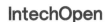

physicians not only in clinical medicine but also in basic sciences so that the clinical scientists could investigate the bedside clinical problems in research laboratories and to understand the basic mechanisms involved in clinical disorders [1–4].

Following the completion of my training under Dr. Watson in 1958, I was contacted by Professor Hobart Reimann, Chief of Medicine, Jefferson Medical College in Philadelphia. Professor Reimann who was a personal friend of the Shah of Iran had just accepted a position as Chief of Medicine at Shiraz University, Iran, and he offered me a position at the Shiraz Medical School to set up a medical curriculum for students and physicians in training on an American pattern. Although I was initially very reluctant, I did accept this offer and arrived in Shiraz, Iran, in July 1958.

The story of zinc began when an Iranian physician presented to me a severely anemic 21-year-old male, who looked like a 10-year-old boy, at the medical school grand round. His genitalia were infantile. He had rough and dry skin, was mentally lethargic, and had hepatosplenomegaly. He ate only bread made of whole wheat flour, he had no intake of animal protein, and in addition he ate 1 pound of clay every day. His severe anemia was due to iron deficiency but he had no blood loss. Iron deficiency in adult males without blood loss is a very unusual phenomenon.

Iron deficiency alone could not account for the severe growth retardation and infantile genitalia as these features are not seen in iron-deficient experimental animals. An examination of the periodic table suggested to me that deficiency of another transitional element, perhaps zinc, may also have been present, which could account for growth retardation and hypogonadism. We considered the possibility that a high phosphate content of the diet and clay may have decreased the availability of both iron and zinc which resulted in their deficiencies [3].

Our studies in Egypt later documented that zinc deficiency occurred in humans and that zinc supplementation resulted in 5–6 in. of longitudinal growth in 1 year and the genitalia became normal within 3–6 months of zinc supplementation [5].

The details of circumstances leading to the discovery of human zinc deficiency have been published recently [6].

2. Clinical manifestations of human zinc deficiency

The clinical manifestations of a moderate deficiency of zinc as described in the Middle East included growth retardation, hypogonadism in the males, rough skin, poor appetite, mental lethargy, delayed wound healing, cell-mediated immune dysfunctions, and abnormal neuro-sensory changes. These manifestations were reported in subjects with nutritional deficiency of zinc [5, 6] and in subjects with conditional deficiency of zinc [7, 8].

It is now apparent that a nutritional deficiency of zinc in humans is globally widespread, particularly in areas where cereal proteins are primarily consumed. Their diets are high in phytate, an organic phosphate compound which complexes both zinc and iron, and this deficiency may be affecting nearly 2 billion subjects in the world [7, 8].

Zinc deficiency is also prevalent in females in the developing world. Cavdar et al. [9] observed decreased plasma zinc levels in almost 30% of the low-socioeconomic-status pregnant women in Turkey. Maternal zinc deficiency was associated with severe congenital malformation of the central nervous system in the fetuses and increased maternal morbidity [9].

In 1973, Barnes and Moynahan [10] reported a 2-year-old girl with severe acrodermatitis enteropathica (AE) who was being treated with diiodohydroxyquinoline and a lactose-deficient synthetic diet, but she was unresponsive to this management. The serum zinc level was low and this prompted the physicians to administer zinc sulfate. Surprisingly this resulted in complete recovery of this patient. This observation was quickly confirmed by others throughout the world, and many lives were saved by zinc therapy of AE patients.

AE used to be a lethal disease. This is caused by an autosomal recessive genetic disorder which usually occurs in infants of Italian, Armenian, or Iranian lineage [7, 8]. The disease manifests in the early months of life soon after weaning from breastfeeding. The dermatologic manifestations of severe zinc deficiency in AE patients include bullous pustular dermatitis of the extremities and the oral, anal, and genital areas around the orifices, paronychia, and alopecia. Ophthalmic signs include blepharitis, conjunctivitis, photophobia, and corneal opacities. Neuropsychiatric signs include irritability, emotional instability, tremors, and cerebellar ataxia. Other manifestations include growth retardation, weight loss, and male hypogonadism. Congenital malformation of fetuses and infants born of pregnant women with AE has been frequently observed [7, 8].

AE patients have increased susceptibility to infections. Immune dysfunction is due to abnormal Th1 functions. Clinical course is downhill with failure to thrive and complicated by intercurrent bacterial, viral, fungal, or parasitic infections. The disease if unrecognized is fatal. Zinc therapy is very effective and is curative.

AE gene has been identified as SCL39A4 and is localized to a ~3.5cm region on 8q24.3 chromosome. The gene encodes a histidine-rich protein which is now referred to as ZIP-4, which is a member of a large family of transmembrane proteins, known as zinc transporters. In patients with AE, mutations in this gene have been demonstrated [11]. So far 31 different mutations or variants of the SCL39A4 gene have been identified in AE patients throughout the world [12–14].

Covering about 4.5 kb of chromosomal region 8q24.3, the human SLC39A4 gene is composed of 12 exons ranging from 55 bP (exon 9) to 292 bP (exon 1) in size and 11 introns ranging from 76 bP (intron 7) to 506 bP (intron 1). The SLC39A4 gene encodes a 647-amino acid protein of about 68 kDa. This protein, which is designated as ZIP-4, belongs to the family of 14 members of specific ZIP zinc transporters (for zinc-/iron-regulated transporter-like protein) which facilitate zinc influx from outside the cell to cellular compartments into the cytoplasm [11–14]. We have previously reported a new mutation in exon 3 of the SCL39A4 gene in a Tunisian family with severe AE [14], and recently we have observed two new mutations (unpublished), one in a United Arab Emirate (UAE) family, which showed a mutation in exon 7, Gly 409→Arg, and the other in a patient from Turkey, which showed the mutation in exon 7 Leu 415→Pro.

3. Severe zinc deficiency in total parenteral nutrition (TPN) patients

Kay and Tasman-Jones reported the occurrence of severe zinc deficiency in subjects receiving TPN without zinc for prolonged periods [15]. Okada et al. [16] also reported similar observations in 1976. The clinical features were similar to those reported in AE patients. These complications of TPN fluids were completely prevented after 1978 when it was made mandatory to include zinc in TPN fluids. In 1976 we reported a severe deficiency of zinc in a patient with Wilson's disease who was treated with penicillamine and eventually became severely deficient of zinc due to chelation therapy. The manifestations were similar to AE patients [17].

We developed an experimental model of mild deficiency of zinc in human volunteers in 1978 [18]. The details of dietary preparation and experimental model studies have been published in detail before [18]. A semi-purified diet which supplied all essential nutrients in RDA amounts except zinc which was restricted to approximately 3.0–5.0 mg of zinc daily was used to induce zinc deficiency [18].

In this model as a result of specific mild deficiency of zinc, we observed decreased serum testosterone level, oligospermia, decreased natural killer (NK) cell activity, decreased IL-2 (interleukin-2) activity of T helper cells, decreased serum thymulin activity, hyperammonemia, hypogeusia, decreased dark adaptation, and decreased lean body mass [18–21]. Our study clearly established that even a mild deficiency of zinc in humans adversely affects clinical, biochemical, and immunological functions.

4. Biomarkers of zinc deficiency

In the Middle East, we assayed zinc in plasma, red blood cells, 24-h urine, and hair by dithizone technique [4]. This technique was very difficult and labor intensive but there was nothing easier available. Extreme precautions were taken to avoid contamination. We also utilized Zn^{65} to study zinc metabolism in our subjects [4].

Zinc levels were decreased in plasma, red blood cells, 24-h urine, and hair in the growth-retarded subjects in comparison to the controls. The plasma zinc turnover rate was greater, and the 24-h zinc exchangeable pool was decreased significantly in the dwarfs. The cumulative excretion of zinc in urine and stool in 13 days was decreased in the dwarfs, in comparison to the controls, indicating body conservation of zinc in the zinc-deficient subjects. We concluded from these results that the dwarfs were zinc deficient. This was the first demonstration that zinc deficiency in humans occurred [4].

On daily oral supplementation with 15 mg zinc as sulfate, the growth rate was 5–6 in. per year in the dwarfs, and the external genitalia became adult like within 6 months of supplementation [5].

5. Atomic absorption spectrophotometric assay for zinc (AAS)

In 1965 we published the first technique of zinc measurement in plasma and blood cells by the use of atomic absorption spectrophotometer (AAS), and this technique is currently being used all over the world [22].

At present plasma zinc by AAS is being widely used as a biomarker of zinc deficiency globally. The machine is expensive, needs careful maintenance, and is not easily available in developing countries. Furthermore, plasma zinc assay is not a specific biomarker of zinc deficiency in humans inasmuch as the plasma zinc pool changes as a result of infections, exercise, and stress. Also, even slight hemolysis increases the plasma zinc inasmuch as the red cells are very rich in zinc.

6. Biomarkers of zinc deficiency in experimental human zinc deficiency model

We used a semi-purified diet based on texturized soy protein which provided all nutrients in RDA amounts except for zinc which was 3–5 mg/d. The RDA for zinc is 12–15 mg/d. The details of experimental model studies have been published before [18].

In this model we studied the effect of zinc deficiency on zinc levels in plasma, blood cells, zinc-dependent enzymes, and immunological functions.

We observed that the assay of ecto 5′ nucleotidase (5′NT), a zinc-dependent enzyme, which is present in plasma membrane of lymphocytes and is a marker of cell maturity, was a very sensitive test for human zinc deficiency [23]. We observed that the activity of 5′NT decreased during early zinc depletion phase (4–8 weeks). Plasma zinc did not change until 24 weeks of zinc restriction.

We also assayed serum zinc thymulin activity in our experimental model of human zinc deficiency subjects [21]. Thymulin is a thymic hormone which requires zinc for its activity. Thymulin is required for the development and differentiation of T helper cells. In our subjects, we observed that serum thymulin activity decreased within 8–12 weeks following zinc-restricted diet, suggesting that this test was also a very sensitive biomarker of zinc deficiency. This correlated well with our observation that the generation of IL-2 and its mRNA were also decreased during the early zinc depletion phase, 8–12 weeks after initiation of zinc-restricted diet [20, 24, 25].

Thus, our studies revealed that the assay of immunological markers is perhaps the most sensitive biomarker of human zinc deficiency. We have published that the assay of IL-2 mRNA in peripheral blood mononuclear cells by RT-PCR was a very good indicator of zinc deficiency in humans [25].

7. Endogenous excretion of zinc as a biomarker of zinc deficiency

Humans maintain zinc homeostasis by increasing efficacy of zinc absorption and decreasing endogenous excretion of zinc when they are subjected to short-term dietary zinc restriction. However, a mild deficiency of zinc in humans is usually an outcome of chronic exposure to low dietary zinc for many months and years.

We, therefore, assessed the efficiency of zinc absorption as well as endogenous zinc excretion during a 6-month period of dietary zinc restriction by the use of Zn^{70}. Our studies showed that the efficiency of zinc absorption was not sustained and decreased in the volunteers when the zinc-restricted diet was continued for 6 months [26]. On the other hand, prolonged dietary zinc restriction did not impair the functional role of endogenous zinc excretion in zinc homeostasis. We observed a significant reduction of endogenous zinc excretion by restricting dietary zinc for 6 months. Our studies thus showed that the measurement of endogenous zinc excretion may also be a sensitive biomarker of human zinc deficiency.

In collaboration with Dr. Chris Fredrickson, we are currently developing a cost-effective, exportable instrument which uses laser-induced background spectroscopy (LIBS) for the measurement of zinc in tissue, plasma, and blood cells. Our preliminary studies have shown that measurement of zinc by LIBS technique in nails is an excellent technique for assessing chronic zinc deficiency in humans.

8. Therapeutic impact of zinc

8.1. Acute diarrhea in children

Zinc supplementation has been shown to prevent and treat diarrhea in children under 5 years of age decreasing both diarrhea and mortality [27, 28]. Zinc deficiency is also correlated with risk of respiratory tract infections, but the benefits of supplementation appears to be limited to more severe episodes and in populations with high incidence of zinc deficiency [28].

Diarrhea causes damage to absorptive mucosa of the intestines and decreases absorption of nutrients including zinc. Children with low plasma zinc were observed to be more susceptible to diarrhea, thus resulting in a vicious cycle of zinc deficiency and infection.

In 2004 the World Health Organization (WHO) issued a global recommendation for the daily supplementation of 20 mg zinc in children ≥6 months for 10–14 days upon diarrheal onset [28].

Meta-analysis of routine supplementation for up to 3 months in seven studies providing one to two times RDA elemental zinc five to seven times per week found an 18% reduction in diarrheal incidence, or 25% decrease in diarrhea prevalence, and a 33% reduction in persistent diarrhea episodes among supplemented children in comparison to those who received placebo [28]. A meta-analysis of three randomized controlled trials providing short course of zinc supplementation with two to four times the daily RDA for 2 weeks following the onset of acute or persistent diarrhea was also reported. The pooled analysis showed an 11%

decrease in diarrhea incidence and a 34% decrease in diarrhea prevalence during 3 months of observation.

8.2. Zinc for the treatment of common cold

Common cold is one of the most frequently occurring diseases in the world [29]. More than 20 viruses cause common cold, and these include rhinoviruses, corona viruses, adenoviruses, respiratory syncytial viruses, and parainfluenza viruses. In the USA, adults may suffer of common cold two to four times and children six to eight times per year. The morbidity and subsequent financial loss resulting from absenteeism from work are considerable. Previous treatments have not resulted in a consistent relief of symptoms.

We tested the efficacy of zinc acetate lozenges in common cold in 50 volunteers who were recruited within 24 h of the onset of common cold symptoms, and we carried out a double-blind placebo-controlled trial [29]. Participants took one lozenge containing 12-8 mg zinc (as acetate) or placebo every 2–3 h while awake as soon as they developed common cold symptoms. Subjective symptom scores for sore throat, nasal discharge, nasal congestion, sneezing, cough, scratchy throat, hoarseness, muscle ache, fever, and headache were recorded daily for 12 d. Plasma zinc and pro-inflammatory cytokines were assayed on day 1 and at the end when subjects were well.

Compared to the placebo group, the zinc group had shorter overall duration of cold symptoms (4.5 d vs 8.1 d, $p < 0.01$), nasal discharge (4.1 d vs 5.8 d, $p = 0.02$), and decreased total severity scores for all symptoms ($p = 0.02$).

In another study, we recruited 50 ambulatory volunteers within 24 h of the onset of common cold for randomized placebo-controlled trial of zinc lozenges [30]. Each lozenge contained 13.3 mg of zinc as acetate. Plasma zinc, soluble interleukin (IL-1) receptor antagonist (sIL-1ra), soluble tumor necrosis factor receptor-1, and soluble vascular endothelial cell adhesion molecule (SICAM)-1 were assayed on days 1 and 5 [30].

Compared with the placebo group, the zinc group had a shorter mean duration of common cold (4.0 d vs 7.1 d, $p = 0.001$), shorter duration of cough (2.1 d vs 5.0 d, $p < 0.001$), and nasal discharge (3.0 d vs 4.5 d, $p = 0.02$). The mean changes between zinc and the placebo groups (before vs after therapy) showed significant difference in sIL-1-ra (interleukin-1 receptor antagonist) ($p = 0.033$) and sICAM-1 ($p = 0.04$). Both decreased in the zinc group, and the mean changes between zinc and placebo group (before vs after therapy) showed significant differences ($p < 0.001$). Our results suggest that zinc decreased oxidative stress of monocytes and macrophages induced by the common cold viruses.

Human rhinovirus type 24 "docks" at ICAM-1 on the surface of the somatic cells [30]. Our results showed that zinc may have acted as an antiviral agent by reducing the ICAM-1 levels. We have also reported earlier that zinc downregulates NF-κB activity which is involved in gene regulation of ICAM-1 [30].

We conclude that zinc acetate lozenges are effective in decreasing the duration and severity of common cold symptoms. We also conclude that these beneficial effects of zinc on common cold symptoms are due to the anti-inflammatory and antioxidant effect of zinc. A meta-analysis published by Cochrane has confirmed our results and conclusions [31].

8.3. Zinc deficiency in sickle cell disease (SCD)

Our extensive studies have documented the occurrence of zinc deficiency in SCD adult patients [31]. Growth retardation, male hypogonadism, hyperammonemia, abnormal dark adaptation, and cell-mediated immune dysfunctions in SCD patients have been related to a deficiency of zinc. Zinc deficiency was associated with decreased levels of zinc in plasma, erythrocytes, lymphocytes, and hair; hyperzincuria; decreased activity of zinc-dependent enzymes such as carbonic anhydrase activity in erythrocytes, alkaline phosphatase activity in granulocytes, and deoxythymidine kinase activity in newly synthesizing collagen connective tissue; and hyperammonemia [32]. Zinc supplementation to SCD patients resulted in significant improvement in growth; secondary sexual characteristics; normalization of plasma ammonia levels; correction of dark adaptation; increased zinc levels in plasma, erythrocytes, lymphocytes, and granulocytes; and expected response of zinc on zinc-dependent enzymes [32, 33]. Zinc supplementation also corrected impaired delayed-type hypersensitivity (DTH).

A recent Cochrane review has concluded that zinc is the only therapeutic modality which results in decreased incidence of infections and pain crises [34].

8.4. Zinc therapy for Wilson's disease (WD)

Wilson's disease is an inherited autosomal disorder due to copper accumulation. The excretion of liver copper in the bile is deceased which leads to the decreased loss of copper in the stool. This leads to accumulation of copper in the liver. Eventually copper accumulates in the brain, kidneys, and other organs. Patients present with liver disease, neurological disease (movement disorder), or psychiatric disturbance in the second to fourth decades of life. In many cases the diagnosis is missed by the physician [35].

The genetic mutation of Wilson's disease gene leads to a defective generation of a protein called ATP 7B which is responsible for a key step in biliary excretion of copper [35–37]. The disease is recessive, and thus both copies of the ATP 7B gene have to be mutated to cause the disease. A large number of mutations in this gene causing Wilson's disease have been reported.

Early diagnosis of Wilson's disease is important inasmuch as effective therapy may prevent toxic accumulation of copper and damage to organs.

Ninety percent of the WD patients have low levels of ceruloplasmin and ceruloplasmin-bound copper, but non-ceruloplasmin copper is elevated in the plasma. Twenty four hour urinary copper is markedly elevated and this is a helpful diagnostic tool. Urinary copper, however, may be elevated also in patients with obstructive liver disease.

A slit lamp examination for copper deposits in the cornea (Kayser-Fleischer rings) is a very useful noninvasive diagnostic test for WD. This is positive in nearly 50% of the cases.

Several years ago, we were using 150 mg elemental zinc in six divided doses as an effective anti-sickling agent for the treatment of patients with sickle cell disease (SCD) [38]. At this level of zinc therapy, we observed that we induced copper deficiency in SCD patients [38]. This led Brewer et al. [35–37] to develop zinc as an effective anti-copper drug for WD.

Zinc competes with copper for similar binding sites, and oral doses of zinc efficiently decrease the uptake of copper [39]. Zinc may act by inducing intestinal metallothionein (MT) which has a high affinity for binding copper. This prevents the serosal transfer of copper into the blood pool. The intestinal cells turn over rapidly and take the complexed copper in stool for excretion. Zinc not only blocks food copper but also the copper which is endogenously excreted via salivary, gastric, and other gastrointestinal juices. Thus zinc is effective in producing a negative balance of copper.

Fifty milligrams of zinc (as acetate) is given orally three times a day to WD patients. Zinc must be given in a fasting or post absorptive state. The only side effect of zinc is that nearly 10% of the subjects may experience mild gastric discomfort. This can be avoided if zinc is administered between breakfast and lunch or after dinner before going to bed.

Zinc is the drug of choice for maintenance therapy. Zinc has no toxicity and is non-teratogenic, and it can be prescribed to subjects of all ages and even to pregnant women. Zinc has been approved by the FDA for the treatment of WD patients.

8.5. Zinc and age-related macular degeneration (AMD)

Age-related macular degeneration (AMD) affects nearly 25% of the subjects over 65 years of age, and late stage of disease accounts for nearly 50% of legal blindness in Europe and North America [40]. Newsome et al. [40] reported for the first time that zinc concentration is reduced in the human eye in patients with AMD, and they suggested that zinc deficiency may have led to oxidative stress and retinal damage.

The Age-Related Eye Disease Study (AREDS) group, supported by the National Eye Institute, NIH, conducted a double-blind clinical trial in patients with dry-type AMD in 11 centers [41]. They enrolled 3640 patients for trial. Their ages ranged from 55 to 80 years, and the average follow-up period was 6.3 years. Participants were assigned randomly to receive orally one of the following: (1) antioxidants (vitamin C, 500 mg; vitamin E, 400 IU; and beta carotene, 15 mg); (2) zinc 80 mg as zinc oxide and copper 2 mg as copper oxide, to prevent copper deficiency induced by zinc; (3) antioxidants plus zinc; or (4) placebo.

The group taking the antioxidant plus zinc reduced the risk of developing advanced AMD by about 25% and the vision loss by 19%.

The group taking zinc alone reduced the risk of developing advanced AMD by about 21% and the vision loss by 11%. In the group taking the vitamins alone, the risk of developing advanced AMD was decreased by 17%, and the vision loss was decreased by 10%. Only the zinc-supplemented group showed increased longevity [42, 43]. The risk of mortality was reduced by 27% in subjects who received only zinc. In a later publication, the AREDS group reported that a decrease in mortality was due to a decrease in the adverse cardiovascular events [43]. These results of zinc supplementation in the elderly are remarkable and suggest that the anti-inflammatory effect of zinc may be beneficial in patients with atherosclerosis.

8.6. Zinc deficiency in the elderly

The daily intake of zinc in the elderly in the Western world including the USA is only approximately 8–10 mg, whereas the RDA as reported in 1974 is 15 mg [44]. Frequently the elderly do not routinely eat three meals a day. Many live alone and do not cook a proper meal.

Our study in Detroit showed that 35% of the well-to-do ambulatory elderly subjects may have a deficiency of zinc [44–46]. Results of the third National Health and Nutrition Examination Survey (1988–1994) also reported that the elderly subjects >71 years were at great risk of inadequate zinc intake.

Oxidative stress and increased inflammatory cytokines have been recognized as important contributing factors for several chronic diseases attributed to aging, such as atherosclerosis and related cardiovascular disorders, mutagenesis and cancer, neurodegenerative disorders, type 2 diabetes, and Alzheimer's disease. Together, O^{2-}, H_2O_2, and $OH\cdot-$ radicals are known as reactive oxygen species (ROS), and excessive generation of ROS causes oxidative stress. Inflammatory cytokines such as TNF-α, IL-1β, and IL-6 generated by activated monocytes and macrophages are also known to generate excessive ROS.

We have shown that zinc supplementation to subjects ages 20–50 decreased oxidative stress markers such as malondialdehyde (MDA), 4-hydroxy-alkelans (HAE), and 8-hydroxydeoxy-guanine in the plasma and downregulated the ex vivo induction of TNF-α and IL-1β mRNA in mononuclear cells (MNCs) by decreasing TNF-α induced NF-κB induction [46]. We have also reported that in the promyelocytic leukemia cell line HL60, which differentiates to the monocyte and macrophage phenotype in response to phorbol-12-myristate-13 acetate (PMA), zinc upregulated the expression of A20 and the binding of A20 to trans-activating factor to DNA which resulted in the inhibition of NF-κB activation [45, 46].

We carried out a randomized placebo-controlled trial of zinc supplementation in 50 healthy elderly subjects (55–87 y) of both sexes and all ethnic groups in Detroit, MI. Exclusion criteria were life expectancy of <8 mo, progressive neoplastic disease, severe cardiac dysfunction, significant renal disease, significant liver disease, and subjects who were mentally incompetent. Zinc supplementation consisted of 45 mg elemental zinc as gluconate daily for 12 mo.

A comparison of our baseline data in the elderly with the younger adults showed that in the elderly, plasma zinc was lower and the percentage of cells producing IL-1β and TNF-α and the generated cytokines were significantly higher [45, 46]. IL-10 generated by Th2 cells which is known to downregulate IL-2 generation from Th1 cells was significantly higher in the elderly. The oxidative stress markers were also significantly higher in the elderly than the younger adults [45].

The mean incidence of infections was lower ($p < 0.01$) in the zinc-supplemented group (1.4 ± 0.95) vs placebo group (20.29 ± 0.46). The plasma zinc increased, and ex vivo generation of TNF-α and IL-10 significantly decreased in the zinc group in comparison to the placebo group [45, 46]. Oxidative stress markers in the plasma also decreased in the zinc group in comparison to the placebo group [46].

In MNCs isolated from zinc-deficient elderly subjects, zinc supplementation increased the ex vivo PHA induced IL-2 mRNA expression and plasma zinc concentration when compared to the placebo group.

Thus our study showed that zinc supplementation to the elderly subjects decreased the incidence of infection by nearly 66%. Following zinc supplementation the oxidative stress markers and the generation of inflammatory cytokines which were increased prior to supplementation significantly declined. These are very significant effects of zinc supplementation and may imply that zinc may prove to be an excellent agent for prevention of some of the chronic diseases in the elderly.

8.7. Biochemical mechanisms of zinc

When I started my studies in zinc metabolism in the early sixties, I knew of only three enzymes which required zinc for their functions. These were carbonic anhydrase, carboxypeptidase, and alcohol dehydrogenase. Now we understand that there is hardly any cellular process that does not depend upon zinc in some way. Zinc is a constituent of at least 2800 human protein structures, enzymatic catalysis, and cellular regulation. The largest group of zinc metalloenzymes is proteinases [47]. Zinc has a major role in the structural organization of protein domains that interact with DNA/RNA, other proteins, and lipids. Several dozen proteins control cellular and subcellular zinc homeostasis and redistribution. This control is essential for regulatory functions of free zinc (II) ions.

Free zinc intracellularly regulates the activity of several kinases, phosphatases, phosphodiesterases, caspases, and transcription factors.

8.8. Zinc and growth

IGF-1 is a zinc-dependent growth factor. Zinc is required for generation of IGF-1, and its receptor tyrosine kinase requires zinc for phosphorylation. IGF-1 intracellularly upregulates thymidine uptake by the nucleus which is converted to dTMP and dTTP for DNA synthesis. The enzyme deoxy thymidine kinase (TK) is required for the synthesis of TTP. Our studies have shown that zinc is required for the gene expression of TK. Thus zinc is involved at various steps for DNA synthesis and cell proliferation. Other enzymes such as DNA polymerase and RNA polymerase are also zinc dependent.

8.9. Zinc and immune cells

Zinc is a second messenger for immune cells, and intracellular zinc participates in signaling events [21, 48–51]. Hirano et al. [48, 49] have shown that a decrease in intracellular free zinc in T cells is essential for LPS-mediated CD4+ activation by dendritic cells (DCs). LPS binds to TLR-4 on DCs and activates Myd88 and TRIF-mediated signaling [48]. TRIF-mediated signaling upregulates ZnT-5 mRNA and downregulates ZIP-6 mRNA, resulting in a decrease of intracellular free zinc in DCs. Reduction in intracellular free zinc increases the expression of MHC class II molecules which is required for the activation of CD4+ T cells [48].

Zinc activates monocytes-macrophages in several ways. Zinc is required for the development of monocytes-macrophages and regulates its functions such as phagocytosis and pro-inflammatory cytokine production [50, 51]. LPS stimulation of zinc-sufficient monocytes results in downregulation of inflammatory cytokines such as TNF-α, IL-6, IL-1β, and IL-8. Zinc inhibits the cell membrane phosphodiesterase (PDE), which results in elevated levels of second messenger cGMP, which is followed by decreased activation of NF-κB and decreased generation of inflammatory cytokines [50, 51]. We have shown that zinc induces A-20, a zinc finger transcription factor protein, which inhibits NF-κB signaling via TNF receptor-associated pathways, resulting in downregulation of mRNAs of inflammatory cytokines [52, 53]. Based on these we propose that zinc is an important anti-inflammatory agent.

Infection or other stresses activate NADPH oxidase in monocytes-macrophages, which upregulates the generation of free radicals ($O\bullet^-_2$). Zinc is an inhibitor of NADPH oxidase. In the next step, the free radical is converted to H_2O_2, and the enzyme involved in this process is superoxide dismutase, a zinc- and copper-dependent enzyme. H_2O_2 generates •OH ions. Free radicals, H_2O_2 and •OH ions, are known as collectively reactive oxygen species (ROS). By the above mechanisms, zinc functions as an important antioxidant.

Zinc deficiency adversely affects Th1 functions [29]. Serum thymulin activity and generation of Th1 cytokine IL-2 and IFN-γ were adversely affected within 8–12 weeks of institution of zinc-restricted diet (3–5 mg daily) in human volunteers, whereas plasma zinc decreased later after 20–24 weeks of the institution of the experimental diet. These studies showed that Th1 cells are very sensitive to zinc restriction. Th2 cytokines were not affected in subjects who received experimental zinc-deficient diet. Thymulin is a zinc containing nonapeptide and is essential for the development and proliferation of Th cells.

Our studies also showed that several transcription factors such as NF-κB, AP-1, and SP-1 were zinc dependent and their binding to the DNA of IL-2 gene were decreased, resulting in decreased generation of IL-2 [24, 25]. A similar effect of zinc was also seen in generation of IFN-γ. Decreased IL-2 resulted in decreased NK and cytolytic T cell activity. Decreased IFN-γ along with decreased IL-12, another zinc-dependent cytokine generated by monocyte-macrophages, results in decreased phagocytosis by monocyte-macrophages.

In Th0, a human malignant lymphoblastoid cell line HUT-78, we showed that in zinc-sufficient cells, mRNA levels of IFN-γ, IL-12 Rβ2, and T-bet in PMA-/PHA-stimulated cells were increased in comparison to zinc-deficient cells [54]. Although intracellular free zinc increased only slightly in PMA-/PHA-stimulated cells, in Con-A stimulated cells in zinc-sufficient medium, there was an increased and sustained level of intracellular free zinc in comparison to the zinc-deficient cells [54]. We hypothesized that in stimulation of cells by Con-A via TCR, there was a release of intracellular free zinc which resulted in signal transduction for generation of IFN-γ and T-bet, IL-12 Rβ2, and STAT-4 mRNAs which participated in Th-1 cell differentiation.

8.10. Zinc transporters

Zinc transporters maintain intracellular zinc homeostasis very tightly. Ten ZnT (SLC 30) family of zinc transporters lower intracellular zinc concentration through export of zinc or by import into cellular compartment organelles such as Golgi, intracellular vesicles, mitochondria, or nucleus.

Fourteen ZIP (SLC 39) transporters are responsible for increasing intracellular zinc concentration through zinc import into cells or export from intracellular organelles.

In humans, ZIP 4 mutation in AE is known to result in severe deficiency of zinc, which is fatal if not recognized and properly treated with zinc. This entity has been discussed in a previous section.

A detailed study of Ehlers-Danlos syndrome characterized by progressive kyphoscoliosis, joint hypermobility, hyperelasticity of the skin, and severe hypotonicity of skeletal muscles has shown that these patients are homozygous for a 9 bp in-frame deletion of exon 4 of SLC 39 A 13 [55].

Bone morphogenetic protein (BMP)/transforming growth factor β (TGF-β) enters the mesenchymal cells, fibroblasts, osteoblasts, chondrocytes, etc. for generation of collagen, Max 2, hard connective tissue of bone, teeth, and cartilage, etc. Intracellularly BMP/TGF-β activates Smad which is then involved in gene expression of collagen, bone, and cartilage. Zinc is required for activation of Smad. ZIP-13 mutation, however, affects the activation of Smad by zinc, and these results in Ehlers-Danlos syndrome.

In prostate cancer cells, ZIP-1 and ZIP-2 are mutated, and this decreases the intracellular zinc concentration of prostate cancer cells. This results in activation of NF-κB, which leads to upregulation of anti-apoptotic genes and growth factors and proliferation of cancer cells, which leads to progression of prostate cancer. It is possible that proper supplementation of zinc in these patients may have a beneficial effect in patients with prostate cancer.

9. Conclusion

The essentiality of zinc for humans was established in 1963. The National Academy of Sciences and the US Congress established recommended dietary allowance for zinc in 1974, and the FDA made it mandatory to include zinc in the total parenteral nutrition in 1978.

The major clinical effects of zinc deficiency in humans include growth retardation in young ages, cell-mediated immune dysfunction, neurosensory disorders, delayed wound healing, and cognitive impairment. Currently it is the estimate of the WHO that nearly 2 billion subjects in the developing world may be zinc deficient. This is due to the fact that these populations mainly subsist on cereal proteins mainly and their diet has high levels of phytate which makes zinc unavailable for absorption.

Over 300 enzymes require zinc for their structure stability and activity, and over 2000 transcription factors are zinc dependent. Zinc is a molecular signal for immune and neuronal cells. Zinc is essential for thymulin, a thymic hormone which is required for T helper cell differentiation and proliferation. Zinc is essential for gene expression of Th1 cytokines. We have now documented that several transcription factors such as NF-κB, AP-1, SP-1, A20, T-bet, and STAT 4 are zinc dependent and are adversely affected by zinc deficiency. Zinc is required for DNA synthesis and cell proliferation, and we have shown that the gene expression of deoxy thymidine kinase (TK) is zinc dependent. Zinc not only improves cell-mediated immune functions, but it is also an antioxidant and anti-inflammatory agent.

Currently plasma zinc assay by AAS is used globally as a biomarker of zinc deficiency in humans. In our experience, this assay is not very sensitive nor specific for zinc deficiency. The immunological assays such as measurement of thymulin activity, assay of IL-2 mRNA and protein following PHA stimulation of mononuclear cells, and assay of lymphocyte ecto 5′ nucleotidase are very specific and sensitive biomarkers of zinc deficiency.

Therapeutic impact of zinc has been tremendous in several conditions. These include treatment of diarrhea in infants and children globally resulting in saving millions of lives, development of zinc therapy for Wilson's disease, common cold, prevention of blindness in elderly subjects with AMD, decreasing the incidence of infections and the incidences of adverse cardiovascular events in the elderly, successful treatment of carbon-monoxide poisoning, and decreasing the incidences of infection and pain crisis in patients with SCD.

Abbreviations

Con-A	concanavalin-A
dTMP	deoxythymidine phosphate
dTTP	deoxythymidine tetra phosphate
IGF-1	Insulin-like growth factor 1
IL-1β	Interleukin-1β
IL-6	Interleukin 6
IL-10	Interleukin-10
LPS	lipopolysaccharide
MHC	major histocompatibility complex
MMP	matrix metalloproteinases
MyD88	myeloid differentiation primary response 88 (human)
NADPH	nicotinamide adenine dinucleotide phosphate
TCR	T-cell receptor
TLR 4	toll-like receptor 4

Author details

Ananda S. Prasad

Address all correspondence to: prasada@karmanos.org

Department of Oncology, Wayne State University School of Medicine and Barbara Ann Karmanos Cancer Institute, Detroit, Michigan, USA

References

[1] Raulin J. Chemical studies on vegetation. Annals des Sciences Naturells. 1869;**11**:93-99 (in French)

[2] Todd WR, Elvehjem CA, Hart EB. Zinc in the nutrition of the rat. American Journal of Physiology. 1933;**107**:146-156

[3] Prasad AS, Halsted JA, Nadimi M. Syndrome of iron deficiency anemia, hepatospleno-megaly, hypogonadism, dwarfism, and geophagia. American Journal of Medicine. 1961; **31**:532-546

[4] Prasad AS, Miale A, Farid Z, Schulert A, Sandstead HH. Zinc metabolism in patients with the syndrome of iron deficiency anemia, hypogonadism and dwarfism. Journal of Laboratory and Clinical Medicine. 1963;**61**:537-549

[5] Sandstead HH, Prasad AS, Schulert AR, Farid Z, Miale A Jr, Bassily S, et al. Human zinc deficiency, endocrine manifestations and response to treatment. American Journal of Clinical Nutrition. 1967;**20**:422-442

[6] Sandstead HH. Zinc nutrition from discovery to global health impact. Advances in Nutrition. 2012;**3**:718-719

[7] Prasad AS. Biochemistry of Zinc. New York: Plenum Press; 1993

[8] Prasad AS. Discovery of human zinc deficiency: Its impact on human health and disease. Advances in Nutrition. 2013;**4**:176-190

[9] Cavdar AO, Babacan E, Arcasoy A, Ertein U. Effect of nutrition on serum zinc concen-tration during pregnancy in Turkish women. American Journal of Clinical Nutrition. 1980;**33**:542-544

[10] Barnes PM, Moynahan EJ. Zinc deficiency in *Acrodermatitis enteropathica*. Proceeding of the Royal Society of Medicine. 1973;**66**:327-329

[11] Wang K, Zhou B, Kuo YM, Zemansky J, Gitschier J. A novel member of a zinc transporter family is defective in *Acrodermatitis enteropathica*. American Journal of Human Genetics. 2002;**71**:66-73

[12] Kury S, Dreno B, Bezieau S, Kharfi M, Kamoun R, Moisan JP. Identification of SLC 39A4, a gene involved in *Acrodermatitis enteropathica*. Nature Genetics. 2002;**31**:239-240

[13] Schmitt S, Kury S, Giraud M, Dreno B, Kharfi M, Bezieau S. An update of muta-tions of the SLC39A4 gene in *Acrodermatitis enteropathica*. Human Mutations. 2009;**30**:926-933

[14] Meftah SP, Kuivaniemi H, Tromp G, Kerkeni A, Sfar MT, Ayadi A, et al. A new mutation in exon 3 of the SLC39 A4 gene in a Tunisian family with severe *Acrodermatitis entero-pathica*. Nutrition. 2006;**22**:1067-1070

[15] Kay RG, Tasman-Jones C. Zinc deficiency and intravenous feeding. Lancet. 1975;**2**:605-606

[16] Okada A, Takagi Y, Itakura T, Satani M, Manabe H. Skin lesions during intravenous hyperalimentation: Zinc deficiency. Surgery. 1976;**80**:629-635

[17] Klingberg WG, Prasad AS, Oberleas D. Zinc deficiency following penicillamine therapy. In: Prasad AS, editor. Trace Elements in Human Health and Disease. Vol. 1. New York: Academic Press; 1976. pp. 51-65

[18] Prasad AS, Rabbani P, Abbasi A, Bowersox E, SpiveyFox MR. Experimental zinc deficiency in humans. Annals of Internal Medicine. 1978;**89**:483-490

[19] Beck FWJ, Kaplan J, Fine N, Handschu W, Prasad AS. Decreased expression of CD73 (ecto-5'-nucleotidase) in the CD8+ subset is associated with zinc deficiency in human patients. Journal of Laboratory and Clinical Medicine. 1997;**130**:147-156

[20] Beck FWJ, Prasad AS, Kaplan J, Fitzgerald JT, Brewer GJ. Changes in cytokine production and T cell subpopulations in experimentally induced zinc deficient humans. American Journal of Physiology Endocrinology Metabolism. 1997;**272**:1002-1007

[21] Prasad AS, Meftah S, Abdallah J, Kaplan J, Brewer GJ, Bach JF, et al. Serum thymulin in human zinc deficiency. Journal of Clinical Investigation. 1988;**82**:1202-1210

[22] Prasad AS, Oberleas D, Halsted JA. Determination of zinc in biological fluids by atomic absorption spectrophotometry in normal and cirrhotic subjects. Journal of Laboratory and Clinical Medicine. 1965;**66**:508-516

[23] Meftah S, Prasad AS, Lee D-Y, Brewer GJ. Ecto 5' nucleotidase (5'NT) as a sensitive indicator of human zinc deficiency. Journal of Laboratory and Clinical Medicine. 1991;**118**:309-316

[24] Prasad AS, Bao B, Beck FWJ, Sarkar FH. Zinc enhances the expression of IL-2 and IL-2 receptors in HUT-78 cells via NF-kB activation. Journal of Laboratory and Clinical Medicine. 2002;**140**:272-289

[25] Prasad AS, Bao B, Beck FWJ, Sarkar FH. Zinc activates NF-kB in HUT-78 cells. Journal of Laboratory and Clinical Medicine. 2001;**138**:250-255

[26] Lee D-Y, Prasad AS, Hydrick-Adair C, Brewer GJ, Johnson PE. Homeostasis of zinc in marginal human zinc deficiency: Role of absorption and endogenous excretion of zinc. Journal of Laboratory and Clinical Medicine. 1993;**122**:549-556

[27] Sazawal S, Black RE, Bhan MK, Bhandari N, Sinha A, Jalla S. Zinc supplementation in young children with acute diarrhea in India. New England Journal of Medicine. 1995;**333**:839-844

[28] Fisher, Walker CL, Lamberti L, Roth D, Black RE. In: Rink L, editor. Zinc in Human Health. Amsterdam: IOS Press; 2011. pp. 234-253

[29] Prasad AS, Fitzgerald JT, Bao B, Beck WJ, Chandrasekar PH. Duration of symptoms and plasma cytokine levels in patients with the common cold treated with zinc acetate. Annals of Internal Medicine. 2000;**133**:245-252

[30] Prasad AS, Beck FWJ, Bao B, Snell D, Fitzgerald T. Duration and severity of symptoms and levels of plasma interleukin-1 receptor antagonist, soluble tumor necrosis factor receptor, and adhesion molecule in patients with common cold treated with zinc acetate. Journal of Infectious Disease. 2008;**197**:795-802

[31] Singh M, Das R. Zinc for the common cold. Cochrane Database of Systematic Review. 2011;**2**:1-58

[32] Prasad AS, Beck FWJ, Kaplan J, Chandrasekar PH, Ortega J, Fitzgerald JT, et al. Effect of zinc supplementation on incidence of infections and hospital admissions in sickle cell disease (SCD). American Journal of Hematology. 1999;**61**:194-202

[33] Bao B, Prasad AS, Beck FWJ, Snell D, Sunega A, Sarkar FH, et al. Zinc supplementation decreased oxidative stress, incidence of infection and generation of inflammatory cytokines in sickle cell disease patients. Translational Research. 2008;**152**:67-80

[34] Swe KMM, Abas ABL, Bhardwaj A, Barua A, Nair NS. Zinc supplementation for treating Thalassemia and sickle cell disease. Cochrane Review. 2013:1-36

[35] Brewer GJ, Yuzbasiyan-Gurkan V. Wilson disease. Medicine. 1992;**71**:139-164

[36] Brewer GJ. Practical recommendations and new therapies for Wilson's disease. Drugs. 1995;**2**:240-249

[37] Brewer GJ, Schoomaker EB, Leichtman DA, Kruckleberg WC, Brewer LF, Myers N. The uses of pharmacologic doses of zinc in the treatment of sickle cell anemia. In: Brewer GJ, Prasad AS, editors. Zinc Metabolism: Current Aspects in Health and Disease. New York, NY: Allan R. Liss, Inc.; 1977. pp. 241-258

[38] Prasad AS, Brewer GJ, Schoomaker EB, Rabbani P. Hypocupremia induced by zinc therapy in adults. Journal of the American Medical Association. 1978;**240**:2166-2168

[39] Hall AC, Young BW, Bremner I. Intestinal metallothionein and the mutual antagonism between copper and zinc in the rat. Journal of Inorganic Biochemistry. 1979;**11**:57-66

[40] Newsome DA, Miceli MV, Tats DJ, Alcock NW, Oliver PD. Zinc content of human retinal pigment epithelium decreases with age and macular degeneration but superoxide dismutase activity increases. Journal of Trace Elements and Experimental Medicine. 1996;**8**:193-199

[41] Age-Related Eye Disease Study Research group (AREDS Report No. 8). A randomized, placebo controlled, clinical trial of high-dose supplemented with vitamins C and E, beta-carotene, for age-related macular degeneration and vision loss. Archives of Ophthalmology. 2001;**119**:1417-1436

[42] AREDS Report No. 13. Association of mortality with ocular disorders and an intervention of high dose antioxidants and zinc in the age-related eye disease study. Archives of Ophthalmology. 2004;**122**:716-726

[43] Age-Related Eye Disease Study Research Group (AREDS Report No. 35). Long term effects of vitamins C, E, beta-carotene and zinc in age related macular degeneration. Ophthalmology. 2013;**120**:1604-1611

[44] Prasad AS, Fitzgerald JT, Hess JW, Kaplan J, Pelen F, Dardenne M. Zinc deficiency in the elderly patients. Nutrition. 1993;**9**:218-224

[45] Prasad AS, Beck FWJ, Bao B, Fitzgerald JT, Snell DC, Steinberg JD, et al. Zinc supplementation decreases incidence of infections in the elderly: Effect of zinc on generation of cytokines and oxidative stress. American Journal of Clinical Medicine. 2007;**85**:837-844

[46] Bao B, Prasad AS, Beck FWJ, Fitzgerald JT, Snell D, Bao GW, et al. Zinc decreases C-reactive protein, lipid peroxidation, and implication of zinc as an atheroprotective agent. American Journal of Clinical Nutrition. 2010;**91**:1634-1641

[47] Maret W. Human zinc biochemistry. In: Rink L, editor. Zinc in Human Health. Amsterdam: IOS Press; 2011. pp. 45-62

[48] Hirano T, Murakami M, Fukada T, Nishida K, Yamasaki S, Suzuki T. Roles of zinc and zinc signaling in immunity: Zinc as an intracellular signaling molecule. Advances in Immunology. 2008;**97**:149-176

[49] Kitamura H, Morikawa H, Kamon H, Iguchi M, Hojyo S, Fukada T, et al. Toll-like receptor-mediated regulation of zinc homeostasis influences dendritic cell function. Nature Immunology. 2006;**7**:971-977

[50] Haase H, Rink L. Signal transduction in monocytes: The roll of zinc ions. Biometals. 2007;**20**:579-585

[51] Rosenkranz E, Prasad AS, Rink L. Immunobiology and hematology of zinc. In: Rink L, editor. Zinc and Human Health. Amsterdam: IOS Press; 2011. pp. 195-233

[52] Prasad AS, Bao B, Beck FWJ, Kucuk O, Sarkar FH. Antioxidant effect of zinc in humans. Free Radical Biology Medicine. 2004;**37**:1182-1190

[53] Prasad AS, Bao B, Beck FWJ, Sarkar FH. Zinc-suppressed inflammatory cytokines by induction of A20-mediated inhibition of nuclear factor-κB. Nutrition. 2011;**27**:816-823

[54] Bao B, Prasad AS, Beck WJ, Bao GW, Singh T, Ali S, et al. Intracellular free zinc up-regulates IFN-γ and T-bet essential for Th1 differentiation in Con-A stimulated HUT-78 cells. Biochemical and Biophysical Research Communications. 2011;**407**:703-707

[55] Fukada N, Civic T, Furuichi S, Shimode K, Mishima H, Higashiyama Y, et al. The zinc transporter SLC3913/ZIP 13 is required for connective tissue development. Its involvement in BMP/TGF-beta signaling pathways. PLoS One. 2008:36-42